NURSING THEORY

IN AUSTRALIA

DEVELOPMENT & APPLICATION

NURSING THEORY

IN AUSTRALIA

DEVELOPMENT & APPLICATION

EDITED BY JENNIFER GREENWOOD

RN, RM, DipN, RNT, DipEd, MEd, PhD, FRCNA
Professor of Nursing
Western Sydney Area Health Service/University of Western Sydney, Nepean

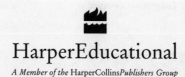

HarperEducational
A Member of the HarperCollinsPublishers Group

To the late Irene Greenwood

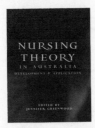

Cover photo by Paula Marchant

HarperEducational*Publishers*

First published in Australia in 1996

Acquisitions Editors: Yasminka Nemet & Belinda Forrest
Publishing Manager: Marah Braye
Project Editors: Katie Millar & Colette Vella
Cover Design: Paula Marchant
Internal Design: Eilish Bouchier

HarperEducational*Publishers*
HarperEducational (Australia) Pty. Limited
ACN 000 772 967
A Member of the HarperCollins*Publishers* (Australia) Pty. Limited Group
25 Ryde Road, Pymble, NSW 2073, Australia

HarperCollins*Publishers*
25 Ryde Road, Pymble, Sydney, NSW 2073, Australia
31 View Road, Glenfield, Auckland 10, New Zealand
77–85 Fulham Palace Road, London W6 8JB, United Kingdom
Hazelton Lanes, 55 Avenue Road, Suite 2900, Toronto, Ontario M5R 3L2
and 1995 Markham Road, Scarborough, Ontario M1B 5M8, Canada
10 East 53rd Street, New York NY 10032, USA

National Library of Australia Cataloguing-in-Publication information:
Greenwood, Jennifer
   Nursing Theory in Australia: Development and Application.
   Bibliography.
   Includes index.
   ISBN 0 06 312167 0.
   1. Nursing – Australia – Philosophy. I. Greenwood, Jennifer.
610.7301

Set in New Baskerville 10/13
Printed in Australia by Southwood Press on 80 gsm precision offset

FOREWORD

This text will join the ever-expanding list of outstanding Australian nursing textbooks. We are fortunate to be able to access material of this standard which has been written specifically for the Australian health care context, by the nurses, academics and clinicians who work within that context.

Although this textbook has been written primarily for students in undergraduate nursing programmes, it has much to offer registered nurses working within the health care sector, as well as those who are undertaking further postgraduate study. It will prove a useful addition to the collections of nursing academics and a valuable teaching resource in the complex area of the application and development of nursing theories.

The book will provide a clear understanding of many of the current debates about nursing theory and how they apply to practice and/or the development of the discipline of nursing. Whether students read the whole book or concentrate on chapters of particular interest, they will find the use of Australian examples of theory development and application add greatly to its value.

Differing perspectives about nursing theories have been brought together in this one volume. Material that is difficult if not impossible to come to terms with for many undergraduate nurses—and graduate nurses too—has been made interesting and highly readable by the contributors. Learning aids throughout the textbook such as the objectives at the beginning of each chapter and the stimulating discussion questions and recommendations for further reading at the end, all provide the reader with useful guidance for exploring the many interesting issues raised.

The contributions have been divided into two main categories: first the development of nursing theories; and secondly the application of these theories in practice. The reader can look in depth at how nursing theories developed as well as studying examples of their application in practice. The illustrations relating to the practical application of nursing theories within the Australian health context are of particular value as this is an area in which there has been much criticism of nursing theories.

I commend this book to readers as one which will make a major contribution to the many debates both within our own health context and throughout the world that have surrounded nursing theories and their development and application over the past two decades. The book is an important addition to the ever-growing number of Australian nursing textbooks which continue to increase our understanding of the discipline of nursing and how this discipline is practised both within our own clinical settings and internationally.

Professor R. Lynette Russell
Dean
Faculty of Nursing
The University of Sydney
Sydney

FOREWORD

This is one of the most important books yet written about Australian nursing. It is the first volume devoted to nursing theory published by Australian nurses. It addresses the state of our nursing theory development and usage and challenges those who believe that nursing is not theory based. It validates nursing as a human profession, art, science and discipline, based on its own body of knowledge. Indeed, one of the strengths of this volume is the emphasis on the *human* dimension of nursing practice with its subsequent fluctuating complexity, changing context and often relative conceptual 'fuzziness'. The clear exposition of this approach in the early chapters challenges the fiercely argued position within nursing that there is a need for *one* particular theory. There is a strong emphasis throughout on the need to theorise about nursing practice rather than to try to capture the elusiveness of effective nursing interactions and outcomes within one framework.

The volume is wide ranging, and has been faithful to the title of offering both 'development' and 'application'. It addresses what is clearly one of the most pressing application issues: the theory–practice gap. The authors discuss the reluctance of nurses to apply theory to practice and they demonstrate the interdependence of nursing theory and practice. In showing how nursing theory can be both applied to practice and derived from it in a meaningful and relevant way, they help to bridge the gap. Both the student nurse and the graduate clinician will improve their practice through application of the material in this volume, with a consequent benefit to their clients.

This book is a benchmark that will establish the place of nursing theory in the Australian nursing profession and as such is a welcome addition to both the national and international discourse on the theoretical nature of nursing.

Barbara Hayes
Professor of Nursing
James Cook University

Kathryn L. Roberts
Professor of Nursing
Northern Territory University

CONTENTS

CHAPTER 3

WAYS OF KNOWING IN NURSING

BEVERLY O'CONNELL

CHAPTER 4

NURSING PROCESS:
A Systematic Approach to Patient Care

BEVERLY O'CONNELL

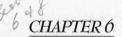

CHAPTER 5

NURSING THEORISING IN THE UNITED STATES AND AUSTRALIA:
Social and Professional Contexts
JUDITH CONDON

CHAPTER 6

CONSIDERATIONS OF CONTEXT:
The Crucial Moderator
ROSALIE PRATT

CHAPTER 7

SELECTING A NURSING THEORY
FOR CLINICAL PRACTICE:
Analysis and Critique
KAREN WOTTON

CHAPTER 8

OREM'S SELF-CARE MODEL
IN DIABETES HEALTH CARE:
An Exemplar
MERILYN KING AND LYN GREEN

CHAPTER 9

PARSE'S HUMAN BECOMING THEORY OF NURSING
JOHN DALY AND JENNIFER WATSON

CHAPTER 10

USING THE NEUMAN SYSTEMS MODEL AS A CURRICULUM ORGANISER
ALISON BALLANTYNE AND ANITA LANGE

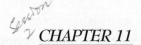

CHAPTER 11

DEVELOPING A PRACTICE-BASED MODEL OF NURSING

BART O'BRIEN

CHAPTER 12

PRESERVING INTEGRITY:
A Theory of Nursing
VERA IRURITA

CHAPTER 13

NURSING THEORY AND PRACTICE MODEL
OF PUBLIC PARTICIPATION
ROBYN WATTS

CHAPTER 14

THEORY GENERATION THROUGH REFLECTIVE PRACTICE
JUDY LUMBY

CHAPTER 15

FEMINISM FOR NURSING
JAN HORSFALL

CHAPTER 16

NURSING THEORY:
Whose Interests are Being Served?
SANDRA SPEEDY AND STEPHEN KERMODE

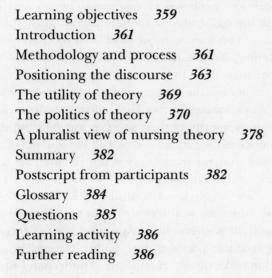

PREFACE

The idea for this book was conceived three years ago in Brisbane when, by chance, both the acquisitions editor from HarperEducational and I happened to be visiting the same School of Nursing. We were both in the staff common room when two nursing lecturers were recounting how badly their lecture on nursing theory had been received by a group of undergraduates the previous evening. No one present was surprised by this—nursing theory has been, and remains, problematic both to learn and to teach.

Undergraduates, it is claimed, cannot see the relevance of nursing theory to nursing practice. There seems to be a number of reasons for this. First, nursing students rarely see evidence of experienced clinical nurses informing their practice with nursing theories, either with insights from nursing models as they are known or with the findings of nursing research. This, in effect, tells nursing students that theory is not required for practice. Secondly, much of the published material on nursing theory has, hitherto, been written by North American or British scholars largely for American and British markets; this means that their applicability in the Australian health context may not always be obvious and, indeed, may even be questioned. In addition, many American nursing theories are difficult to comprehend and, given the previous two points, Australian nursing undergraduates may be disinclined to make the effort required to understand and utilise them. And lastly, generally speaking, 'nursing theory' is not an exciting read!

This book attempts to address these issues, mainly for undergraduate nurses but also for their teachers, postgraduate nurses and nurse academics. It is intended that nurses reading it will be given a sound understanding of nursing theory and that, as their understanding develops, they will come to appreciate the profoundly theoretical nature of nursing practice. It is also intended that they should come to a deeper appreciation of the complexity of nursing practice and find the theories that inform it of increasing interest.

Contributors to this collection were selected on the basis of their experience and specialist expertise in either developing/applying theory or teaching courses on nursing theory. Contributors were asked to write chapters that were both scholarly and understandable. To the author's credit I think they have achieved this, although some chapters may appear more challenging than others. While many of the concepts in nursing theory are abstract and challenging, some understanding of them is essential if nurses are to appreciate the relationships and the processes underpinning theory generation and professional nursing practice. Undergraduates and even postgraduates should not be daunted by this. The book was written as a test for courses such as Nursing Theory, Nursing Knowledge, Nursing Constructs and Professional Nursing Studies and its structure reflects this purpose. It is intended that readers will discuss the material in tutorial/seminar situations. It is a book written as much for group learning as for individual learning and each chapter is structured to facilitate both these types of learning.

The chapters begin with two or three learning objectives and end with discussion questions, learning activities, further reading and a glossary. The learning objectives are meant to prime the expectations of readers as they begin the chapter. The discussion questions and learning activities aim to promote readers' critical reflection on each chapter's contents and to stimulate interaction and dialogue between students of nursing and their teachers. Recommendations for further reading provide pointers to additional useful information related to chapter contents and individual glossaries are included to accommodate the different interpretations of common concepts which different contributors hold. Readers should expect that the authors differ to some extent in both perspective and the terminology they use. This is because, at the present time, a range of different but equally acceptable views related to nursing theory prevail. Additionally, because the book is a collection of chapters written by a number of authors, readers will experience a range of writing styles. Each chapter is meant to both stand alone and comprise an element in a comprehensive and cohesive text on nursing theory; readers should also expect some overlap, therefore, but not to the point of tedium. The book is meant to be 'dipped into' as coursework demands but also read cover to cover by those sufficiently interested to do so.

In general, the collection focuses on the development and application of nursing theory in Australia. The chapters cover theory–practice gaps; the relationship of research to theory; knowing in nursing; nursing process; the contextual and sociohistorical influences on nurse theorising; the critical application of 'imported' theories to Australian nursing practice; and the development of nursing theory from Australian nursing practice. There is even a chapter (written especially for nurse academics and curriculum developers) on the use of one nursing model in curriculum organisation. Whenever appropriate, contributors have illustrated their material with examples from their own practices and this brings their chapters alive. The important themes running through the book are that theory is always historically and contextually embedded; that it changes as views on what counts as valid knowledge changes; that it is constructed both 'bottom-up' (from practical experience) and 'top-down' (from conceptual thinking); and that it always reflects a partial view of reality.

Three years ago I had only the vaguest idea of how the book would shape up. I hardly dared hope that it would turn out to be the innovative and intellectually stimulating collection that it has. Such a collection, I believe, could only be written in Australia. Australian nursing scholarship at the present time has a breadth and freshness found nowhere else in the world and I am delighted that some of its vitality is captured in this book.

This is a unique collection. Many of its chapters are ground breaking and all have been written by nurse scholars in Australia. It is not just *about* nursing theory; I believe it makes a significant contribution *to* nursing theory. As such, it is an important contribution to Australian and international nursing literature.

I do hope you will enjoy reading this book and that you will find its content stimulating and challenging. I hope, too, that it will help you understand, critique and further develop the theoretical bases of your own nursing and teaching practices.

I am indebted to Jim Davidson, Yasminka Nemet and Belinda Forrest from HarperEducational for their enthusiastic support throughout the preparation of this collection. I am also hugely indebted to Rosali Harland, secretary extraordinaire, who not only typed and retyped my contributions to the book, often within seemingly impossible timeframes, but liaised directly with HarperEducational and the chapter writers to ensure that we kept to publication schedule.

Jennifer Greenwood

1

NURSING THEORIES

An Introduction
to their Development
and Application

JENNIFER GREENWOOD

LEARNING OBJECTIVES

When you have read this chapter you should be able to:

1 Understand that no human action, including nursing action, is atheoretical.

2 Explain why and how the theory–practice gap in nursing is constructed.

3 Understand how both intelligent, humane nursing practice and the development of practically relevant nursing theories may be promoted.

Jennifer Greenwood, RN, RM, DipN, RNT, DipEd, MEd, PhD, FRCNA, has 25 years' experience teaching nursing in both hospital-based and tertiary-based programs in Australia and the United Kingdom. She also has 12 years' experience in education management, at operational and strategic levels, in both health and education sectors. Throughout her career, Jennifer has strived to maintain the strongest possible links with colleagues working in and managing clinical facilities. Her own practice interests focus on the development of clinical nursing leadership especially in the context of Nursing Development Units.

Jennifer's main research interests focus on cognition and action, particularly in relation to human skills development, verbal protocols and protocol analyses, clinical education and action research. She is a Fellow of the Royal College of Nursing, Australia, a member of the Management Committee of RCNA Research Society and Editor of the Research Society's Bulletin.

INTRODUCTION

This first chapter aims to set the scene for the chapters that follow. It deals with the purposes of concepts, which are the building blocks of theory, and how they are acquired. I intend to show that all human action is theory driven, irrespective of whether or not the person is aware of it. If I am successful in this I will explode the myth that theory is irrelevant to practice.

The view of theory, or theories, reflected in this chapter is that theories comprise the beliefs and values that everyone possesses in relation to the world and their subjective experiences of it. We all possess 'theories' to explain (even unconsciously) or render meaningful (even unconsciously) salient aspects of our lives. It is simply not possible to avoid these 'theories', as I shall try to show in this chapter. It is possible, however, for us to make serious attempts to ensure that our 'theories' represent the important aspects of our lives as adequately and accurately as possible; this will enable us to control them more systematically and more strategically.

What follows is an account of my theories relating to nursing—that is, its nature, purposes and how it is learned. Of course, these theories are not only mine; they are shared by scholars who studied at the same institutions and with the same academic mentors as myself. I learned them from, and with, other scholars; people with different views of nursing and how it is learned acquired their views from, and with, different scholars and probably in different educational institutions. (See Chapter 3 for a detailed discussion on knowing in nursing and Chapter 5 for an examination of the sociopolitical influences on nursing theorising.)

My view of nursing is that it is an intensely theoretical practice discipline and profession which is learned through feedback-governed practice in relevant situations and settings. I believe that situations and settings are both clinical and academic, that these promote the development or construction of different theories of nursing in the minds of nurses and that this can impede the delivery of high quality nursing care. In this chapter, therefore, I will describe the processes underpinning the construction of these different theories and offer some suggestions for their possible remediation. I will argue that the development of relevant practice theories and the promotion of rational, humane nursing practice depends on such remediation.

THE NATURE OF NURSING AND NURSING SKILL

Whatever else it might be, nursing is directed towards improving the health status of people, both individuals and communities; this is what professional nursing claims to do and what the larger community, or 'society', licenses it to do. Nursing activities, therefore, are enormously diverse in that they include promoting health, preventing disease, aiding and supporting people during recovery and rehabilitation, and helping people die comfortably and with dignity (Henderson 1966). Given this, the theoretical underpinnings of nursing are derived from nursing science and a range of behavioural and biological sciences. In addition, nursing activities take place in, affect and are affected by particular physical and social environments, which evolve and change in response to many complex and interrelated factors. (See Chapter 6 for a discussion of the effects of context on nursing practice.) Knowledge of such factors is also biologically and/or behaviourally derived as these factors can be examined and explained from perspectives such as biochemistry, sociology and ecology.

Since nursing is directed towards changing (or enabling the changing of) the health status of people, it is clearly a practical activity. In an important sense, it is what nurses do in relation to these complex and interrelating physical and social factors that renders nursing interventions successful or unsuccessful. This means that nurses require both an understanding of the nature of these factors and their interrelationships, and the intellectual, practical and interpersonal skills to deal readily and appropriately with their implications, if health care aims are to be achieved.

The demands of nursing are clearly complex, because nurses provide care in situations which are relatively unpredictable and, in a sense, are always unique. For in each situation it is the needs of *this* patient, *here* and *now*, which demand attention. Nurses respond to these demands in two complementary ways. First, they deploy an intuitive or unconscious repertoire of strategies for interpreting, judging and responding to needs, situations and events that are relatively familiar. Second, they consciously use knowledge and understanding to solve problems in situations that are relatively unfamiliar and demanding. Importantly, however, it is the ability of nurses to respond unconsciously to much that is familiar in their clinical world that frees them to focus on conscious problem-solving in, or in anticipation of, novel and exacting situations (Tomlinson 1995).

Thus, for instance, a nurse can consciously review options and then decide which new interventions he or she will implement once he or she gets to work, in relation to the care of patients with complex health problems, while she or he is 'unconsciously' driving (accelerating, decelerating, negotiating traffic lights) to the workplace. Nursing expertise, therefore, is a function of the skills with which nurses deal with information both consciously and unconsciously. This information constitutes nurses' theories of nursing which are, as I have already indicated, built with concepts.

CONCEPTS CENTRAL TO NURSING

Since nursing is undertaken in the pursuit of aims, it is a purposeful or intentional activity; this means that when nurses are nursing they necessarily require some internal belief or theory, however vague or unconscious, of the purposes of their activities and the means to their achievement. For without such beliefs or theories, nursing could not be purposeful.

These theories are constructed by individual nurses; it is they, the subjects, who construct in their own minds the objects of their experience and their subjective experiences of such objects. This means that nurses will tend to construct similar theories or belief systems since their personal, and especially their professional, experiences will be similar. Importantly, however, many of the more everyday theories of nurses appear to be constructed in the same way as much of their everyday reality is experienced—that is, without their conscious awareness. This is particularly true of the learning of values (Tomlinson 1988).

The construction of theories begins before children learn to speak (Eysenck & Keane 1990) and, according to at least one eminent scholar (Polanyi 1958), some forms of theory are unspecifiable in principle. This means that we may not be aware of our own beliefs, or even that we possess them, and we may not be able to express them verbally; this, in turn, implies that they may not be consistent or readily modified. And, indeed, there is now evidence that the concepts central to nursing 'in theory' and nursing 'in practice' can be inconsistent. The discrepancies between nursing theory concepts and nursing practice concepts result in nursing's now almost celebrated **theory–practice gap** (McCaugherty 1991), and it is to a brief examination of these that I now turn.

NURSING 'IN THEORY'

'Nursing theory' appears to mean at least three distinctive and interrelated things to nursing students: it can refer to the part of their training that takes place in the school of nursing, and in this respect is distinguished from practice (Melia 1981); it can also mean the conceptual models of nursing that have proliferated in the last two to three decades; and it can mean knowledge derived from research.

It is interesting to note that undergraduate nurses tend to categorise all the learning and teaching activities that go on in universities as 'theory' though some of them, strictly speaking, are not theory. An example of 'practice' learning is the learning of clinical nursing skills in nursing laboratories. These divided (and divisive) categorisations, however, reinforce the distinction that students of nursing make between the theoretical and practical aspects of their professional education.

Conceptual models of nursing can be categorised according to their primary focus (Salvage & Kershaw 1986). They represent different views and explanations about:

- the person receiving nursing care;
- the environment in which the person exists;

* the health–illness continuum within which the person falls at the time of the interaction with the nurse; and

* nursing actions themselves.

Thus even though they reflect different views of patient, environment, health and nursing interventions, conceptual models all address these concepts.

Models of nursing, or conceptual models as they are sometimes termed, fall into two categories—totality paradigm models and simultaneity paradigm models. *Totality paradigm models* view the person as a total summative organism (hence the name) whose uniqueness is a function of biopsychosocial–spiritual features. These models view the environment as something in which people live and interact and which is experienced by them as internal and external stimuli. Totality paradigm models can be usefully classified into five groups (Salvage & Kershaw 1986):

* developmental

* systems

* interactionist

* self-care

* activities of daily living.

(See Chapter 8 for a detailed analysis of Orem's self-care theory and an interesting application of it to diabetes nursing practice.)

Simultaneity paradigm theorists view the person as being in mutual process with the environment or universe (Parse 1992). This concept may be difficult to grasp; it merely implies, however, that the human being is merged or immersed in all that is living. It is this view of the relationship of person and environment/universe which differentiates simultaneity models from totality models. In simultaneity models, the environment and the person exist as one and change mutually. (Parse's theory of nursing is discussed fully in Chapter 9.)

Nursing models share certain interrelated and important features, because they all reflect the currently dominant professional values concerning the person, health and nursing activities.

* They are all holistically oriented, in that they take account of the whole person.

* Related to this, health is seen as more than simply a disease-free state.

* They all imply that nurses are autonomous professionals who make judgements independently of medical prescription. Nurses are thinkers as much as, or even more than, they are 'doers' and nursing is thoughtful and theoretically based.

* People are viewed as idiosyncratic individuals and nursing care should reflect this.

It is important to note that these models exhibit dissimilarities as well as similarities, and this reflects a range of differing perspectives or 'theories'; this is in addition to the range of 'commonsense' theories of nursing that different individuals hold. What this means, rather obviously, is that there is not any one theory of nursing, only theories of nursing. Nevertheless, the fact that such theories are both similar and dissimilar in certain respects permits dialogue between nurses who construct them.

Readers will have noticed that, along with Meleis (1991), I use nursing theory and conceptual model interchangeably. This is because both conceptual models and 'my' theories deal with the relationship of concepts (at differing levels of generality and complexity) of the phenomena with which nursing is centrally concerned. Because of this, they both provide a description of what nurses do, or a prescription of what nurses should do, to the recipients of their care, in or with particular physical and social environments, to optimise their health status.

A further theory, one that describes how nurses should approach and structure their practices, gained popularity in the 1960s, 1970s and early 1980s. This theory is known as the nursing process approach to care. Nursing process aims to individualise care through 'scientific problem solving' (Marriner 1979) and, as such, should incorporate nursing research findings. (An analysis of the nursing process approach to care is provided in Chapter 4.)

The concepts underpinning theories or models of nursing and the nursing process approach to care are components of the **espoused theories** of nursing theorists and academics—that is, they are the theories they claim to hold (Argyris and Schön 1974). Unremarkably, therefore, they are also the espoused theories of nursing undergraduates and graduates. They are acquired consciously by undergraduate nurses, largely through formal classroom teaching and from reading nursing literature. They are strikingly different, however, from nurses' **theories-in-use** (Argyris & Schön 1974)—that is, those concepts or theories that manifest in action. These they learn from clinical nurses who use them constantly in everyday nursing practice.

NURSING 'IN PRACTICE'

The nursing theories with which undergraduate and newly graduated nurses are equipped by nurse academics and through nursing literature—that is, their espoused theories of nursing—are of questionable assistance to them when they encounter the real world of nursing. Nursing's 'real world' is the clinical facilities to which undergraduates and graduates are allocated and where they are required to render service to a range of patients and clients with a number of competing demands. In such facilities, undergraduate and newly graduated nurses discover that care is still largely task-centred, despite nursing theory and thinly disguised pretensions to the contrary. 'Primary nursing' and 'total patient care' are the new labels for what amounts to one nurse, or a small team of nurses, performing all the required tasks for a limited number of patients. They still 'do obs' and 'do beds', but for their own group of patients. It is now almost a cliché that total patient care is provided whenever workload permits (Greenwood 1993).

In addition, undergraduates and new graduates feel inadequately prepared for their clinical role. They feel that they possess neither the clinical nor the interpersonal skills that are required for nursing (Department of Human Services and Health 1995). Despite their lack of knowledge, however, the workload in clinical facilities is often such as to require the immediate incorporation of undergraduates and new graduates into the clinical team. This is most effectively accomplished by pairing them off with a peer, preceptor or clinical nurse who is already familiar with the way nursing work is typically organised on the ward or unit—that is, the ward routine (Hart 1991).

Ward routines are a means of organising nursing care related primarily to patients' physical needs and they reflect the individual preferences of the senior nursing and medical staff (Proctor 1989; McCaugherty 1991). Undergraduate nurses and new graduates feel they must discover what senior staff expect of them and, thereby, learn to 'fit in' to the team (Melia 1981; Seed 1991; Hart 1991). The organising function of routines allows junior nurses to structure and sequence their nursing tasks; because of this, routines help nurses to 'get through' their workloads (Melia 1981; Seed 1991; Street 1991). 'Getting through' is approved by senior colleagues and helps undergraduates and new graduates to feel accepted and to fit in. Learning the professionals' 'trade secrets' (Moorhouse 1992) allows nurses to fit in more easily.

The urgent need to 'get through' their workload actually justifies skimping tasks and using incorrect procedures (Kelly 1991; French 1992) as far as junior nurses are concerned. If they 'get through', they are seen to be 'pulling their weight' and 'fitting in' (Melia 1981; Seed 1991).

Of course, nurses learn more than just routines and how to get through in their everyday nursing activities in clinical practice; they also learn what 'real' nursing is. 'Real' nursing, unsurprisingly, is what 'real' nurses do—that is, senior clinical nurses. Senior nursing colleagues usually undertake the more technical, medically devolved tasks and teach these more technical aspects of care to junior colleagues. Senior staff tend not to give 'basic' care, nor do they tend to teach it (Gott 1984).

This contrasts sharply with nursing in theory. 'Real nursing', in theory, is that kind of care which is person-centred, related to everyday living activities and independent of medical prescription. 'Real nursing' in practice, however, is technical nursing and everyday nursing activities are just 'basic nursing' (Seed 1991).

To sum up: 'in practice' the focus of nursing is physical care and not the person; nursing consists in getting through the workload at almost any cost; 'real nursing' is technical nursing and everyday nursing activities are just 'basic nursing', which can be undertaken following minimal instruction.

Such are the theories-in-use which operate to structure nursing activities in practice. It is surprising how similar they are to 'commonsense' theories of nursing.

COMMONSENSE THEORIES OF NURSING

It was claimed earlier that concept construction in human beings begins before people learn to speak. This is worth remembering; nursing students are all adults, which means that their personal histories reflect at least 17 years of interacting with their experiences of reality and learning to interpret them and respond appropriately—that is, construct interpretive and action theories related to them. These theories can be clear-cut and explicit or, more likely, relatively implicit and fuzzy. Commonsense theories encompass the stereotypical images characteristic of the parent culture, which are internalised during a person's socialisation. Clearly, these will include gender and occupational stereotypes. This means that nursing recruits will already possess commonsense theories of what nursing is and who does it (Wilson-Barnet 1988); indeed, they could hardly have chosen to become nurses if this were not the case. According to such views, nursing is women's work requiring little in the way of formal training, being instinctively or intuitively derived (Hagell 1989). Additionally, it is complementary and subordinate to medicine; by implication, then, the formal training that nurses require is medically related. It would appear, therefore, that nursing in practice reinforces these commonsense theories, while nursing in theory explicitly rejects them. Nursing theory might well reject them but this hardly counts; nursing theory is perceived to have little to do with practice.

The discrepancies between nursing in theory (nurses' espoused theories) and nursing in practice (nurses' theories-in-use), as they relate to these values aspects, are striking and it is not without interest to note that they are recognised, certainly in a vague and general way, by nurses themselves. The theory–practice divide is now an established element in nursing tradition (McCaugherty 1991), to the extent that there appears to be some compartmentalisation or segmentation (Melia 1987) of 'theory' and 'practice' in the cognitions (or thinking) of nursing students and new graduates. This clearly has important implications for the quality of nursing practice.

COMPARTMENTALISING THEORY AND PRACTICE

Understanding how this compartmentalisation occurs in the minds of nurses presupposes at least some grasp of the nature of human thinking and learning; accordingly, I will begin with some introductory material on human thinking and learning. I will then go on to discuss the role of practice and feedback in these processes.

Human minds will construct mental images, ideas or 'theories'—technically known as concepts, constructs or representations (Tomlinson 1981)—of the objects they experience in the world; for example, articles, events, actions, and the results of actions, and their own subjective or internal experiences of such objects. My own preference is for the term 'representations', because they allow us to re-present to our own minds all that we have experienced. Minds will construct representations quite automatically, simply in response to exposure. Thus, for instance, a mother can call to mind, virtually at will, an image of her newborn baby ('object' of experience) and feel again the sensation of intense joy (experience of 'object') she felt when she first beheld the child.

These representations are what we 'learn' whenever we learn anything; we string together related representations of the different things we experience to construct 'theories' of them, in order to broaden our understanding of the world. Representations are, therefore, the 'contents' of human thinking.

This natural tendency to construct in mind images or representations of the experienced world allows us to recognise the same or similar stimuli when we next encounter them. Importantly, too, because both biological and social survival could well depend on it, this tendency allows us to construct and execute the appropriate response (Sanford 1984).

The ability to recognise the things we encounter as being of a certain sort—for example, a visually impaired patient—allows nurses to render their experiences meaningful. For when a nurse recognises something in the world as a 'visually impaired patient' she or he is really recognising that this particular stimulus means 'visually impaired patient' to him or her. The planning and execution of the appropriate response—'I should remove all potentially dangerous obstructions from the patient's path'—allows him or her to render such stimuli manageable. We construct images or representations of our experiences, therefore, precisely to render them meaningful and manageable. This is the function of human learning and thinking.

The construction of such images or representations need not go on consciously, however. In fact, a great deal of representational construction goes on unconsciously or automatically, so that we are not aware that we have constructed images. This has to be the case; the human mind can attend to only seven (plus or minus two) items or chunks of information at any one time (Miller 1956). The number of digits in your telephone number may be no accident. A vast number of representations are constructed unconsciously, especially those of repetitious everyday experiences, and some, as we already know, are constructed before infants learn to talk. Thus, for example, Japanese and American babies learn to be typical Japanese and American babies (i.e. passive and active babies respectively) by the age of four months (Caudill & Weinstein 1969).

Representations are constructed either consciously or unconsciously in response to experiential stimuli. Consciously constructed representations are acquired typically as a result of teaching, reading and disciplined enquiry; unconsciously constructed representations are acquired through repeated, everyday exposure.

Deliberately constructed representations tend to be 'clear-cut' (Howard 1987) and are presented as 'feature lists'; for example:

. . . activities of daily living are . . .

. . . maintaining a safe environment . . .

. . . communicating . . .

. . . breathing . . .

. . . eating and drinking . . .

. . . etc. . . .

These representations are called 'clear-cut' because what they represent is clearly delineated. Totality and simultaneity paradigm nursing theories and, to a certain extent, the nursing process approach to care are composed of clear-cut representations as, indeed, are the theories generated through nursing research and research in the behavioural and biological sciences. They delineate precisely what their central concepts include and, with respect to nursing theories, they represent their theorists' views of what nursing is or should be.

Incidentally and unconsciously acquired representations are rather different. They are not clear-cut but 'fuzzy' (Howard 1987) and consist, typically, in images because they are constructed in response to real, practical situations. They are called 'fuzzy' because what they represent is not clearly delineated. An example would be your own 'fuzzy' of a $5 note. You can select one from purse or pocket, but probably cannot describe in detail the words that appear on the note. Of course, you do not have to possess this level of detailed knowledge about $5 notes in order to use one. All you need is sufficient knowledge to allow you to select a $5 note from among others and to spend it.

This is a critically important point. It indicates clearly that, as representations are constructed automatically to render subsequent, similar experiences meaningful and manageable, the representations constructed will only be as adequate and accurate as they need to be for people to get by. If clear-cut representations are not required for nursing practice, therefore—and there is evidence that they might not be (Moorhouse 1992; Waters 1994)—they will not be constructed.

Similarly, because representations are constructed automatically to render subsequent similar experiences meaningful and manageable, by allowing the interpretation of subsequent similar stimulation and the planning and execution of appropriate responses, they are activated or triggered by the same or similar environmental cues. What this means is that, potentially, we can possess several representations to represent the same experiential object or stimulus for use in differing situations.

It is entirely possible for a nurse to have one clear-cut representation of nursing as giving holistic, individualised care, for examination and assignment purposes, and another 'fuzzy' concept of nursing as getting through the workload, for use in clinical practice situations (Greenwood 1990). Clear-cut nursing representations (espoused theories) will be activated by examination/assignment cues and nursing academics, and 'fuzzy' representations (theories-in-use) by cues normally found in clinical practice situations, such as patients, clinical nurses and doctors.

It is important to realise that, if we are unaware that we have constructed certain representations, we will also be unaware when we are using them to interpret incoming stimuli and structure action (respond appropriately). It also means that we are unable to surface them, identify them, or examine them for adequacy and accuracy against the realities they were constructed to make meaningful and manageable. We will also be unable to examine them against the clear-cut representations of the same realities reflected in the nursing literature. Their modification and refinement will, therefore, be unlikely.

A further point regarding representations, be they espoused theories or theories-in-use, remains to be made and this relates to their 'holistic' construction.

THE CONSTRUCTION OF EXPERIENTIAL 'WHOLES'

Representations, both clear-cut and fuzzy, are constructed as 'wholes' in just the same way as objects and stimuli are experienced. For when we learn what objects mean in our culture, we normally learn, simultaneously, how they are valued and how we should respond to them. Experience tends to be represented holistically in the mind.

Consider a toddler, Emma, playing in the park. A large labrador bounds up to the child, wags its tail and nuzzles her. The mother joins the child . . .

'. . . doggy, Emma . . . '

'. . . ah . . . nice doggy, Emma . . . '

'. . . Emma stroke doggy . . . '

Thus, at a stroke, Emma learns that certain sorts of objects in the world (or stimuli) are 'dogs' (object), that they are 'nice' (value) and that they should be stroked (action tendency). Emma might well have learned three different things about dogs had her encounter involved a pitbull terrier . . .

From a more professional perspective, Seed (1991) provides a telling illustration of how such 'wholes' are experienced. She described a student nurse's account of the behaviour of a registered nurse on the ward where she was working. This registered nurse held the nose of a patient while pouring fluid into his mouth. The nurse explained that the patient would swallow or choke. From this one experiential exposure the student nurse learned that the characteristics of this patient ('objects of experience') were valued less than those of other sorts of patients by professional nurses (relative value) and warranted different treatment (action tendency). By stringing together representations related to certain kinds of patients, nurses construct 'theories' of them.

To summarise so far: undergraduate and newly graduated nurses are exposed to and, therefore, may acquire two distinct repertoires of concepts—one for 'nursing theory' situations and another for 'nursing practice' situations. The former consists of a range of clear-cut representations, largely learned as feature lists from nurse academics and from nursing literature. This repertoire is the espoused repertoire—that is, it is composed of nurses' espoused theories about nursing, which typically represent nursing as being patient focused, holistic and concerned with activities of daily living. The latter repertoire, that concerned with nursing practice situations, consists of a range of fuzzy representations, learned largely as images through repeated, everyday exposure in clinical nursing settings. This repertoire is composed of nurses' theories-in-use, which typically represent nursing as focused on physical care and concerned with getting through the workload and fitting in to the ward team. Espoused theories are learned in classrooms and libraries, and theories-in-use in clinical settings.

PRACTICE AND FEEDBACK

Representations are constructed in response to experiential stimuli in order to render meaningful and manageable subsequent exposure to the same or similar stimuli. They will be activated and brought to bear in human thinking, therefore, by subsequent exposure to the same or similar stimuli. Emma, for instance, will only need her representation of 'dog' and her concept of an appropriate response to encounters with dogs (stroke them) when she next encounters a dog (or, of course, when she wishes to think about dogs or reflect on her experiences of dogs). Each time she activates her representations, 'dog' and 'stroke', she reinforces their connection and makes their subsequent retrieval easier. In technical terms, she 'chunks' input (sensory) data with output (effector) mechanisms (Eysenck & Keane 1990). Through the repeated activation of her associated representations of 'dog' and 'stroke', Emma will eventually respond automatically to dogs—that is, without thinking consciously that 'this' is a 'dog' and that it should be stroked. The interpretive and executive cognitive processes underpinning her recognition of and responses to 'dog' are eventually undertaken at lightning speed and quite automatically.

In precisely the same way, undergraduate and newly graduated nurses chunk sensory input data (these sorts of patient characteristics) with effector mechanisms (certain sorts of nursing actions) through their repeated activation in everyday clinical practice situations. It is the progressive chunking of component subroutines and skills (and, of course, the representations they reflect) and their eventual automatic or unconscious firing in simple or familiar task situations, that frees nurses for conscious problem solving in more complex or unfamiliar clinical situations. This, then, is the function of practice.

Feedback is nothing more than 'knowledge of results' (Fitts & Posner 1967) and, although it can take a variety of forms, it is unavoidable. Many people fail to realise this.

Every time we activate a representation (or, more likely, a chunk or repertoire of associated representations) to interpret incoming stimuli, and plan and execute an appropriate response , we are, in an important sense, testing it on them for adequacy and accuracy. The feedback we inevitably and unavoidably elicit confirms or disconfirms their usefulness in these respects. Consider Emma's subsequent encounter with a pitbull terrier when she activates her representations of 'dog'. This is a horrendous example, but one that illustrates the point quite beautifully.

Again, from a more professional perspective, the 'looks' that Melia's (1981) and Seed's (1991) nursing students elicited from senior clinical nurses, when they were seen not to be pulling their weight in order to get through the nursing workload, provided feedback to the students concerning their senior colleagues' expectations of their performance. Feedback, therefore, allows the refinement, elaboration and/or modification of representations which, in turn, enable the cogniser to become progressively more discriminating.

CLOSING THE THEORY–PRACTICE GAP

Closing the gap depends on two factors. First, nurse academics who wish undergraduate nurses to use person-centred, holistic concepts in clinical practice settings should teach these concepts in clinical settings (wherever practicable). They will thus ensure that representations of different kinds of patients are chunked with appropriate values and action tendencies. Repeated practice in clinical settings, reinforced by appropriate feedback from teachers and patients, will guarantee, other things being equal, that the activation and deployment of them will become automatic.

Second, nurse academics, clinical preceptors and even their peers should assist undergraduates to surface, identify and examine the 'fuzzies' (or theories-in-use) of nursing that they have incidentally constructed. This will entail sharing clinical experiences with them, as some of these 'fuzzies' will only become apparent in action (use). Surfacing and identifying 'fuzzies' can go on prior to nursing action—that is, nurse academics and clinical preceptors can require students to state what they intend to do (facts), why they intend to do it, how, when and with what resources (facts, values and action tendencies) before giving care. Appropriate feedback derived from nursing and other theory can then be given and, importantly, incorporated into the students' nursing care. Moreover, should inappropriate 'fuzzies' manifest unconsciously during the caregiving, their tutorial colleagues, preceptors or peers can draw attention to them and assist students to examine them for adequacy and accuracy.

'Fuzzies' can be examined in two ways, namely, against the 'realities' they were constructed to render meaningful and manageable, and against the clear-cut representations of nursing and other relevant disciplines.

For instance, observation of the behaviour of some nurses could lead to the assumption, sometimes, that the 'fuzzies' operating to structure their practices represent patients who have suffered a stroke as, typically, deaf and intellectually impaired. There does seem to be a tendency for some nurses to shout at such patients and use unnecessarily simple language when interacting with them.

The 'fuzzies' can be tested against the reality of patients who have suffered a stroke. If such patients can respond, in some terms, to normal speech, they manifestly are not deaf and, probably, not intellectually impaired either. In addition, such 'fuzzies' can be tested against the clear-cut representations, relating to people who have suffered a stroke, that have been constructed through nursing and related research. (To my knowledge, there is no evidence (clear-cut representations) in either nursing or related research that such people are typically deaf and intellectually impaired.)

An additional and important means of examining such 'fuzzies' is against the conceptual models put forward by various theorists (see above). This is not to suggest that all the models are adequate in every respect; clearly they are not. (Chapter 7 provides valuable insights into theory critique and application, and Chapter 10 demonstrates the utility of a nursing model in structuring a preregistration nursing curriculum.)

Conceptual models illuminate how nursing scholars believe nursing should be; this means that they provide the tools with which to criticise and adapt nursing as it is. It is through the sensitive and insightful examination of nurses' fuzzy representations of practice against the clear-cut representations of 'theory' that practice can be improved. Similarly, it is the testing of clear-cut theoretical representations in practical situations that allows theory's development and refinement. This does not relate exclusively to nursing models, of course; it also relates to 'theories' derived from nursing research and from the biological and behavioural sciences. It is through this iterative process that the representations which underpin practice become as accurate and as adequate as they possibly can be; this allows nurses to plan, implement and evaluate the sort of nursing care they have consciously come to consider appropriate and desirable. In addition, it offers a means of closing nursing's theory–practice gap and of developing nursing theory from practice.

Chapters 11 and 14 describe the processes whereby, through systematic and critical reflection on practice—that is, through the surfacing and critical examination of their fuzzy representations—two groups of practising nurses developed their own theories of nursing.

SUMMARY

It has been argued that both nursing 'in theory' and nursing 'in practice' are intensely theoretical but that their theoretical underpinnings are discrepant. Undergraduate and newly graduated nurses learn these two discrepant theoretical repertoires, one for use in 'nursing practice' situations, the other for use in 'nursing theory' situations.

Representations characteristic of nursing theory are typically learned by students in university settings from nurse academics and nursing literature and, because of this, such representations are likely to be clear-cut. The retrieval cues of such representations are likely to reflect those typically used by nurse academics and in student assessments/examinations.

In contrast, practice representations are learned in clinical facilities from working alongside clinical colleagues. And, since routine experiences typically neither elicit nor require clear-cut representations, practice representations are likely to be fuzzy. The retrieval cues of nursing practice representations are likely to be those typically found in practice settings—for example, clinical nurses, patients, and the goals of getting through and fitting in.

The promotion of high-quality nursing care and the development of practically relevant nursing theories, therefore, depend on the mutual and critical examination of the previously surfaced fuzzy representations of practice against the clear-cut representations of nursing models and research and those derived from the behavioural and biological sciences.

GLOSSARY

Espoused theories: the representations of reality (in our case, of nursing reality), which people claim ('espouse') to hold but which may not be expressed in practice. Some nurses claim, for instance, that they provide holistic nursing care when, in fact, their care is predominantly physical in focus.

Theories-in-use: the representations of reality which people express in action or practice (in 'use') but which they may not know they hold or, indeed, may even deny holding. The depth of the sexist representations inherent in statements that claim that 'Man' is a another name for the human species, and thus gender neutral, is a telling example.

Theory–practice gap: a term used to represent the perceived discrepancy between the ideals of nursing as taught in universities and the realities of practice as experienced in clinical units.

QUESTIONS

1   Which patients do you prefer to nurse? Why? What 'theories' do your preferences reflect and what implications do your preferences have for your practice?

2   When you first arrive at the unit at the beginning of a new clinical allocation, what is your main objective? Why?

3   Who teaches you communication skills when you are on clinical placement? In terms of the perceived importance of communication skills, what does this imply?

LEARNING ACTIVITY

Look carefully at the contents of a nursing handover report. What is the ratio of statements relating to physical and psychosocial aspects of care? What representation of nursing makes this ratio understandable?

FURTHER READING

Benner, P. 1984, *From Novice to Expert: Excellence and Power in Clinical Nursing Practice*, Addison-Wesley, Menlo Park, California. This book is a classic and is essential reading for all nurses. Benner effectively illustrates the growth of nursing expertise through five identifiable phases and describes the approach to practice typical of each phase.

Moorhouse, C. 1992, *Registered Nurse: The First Years of a Professional Nurse*, La Trobe University Press, Bundoora, Melbourne. Moorhouse describes the characteristics of 'reality shock' that newly graduated nurses experience when they become health service employees for the first time. He also explains the cause(s) of reality shock.

2

NURSING RESEARCH AND NURSING THEORY

JENNIFER GREENWOOD

LEARNING OBJECTIVES

When you have read this chapter you should be able to:

1 Understand the interrelationship of nursing research and nursing theory.

2 Explain the purposes of nursing theory or theories.

3 Explain the reasoning underpinning the construction of nursing theories.

INTRODUCTION

Some time ago a second-year nursing undergraduate asked me a very interesting question about the purposes of research; I had just given a lecture on the different research paradigms that inform contemporary nursing research. She asked if research made you a better person. I was struck by this penetrating question. It took me a while to articulate what to my mind is a satisfactory answer and it is this: research potentially makes people 'better' because it furnishes them with the sort of information, both factual and ethical, that enables them to take, or have, a justifiable position on issues of salience to them. Their reasoning should become more rational and more humane. The information generated and tested by research is incorporated into theory by human scientists (in the broadest sense) to describe, explain, predict and prescribe important aspects of our lives.

In this chapter, therefore, I intend to discuss the nature and purpose of research, the relationship of research and experience, and the nature of human theorising. These discussions will include some material on the research process and some introductory information relating to contemporary, and general, approaches to research.

THE NATURE AND PURPOSE OF RESEARCH

Research is doing what comes naturally, only doing it better

People construct their knowledge bases on systems of related **concepts**. This is done in two ways. Some concepts are constructed carefully, deliberately and in a highly disciplined way. Other concepts are constructed relatively carelessly and incidentally. Concepts constructed systematically and in disciplined ways are said to be 'scientifically derived' and are produced as a result of **research**. Concepts constructed relatively carelessly and unconsciously are known as 'experientially-derived' concepts and are constructed, as their name implies, in response to exposure to particular experiences.

Human minds will construct concepts or representations quite automatically in response to exposure to experiential stimuli, both 'objects' of experience and subjective experiences of 'objects'. Thus, for instance, nurses can construct concepts of an infected, purulent wound ('object' of experience) and feel again the sensations of repulsion or sympathy (subjective experience of 'object') they felt when they first observed the wound. This natural tendency of human minds to construct concepts automatically is linked to biological survival. It allows us to interpret subsequently experienced stimuli and, because biological survival could depend on this, execute an appropriate response (Sanford 1984). Interpretation of stimuli of the type 'this wound is suppurating' presupposes something in mind with which, or against which, to appraise the stimulus—that is, a representation or concept of it. Such mental images allow us to represent in our own minds the objects we experience and our subjective experiences of them. It would be a mistake, however, to believe that the representations of the reality we experience correspond faithfully to the reality we do experience. It is important to recognise, along with Tomlinson (1981) and Foucault (1972), that representations or concepts are constructed according to cultural convention and, therefore, do not necessarily mirror accurately the object/subject they seek to represent. For instance: are patients who constantly complain attention seeking or attention needing? Or something else . . . ?

The recognition and interpretation of stimuli—for example, 'this wound is suppurating'—allows us to render experiences meaningful, because this interpretive statement implies 'this stimulus means a suppurating wound'. And the execution of the appropriate response 'I should apply extra padding' allows us to render our experiences (or the stimuli that constitute our experiences) manageable. We construct concepts, therefore, precisely to render experience meaningful and manageable; this is true, irrespective of the thinker's relative awareness or their relative **validity**. (See Chapter 1 for a fuller discussion of concept-acquisitive processes.)

Researchers construct their concepts very carefully and systematically using logic and skilled observation. They normally follow a series of steps, recognised as appropriate by relevant research communities and generally termed 'the research process'. This is to ensure, as far as they possibly can, that the concepts they construct are accurate and adequate representations of the 'reality' they seek to understand. For instance, it took many years of painstaking research, conducted according to contemporary views on research process, to construct accurate and adequate concepts of AIDS.

In a nutshell: research aims to construct the most adequate and accurate (or valid) concepts of reality in order to render it meaningful and manageable.

Research constructs concepts of natural and social phenomena

For ease of explanation, natural and social **phenomena** can be distinguished in two ways. To begin with, natural phenomena, as the name implies, are found in the world of nature, the natural world. They are physical entities, like snow; they have shape, size, volume and colour; and they exist independently of anyone's knowledge (concepts) of them. In addition, they are considered to be governed by causal laws of the type: *if A, then B, and B always.* In other words, if certain antecedent conditions, A, obtain—for example, snow is heated to 45°C—the consequences, B, are guaranteed to follow, and follow always; that is, snow will melt.

Social phenomena are rather different. They are not physical entities (except the artefacts or 'products' of social practices) in quite the same way. Social institutions that are, or reflect, traditional human practices convey social meanings and, therefore, they do not exist independently of anyone's knowledge (concepts) of them. A particularly salient example is nursing. Nursing (practice, education, management and research) exists only in nursing behaviour and, rather obviously, people can only behave as nurses when they know how to. 'Know how to' here means 'possess the necessary concepts of what nursing is or should be'. In other words, knowing how to nurse (or behave as a nurse) requires a knowledge of what nurses do, with whom, what for, where and how, and these are functions of what nursing means in any given culture. Knowing what to do, when, why, how, where and to whom, as a nurse, means knowing the rules that govern nursing. And this points to a further distinction between natural and social phenomena. Social phenomena are rule-governed rather than law-governed. Rules, unlike laws, are context-dependent; they permit the management of particular situations where the what, why, to whom, when and where may differ.

Social rules embody the meaning of human behaviour. The rules arise from the shared meanings that operate to create and sustain social situations. They are shared meanings because they are transmitted through cultures in language, skills and practices (Allen, Benner & Diekelmann 1986).

Because natural and social phenomena are now considered by many scholars to be different, they are normally investigated or researched in different ways (see below).

Research proposes relationships between concepts related to both natural and social phenomena, and then tests such propositions

A proposition is a statement of relation (Dickoff & James 1968); it describes the relationship between two or more concepts. It is, quite literally, by stringing concepts together in propositions of increasing generality and inclusiveness that we broaden our understanding of the world:

. . . *when a wound is red* . . .

. . . *and hot* . . .

. . . *and swollen* . . .

. . . *and painful* . . .

. . . *it is infected* . . .

and

. . . *an infected wound* . . .

. . . *is accompanied by pyrexia* . . .

. . . *and flushed skin* . . .

. . . *and sweating* . . .

. . . *and decreased urinary output* . . .

. . . *etc.* . . .

Propositions, that is, statements relating two or more concepts, are tested to assess their validity and, as already indicated, validity is a function of the adequacy and accuracy of concepts and their proposed relationships. What constitutes an appropriate test of validity, however, depends on how the nature of the phenomenon under investigation is construed. 'Construed' is an important word here; there is no way we can 'know' with certainty that the realities we perceive are as we perceive them. Our concepts *are* what we know and, as discussed above, these are constructed according to cultural convention. What this also implies, rather obviously, is that decisions concerning what counts as a test of validity are also a function of social convention.

The 'objects' that are found in the world (e.g. bacteria) are viewed by contemporary scientists as natural phenomena and are considered to be governed by causal laws. The validity of propositions concerning natural phenomena is considered to be appropriately assessed, therefore, through repetitive testing, under highly controlled conditions—that is, 'scientific' experiment. This is to ascertain that it is A that causes B, not C . . . or D . . . or E . . . and causes B, always.

Social phenomena (e.g. nursing 'rules') are a product of the meanings that are more or less shared among members of a cultural group. What these meanings are can be inferred from what people do and say. It is through the identification of these meanings that we come to understand human behaviour. Since many of the social rules and meanings that we learn, however, are learned relatively automatically and carelessly through mundane repetition in any given culture or subculture, close examination may well reveal a range of inconsistencies. In an important sense, therefore, we are uniquely privileged with respect to the contents of our own minds.

Consider, for example, the differing motivations that could account for a nurse watching a patient struggle to get out of bed. (What rule is she observing? Is she promoting mobility . . . or self-care . . . or something else . . . ?) What this implies is that the validity of propositions constructed by researchers, concerning the meanings of social phenomena, should always be checked with the people who constructed/are constructing them. Whenever human action or human behaviour is being researched or studied, the meanings attributed to the behaviour *by the researcher(s)* should be confirmed by the observed (inter)actors as being faithfully representative of their meanings.

It is worth remembering that all propositions and the concepts they relate, irrespective of their relative consciousness or adequacy, are tested repeatedly by the thinker who constructs them. Responsible researchers test their propositions carefully, according to research process and contemporary social convention, taking into account the nature of the phenomenon under investigation. 'Ordinary people' going about their everyday business test their propositions, too, but less carefully. They test their propositions every time they are used to interpret incoming stimulation and to execute a response; the feedback elicited either confirms or disconfirms their validity. (Consider, for instance, the last time you made a mistake socially. What propositions were you operating with at the time? How were they modified as a result of feedback?) This is precisely how undergraduate nurses and beginning practitioners learn nursing 'rules'.

There is another point concerning propositions that needs to be made here. It is this: only propositions can be true or false, that is, validated (confirmed as true) or invalidated (confirmed as false) according to extant social convention. Research tests only the validity of the propositions we construct about reality, because that is all it can test. Research does not, because it cannot, test the existence of anything; reality may or may not exist but it can never be true (or false).

Research is always tentative

It is because things like snow, bacteria and nursing 'rules' can never be true or false that research is always tentative—it requires human reasoning and judgement to construct propositions concerning reality. In addition, and as already pointed out, the tests of validity to which researchers' propositions are subjected are reflective of dominant scientific views or conceptualisations of what counts as acceptable validity tests. It has to be this way, because 'validity' is an abstraction which is socially constructed; what counts as validity, or what validity means to any given scientific community is, again, merely a function of social convention.

Research constructs theories about the natural and social worlds

One final point concerning propositions needs to be made: propositions are formulated and validated to construct theories about the natural and social worlds. Theories are logical systems which organise and group propositions at differing levels of inclusiveness and generality. As Shelley (1984) puts it, 'the creative integration of known facts and observations that, in addition to explaining the phenomenon, predict events to come' (p. 5). She goes on to elaborate on the sources of known facts and observations and identifies research findings, clinical experience and hunches. The construction of logically related propositions (theories) about the natural and social worlds allows us to describe and explain experiential stimuli to render them meaningful, and to predict and prescribe experiential stimuli to render them manageable.

Research is but the tool or instrument of invention; it allows researchers to construct or invent theories about the world to describe, explain, predict and prescribe salient particulars in it (Dickoff & James 1968).

Research is always theory-driven

Research is always theory-driven because, as will be evident by now, the recognition of a problem or an issue, or even the formulation of a question presupposes some recognition of a potential relationship. This, in turn, necessarily presupposes a prior interpretive effort—that is, some effortful relating of incoming stimuli to existing conceptual structures (or, of course, the creative relating of existing, but distinct, conceptual structures in the service of some task). Even when a researcher merely seeks to describe some interesting phenomenon, the recognition that some description is required also presupposes a prior interpretive effort. The passive reception of uncontaminated or raw data, therefore, is not possible.

What researchers already know—that is, their existing conceptual repertoire, the situation they find themselves in, and the purposes to which the research is directed—drives the selection of their research focus; this drives the design of the study and appropriate analysis of data. It is because research is always theory-driven that responsible researchers try to make manifest the theoretical underpinnings of their work and subject their propositions to rigorous tests of validity, however construed, to minimise the possibility of bias.

What constitutes a validity test will depend on dominant views regarding the nature of the reality being investigated, what counts as valid knowledge about it and how to go about collecting this valid knowledge. More technically, questions surrounding conceptions or constructions of the nature of reality are *ontological* questions; those surrounding the validity of knowledge are *epistemological* questions; and those surrounding how knowledge should be collected and analysed are *methodological* questions. You will notice that these questions are logically related. Their logic is captured in theories of science, more commonly known as the philosophy of science.

RESEARCH AND EXPERIENCE

I have been at pains throughout the foregoing discussion to indicate that research and experience are functionally similar; they both permit us to render salient aspects of our lives meaningful and manageable. They do this by exciting the construction of concepts that allow subsequent, similar stimulation to be recognised and interpreted and the appropriate response to it planned and executed. (The planning and execution of the appropriate response may be consciously created, or automatic and habitual, depending on the demands of the task situation—see Chapter 1.) Concepts, as we have already noted, that are invented through consciously disciplined and systematic enquiry (research) are known as 'scientifically derived', and those that are invented incidentally and relatively unconsciously through repeated mundane exposure are known as 'experientially derived'.

Scientifically derived concepts are constructed and presented propositionally, in 'feature lists' (Howard 1987). For instance,

. . . *swelling in skin edges* . . .

. . . *redness in skin edges* . . .

. . . *heat in skin edges* . . .

. . . *pain in skin edges* . . .

. . . *means infection of the wound* . . .

and

. . . *wound infection can result in* . . .

. . . *abscess formation, pointing, bursting* . . .

. . . *raised body temperature* . . .

. . . *raised white cell count* . . .

In contrast, experientially derived representations are normally constructed pictorially—that is, as pictures or images from concrete experiences (Howard 1987); what they include, however, can also be construed as propositional. This is because, as I have already indicated, each time they are triggered and used to render experience meaningful and manageable, they are tested for adequacy and accuracy—that is, validity. Thus, for instance, each time nurses confirm (or validate) that a patient with an infected wound is pyrexial, they confirm their concepts of infection.

Of course, recognition of experientially derived concepts (i.e. becoming aware of their construction) can, and in the case of nursing increasingly frequently does, lead to their scientific investigation. Relationships between clinical phenomena are proposed by enquiring practitioners because, as the signs of wound infection (above) illustrate, such phenomena are frequently observed to occur together. These propositions are then tested systematically to confirm or disconfirm their validity (see p. 24, 'The research process').

Concepts, both scientifically and experientially derived, are stored in memory in highly organised hierarchical frameworks (Sanford 1984; Eysenck 1993) to facilitate retrieval when needed. This hierarchical organisation is a function of chunking (Sloboda 1986) of related 'items' of information. Chunking, in turn, is a function of repeated exposure to related information. Human scientists, therefore, chunk wound redness, swelling, heat and pain under 'infection' or 'sepsis'. In addition, repeated exposure to these signs of wound sepsis and elevated white cell counts leads to the further elaboration of scientists' concepts of wound sepsis. Adequate and accurate concepts of wound sepsis then allow scientists to predict certain things about wound sepsis. If, for instance, scientists observe a wound that is very red and swollen they will make an informed guess (hypothesise) that it will also be hot and painful. And again, if their concepts of wound sepsis include predisposing causal factors (e.g. faecal contamination, long-term steroidal treatment, and lack of sterile precautions) they can also predict that, in the event of any/some/all of these factors obtaining, sepsis is possible/probable. Knowing these predisposing factors will also equip scientists to prescribe certain preoperative interventions (e.g. bowel preparation, cessation of steroid therapy and sterile surgical conditions) to prevent the occurrence of wound sepsis. Their ability to do all these things hangs on the different levels and types of theory that they or someone else have constructed. Theory, therefore, is constructed to describe, explain, predict and prescribe salient aspects of reality (Dickoff & James 1968; Doheny, Cook & Stopper 1987; Meleis 1991).

The description, explanation, prediction and prescription of reality is a function of the ways in which people theorise or reason about their worlds. To theorise *is* to reason.

HUMAN THEORISING

People theorise, or reason, in two ways—that is, theoretically and practically. These two reasonings have different purposes. Before describing these, however, it may be useful to emphasise again that the 'contents' of human theorising—that is, the propositions in relationship that are manipulated in human thinking—are derived scientifically (through research) and/or experientially through everyday experiences. We construct theories, or schemes of logically related propositions, to render our experiences meaningful and manageable.

When we reason, or theorise, theoretically we aim to reach a conclusion about something that interests us or, related to this, some 'truth' about our world. We reason, just as the scientists described above did, from simple or basic observational propositions of a '. . . this is a'. . . and '. . . it is related to'. . . nature, to complex truths or conclusions about the world. We reason inductively, that is, from specific instances to more general conclusions/truths, to describe and explain our experiences. Thus, for instance, we induce the relationships of red, swollen, hot skin edges to wound sepsis in **inductive reasoning**. This knowledge will then allow us to predict the occurrence of red, swollen, hot skin edges when we observe wound sepsis. This prediction is reflective of '. . . if . . . then'. . . reasoning, of the type '. . . *if* this wound is infected *then* red, swollen, hot skin edges are probable . . . '. This is known as **hypothetico-deductive reasoning**, because the scientist can deduce specific propositions from more general, inclusive propositions. These more specific propositions, referred to earlier as informed guesses, are known as hypotheses. **Theoretical reasoning**, then, allows us to describe, explain and predict objective and subjective experiences.

Practical reasoning is rather different. Practical reasoning typically begins in very complex human purposes or goals (e.g. the prevention of postoperative infection) and ends in their successful execution in a surprisingly limited range of simple actions (e.g. manipulating instruments to perform an aseptic dressing) (Carr 1981; Sloboda 1986). Practical reasoning, therefore, allows us to bring about the changes we consider desirable

(Carr 1981). Practical reasoning, just like theoretical reasoning, proceeds logically, but only through the hypothetico-deductive manipulation of propositions of an '. . . if . . . then'. . . nature. In addition, this hypothetico-deductive reasoning proceeds through conceptual structures of decreasing levels of generality and inclusiveness. Thus, for instance, our scientist recognises that faecal contamination of wounds leads to their infection. The scientist theorises thus:

. . . if I want to prevent faecal contamination of this wound . . .

. . . then I must empty the bowel preop . . .

. . . if I want to empty the bowel preoperatively . . .

. . . then I must purge the patient . . .

. . . if I want to purge the patient . . .

. . . then I must prescribe purgatives

. . . etc. . . .

The termination of this chunk of practical reasoning, which aims to prevent postoperative wound infection, is reached when a simple action is performed—that is, the patient is written up for purgatives (or a purgative is administered). Of course, skilled scientists do not need to progress consciously through such reasoning schemes. Practice in a range of situations has facilitated the chunking of much of this information to the extent that patients who are at risk of wound sepsis due to faecal contamination will automatically be prescribed purgatives (or other 'bowel-prep' items). But until automatic responses are perfected, we do have to reason in detail from our intentions to their execution in action. Practical reasoning thus allows us to prescribe our realities—that is, to bring about the changes in our realities that we believe are desirable and appropriate.

Nursing is a practice discipline (Meleis 1991; Pearson 1992); it is directed towards changing positively the health status of individuals and communities. The reasonings that bring about such changes are, therefore, practical. It is important to note, however, that the ability to theorise practically, as the above example illustrates, presupposes a whole raft of previous theoretical reasonings. This is because, in order to change something, we must know what it is that requires changing and also how it should be changed. In the words of Dickoff and James (1968), we must possess a range of related concepts which describe the current state of affairs—that is, the risk of postoperative infection and why the risk exists—and a range of related concepts which prescribe the to-be-brought-about state of affairs—that is, how to prevent it actualising.

The 'truths' and conclusions reached through theoretical reasoning, and the actions reached through practical reasoning, will be the more compelling and appropriate, respectively, when the propositional contents of them are as accurate and as adequate, in their own terms, as we can make them. And it is the accuracy and adequacy of our theorisings that justify our position on any issue. This is why research and theory make people 'better' (see the Introduction to this chapter).

The adequacy and accuracy of the nursing theory, or theories, constructed are dependent on the rigour with which nurse researchers approach their enquiries—that is, the rigour with which they follow the research process. What adequacy and accuracy might mean, however, and how the research process may be differently interpreted, depend critically on the world view of the researchers. It is, therefore, to a discussion of the research process and world views that I now turn.

THE RESEARCH PROCESS

The reflective practitioners among nurses are constantly bombarded with problems and ideas related to their practical (clinical, educational and administrative) concerns that require exploration and clarification. Sometimes, in order to achieve clarification, they need more information than is available; this means they have to construct the information or knowledge they require through research (Shelley 1984).

The process through which nurse researchers pursue their quest for scientifically derived knowledge has three stages (Fox 1982): designing the research plan, implementing it, and reporting and (paradigm depending) applying the findings. Each stage incorporates a series of steps. At the design stage there are 15 tasks the rigorous researcher must consider, at the implementation stage, two, and at the reporting/ applying stage, three. You should note the clear importance Fox accords the design stage. His point is that good (valid) research is meticulously and painstakingly planned. If the research design is sound, the implementation stage, which includes data collection and analysis, should be relatively unproblematic.

RESEARCH DESIGN

What follows is an illustration of the most important features of the design stage of the research process. (I am indebted to Susan Patterson, a BN (Hons) student at the University of Western Sydney, Nepean for granting her kind permission to use this illustration.)

The initiating idea and problem area

A nurse is working in a rehabilitation setting with patients who have sustained a traumatic brain injury and she begins to wonder if the family carers of such patients have needs that are not being met by the nursing staff. She begins to wonder about this because the outward manifestations of anxiety she has been taught to recognise do not seem to decrease in family carers in the rehabilitation setting. She wonders, too, if carer anxiety impacts on the well-being of brain-injured patients. She wonders about this because they appear to behave atypically when family carers appear more anxious. This nurse has induced that anxiety and need are related and, further, that carer anxiety and patient well-being are related.

The initial review of the literature

The nurse researcher, as she is now becoming, reviews the existing literature for scientifically derived concepts related to people who have sustained a traumatic brain injury and their family carers. She reviews the conceptual literature—that is, the theories of recognised authorities on traumatic brain injury, and its effects on patients and families—and also the data-based literature (Fox 1982). The latter refers to the findings of nursing research. Through this extensive literature review the nurse researcher constructs a conceptual framework related to the effects of traumatic brain injury on individuals and families. In other words, she uses the ideas, findings and understandings of other scholars to provide the foundation for her research and the background against which it will be undertaken (Fox 1982). The nurse researcher learns what has been studied in relation to the needs of the family of the traumatic brain-injured patient, by whom, where, when, which family members, how and with what limitations, and with what results. She thus acquires a comprehensive grounding in the contemporary knowledge relating to her area of interest, what gaps exist in this knowledge, which questions are reasonable and significant to nursing practice, and how they might usefully be investigated. Careful analysis of this literature, therefore, allows her to focus her research problem or question.

She now knows that it is the different needs of different family members that she wishes to study in the rehabilitation setting; she knows, too, that she must define (operationalise) 'family member' and 'need'. She decides this because the literature review indicates that no-one, so far, has investigated the different needs of different family members, and no-one has investigated these needs in rehabilitation settings.

The researcher quite rightly decides that the relationship of carer anxiety to patient well-being is a separate issue, one that can be explored at a later date.

The second review of the literature

The researcher reviews the literature a second time, but this time from an informed perspective. This secondary analysis allows her to identify precisely the questions to which she will seek answers, the sample population she will study and how. The questions she now wishes to address are as follows:

- What are the perceived needs of different family members of traumatically brain-injured people in one rehabilitation setting in Western Sydney?

- Do family carers perceive these needs as being met? If so, by whom?

Designing the data collection plan

The nurse plans to use both focus group interviews and individual interviews with different family members to collect her data. The focus groups of family members will furnish her with information related to perceptions of family needs in general in rehabilitation settings; the individual interviews will indicate the extent to which these perceived needs differ between family members. In the same way, the extent to which they are perceived as being met, and by whom, can be canvassed. The data will be analysed for differences in the perceptions of different family members. (Refer to the Further reading section at the end of this chapter for more details on the research process.)

WORLD VIEWS AND NURSING THEORY

If you were to trace the history of nursing theory and nursing research in the past 30 years you would notice that, in general, nurse theorists have espoused the dominant world views of their time (Gortner 1983; Kim 1989; Meleis 1991; Emden 1991; Lawler

1991; Pearson 1992). This is simply because they undertook their research training and postgraduate studies in university departments which also espoused the dominant world views of the period.

Chronologically, these world views were/are scientific, naturalistic and emancipatory. They have other names; the scientific paradigm is known as Analytic Empiricist (Sarantakos 1993) and Empirical Analytic (Allen et al. 1986). Similarly, the naturalistic paradigm is also known as the interpretivist paradigm (Sarantakos 1993), and the emancipatory paradigm, the critical paradigm (Allen et al. 1986; Sarantakos 1993).

Each of these world views, or overarching philosophies, incorporates assumptions about the nature of reality and the purposes of research (Patton 1990), the details of which need not concern us here (see, however, Emden and Sarantakos in the Further Reading section). Suffice to note that such world views reflect conclusions or 'truths' about the nature of reality, knowledge and knowledge acquisition; they are, therefore, in my view, the end products of scientists' theoretical reasonings.

These observations notwithstanding, the *scientific world view*, which was utterly dominant in the 1960s and 1970s, informed the construction of the nursing process, nursing models and theories that were expected to be 'applied' to nursing practice, and also of highly controlled quantitative research studies (Meleis 1991), the results of which were also expected to be 'applied' in nursing practice. These expectations were reflective of an often implicit view of social behaviour or human action as being causally determined—that is, governed by causal laws in much the same way as natural or physical phenomena (see above). They were certainly reflective of the expectation that insights generated in highly controlled experimental conditions could be applied in (or generalised to) the messy and unpredictable world of practice to control it.

The reaction of clinical nurses to these expectations was often stridently unsympathetic. Nursing theories and research findings that were not practically grounded in nursing realities were eschewed by clinical nurses as irrelevant (Greenwood 1984). Human action, it was argued, is context-dependent and reflective of meaning (concepts). Given this, human action should be studied in the contexts (natural settings) where it is meaningful, if its meaning is to be properly understood.

The *naturalistic* or *interpretivist world view* had begun to be appreciated. Part of this movement comprised the 'reflectivist' school, which recognised that many of the concepts underpinning human action are tacit (Polanyi 1958; Schön 1983). These actions can only be identified from the systematic and critical examination, including the self-examination, of action. Systematic, critical reflection on action allows us to induce the concepts that underpin it, to relate such concepts inductively and then hypothetico-deductively to render explicit the tacit meanings of our actions. This is prerequisite to the examination of such meanings for adequacy and accuracy (validity) and their possible elaboration, refinement and revision.

The naturalistic world view recognises that social situations are constructed and maintained through the observation of complementary social rules by all the interactors engaged in them. And, further, that social rules are reflective of the action concepts (or action theories) held by social interactors. These concepts need to be identified and understood—that is, induced and also, in some cases, hypothetico-deduced through qualitative research methods. An inbuilt requirement of these methods is the validation of the researcher's inferences or interpretation of the research subjects' meanings by the subjects themselves.

The *emancipatory* or *critical world view* evolved from the naturalistic movement. Emancipationists, like naturalists, believe that social reality is constructed through the observation of rules, but they also believe that these rules serve the purposes of dominant groups. Emancipatory or critical social science, therefore, seeks to uncover these social rules and the oppressive ideologies they reflect, to enable the emancipation or liberation of oppressed people from them.

Emancipists also induce and deduce the meanings (concepts) operating in the minds of those they are observing, in terms of both individual actions and the sociopolitical influences acting on them. Additionally, critical researchers check the validity of their inferences with the people being observed. They may do something more, however, and that is assist their research subjects to deduce, and implement, means to their (relative) liberation. (See Chapters 13 and 15 for further discussion.) It is interesting to note here what many readers will have already deduced—that is, when emancipists assist research subjects to deduce the means to their liberation they are, in effect, helping them to reason practically.

The point I wish to emphasise is that each world view, and its assumptions about realities and valid means to their investigation, is legitimate *in its own terms*. Aspects of people that we believe do conform to causal laws (e.g. their physiobiochemical aspects) can and should be investigated 'scientifically'; aspects relating to meaningful human action, including 'oppressed' human action, should be studied naturalistically. The important thing is to make clear which world views and assumptions underpin nursing theorising.

The differing world views briefly described above demonstrate clearly that views of what counts as science (and, therefore, nursing science) change in response to growth in knowledge, technological advance and sociopolitical influences. These are not the only world views to feature in contemporary nursing research, however; two others, namely, 'New Generation Research' and postmodernism, are currently relatively powerful. Together with the three world views already discussed, they differ to varying degrees on how research 'subjects' should be viewed and treated, on the relationship of the researcher to the research study, and on the essential nature of the research process through which investigations should be undertaken.

I will deal with these last two world views in reverse order, because I believe it is a little easier to grasp the rationales underpinning 'New Generation' approaches than those of postmodernism.

NEW GENERATION RESEARCH

I suggested above that research generates and tests concepts, propositions and theories to allow us to describe, explain, predict and prescribe salient aspects of our lives; I further suggested that this is most rigorously accomplished by following the stages and steps of the research process. Two assumptions could be read into these suggestions. The first is that the primary goal of research is understanding and the second, that methodology is of critical importance to valid research. Both these assumptions are rejected by New Generation researchers.

New Generation approaches are based on the collective New Generation beliefs that:

■ nursing is both human and technological science;

■ nursing is a practice discipline; and

■ scientific exploration has ethical and moral implications.

Three research goals are derived from these three beliefs. The first is that the apparent competition between quantitative and qualitative methodologies should be deemphasised. This is because nursing, as both humanistic and technological science, requires investigation from as many research approaches as have potential applicability. The second goal is to value research which directly improves nursing practice more than research which simply generates and tests theory. The third goal is that ethical and moral principles should guide all the steps in the research process (Streubert & Carpenter 1995).

Of course, scientists down the ages would claim to espouse these goals. New Generation researchers do not deny this; they simply assert that the pursuit of such goals has traditionally been secondary to theory construction and method.

The implications of New Generation approaches are clearly important. Approaches which ethically demand that research be undertaken *with* rather than *on* research 'subjects' require a radically different research design. The design, however, and the research process through which it is actualised should be as rigorous and systematic, in its own terms, as any other.

POSTMODERNISM

Postmodernism is yet another world view. It is not a specific doctrine and there is not 'one line' in postmodernism; it is an umbrella term for a range of theories which eschew the modernist view of the relevance of philosophy and theory to enlightenment and humanity. According to this postmodern world view, all representations, irrespective of their 'scientific' or experiential derivation, are strategic, not neutral; representations are always tied to political agenda, they are sociohistorically located and value-laden. They are valid or relevant for the immediate present and for certain people only.

These postmodern propositions are based on further propositions related to language. Experiences of the world are determined by language, or at least, by some underlying structure that gives shape to both language and our experiences (Solomon 1988). The construction and validation of knowledge is through the mastery and manipulation of language.

The central strategic device of postmodernisation is deconstruction (Derrida 1983)— that is, the analysis of forms and contents of communications, oral or written, to expose underlying discrepancies in logic and attitude. Deconstruction can, therefore, provide an interesting tool for the critique of nursing texts and theories (Lister 1991).

SUMMARY

Nursing research begins and ends in nursing practice. Questions which arise in nursing practice excite or motivate enquiring nurses to find answers to them; they pursue their answers in a systematic and rigorous way, following the appropriate research process. The answers they construct are logically combined to form theories and these, in turn, are tested for validity in practice. Research is the means by which practical problems may be investigated and ameliorated; it produces theories which indicate or prescribe means of improving practice and patient outcomes. Theories can also provide useful frameworks for reconceptualising problems and issues.

Nursing theory or, more accurately, nursing theories are theories of different levels of specificity and generality that are related to the phenomena with which nursing is centrally concerned (Meleis 1991)—that is, patients, clients, nurses, the environment and health and their interfaces (Fawcett 1984; Stevens Barnum 1994). Nursing theories are, therefore, systems of logically related and hierarchically organised propositions concerning the relationships of patients and clients, nurses, the natural and social environments and health.

These theories may be constructed inductively—that is, from observations of specific instances and their relationships to other specific instances—through theoretical reasoning. The relating of concepts of specific instances (e.g. wound swelling and leucocytosis) allows theorists to infer their further relationship to more general, inclusive concepts (e.g. wound sepsis). They may also be constructed deductively—that is, propositions relating to specific instances may be derived from those of a more general inclusivity.

Nursing theories constructed of propositions which describe, explain and predict the practical realities with which nurses and nursing are centrally concerned allow nurses to render meaningful such realities. Similarly, nursing theories constructed of propositions which prescribe the practical realities with which nurses and nursing are centrally concerned allow nurses to render manageable such realities. Importantly, too, prescriptive nursing theories presuppose descriptive, explanatory and predictive nursing theories.

In short, nursing theories allow nurses to identify health needs, and plan, implement and evaluate therapeutic interventions aimed at fulfilling such needs on behalf of individuals and communities. Nursing theories of differing levels of inclusiveness and generality are the 'contents' of mind manipulated in both theoretical and practical reasoning, using inductive and hypothetico-deductive logic, in the service of health gain. To my mind, therefore, they allow nurses to (potentially) enlighten and humanise lives.

GLOSSARY

Concept: mental representation of what is perceptually experienced (Chinn & Kramer 1995).

Hypothetico-deductive reasoning: reasoning which proceeds by deducing specific instances from more general categories, for example, *if* there is inflammation, *then* hotness, redness and swelling will be apparent.

Inductive reasoning: reasoning which proceeds by inducing relationships of specific instances to more general categories, for example, hotness, redness and swelling indicate infection.

Phenomena: anything that can be perceived.

Practical reasoning: reasoning which begins with complex human purposes and ends in simple or basic actions. It involves the hypothetico-deductive manipulation of concepts at progressively decreasing levels of generality and inclusiveness to bring about whatever we consider desirable (or to construct prescriptive theories).

Research: a disciplined and systematic process of enquiry which seeks to construct adequate and accurate concepts of perceived reality in order to increase our understanding of reality and, thereby, our rational control over it.

Theoretical reasoning: reasoning which begins with simple or basic observational propositions relating to experienced reality, and ends in 'truths' or conclusions about it. It involves the inductive and hypothetico-deductive manipulation of concepts at differing levels of inclusiveness and generality to describe, explain and predict realities (or to construct descriptive, explanatory and predictive theories).

Validity: the extent to which concepts satisfy the criteria for adequacy and accuracy in different research orientations. When used in relation to research instruments, it refers to the extent to which the instrument measures what it is supposed to measure.

QUESTIONS

1 You wish to prevent an 80-year-old, undernourished man from developing pressure sores. What nursing theories would you utilise and what sort of theorising would you engage in to achieve this goal?

2 What particular aspects of clinical practice would you like to investigate? How would you go about doing this?

3 As a nurse, what is more important: your ability to reason theoretically, or your ability to reason practically? Justify your answer.

LEARNING ACTIVITY

Formulate a nursing goal for a real or an imaginary patient. Use practical reasoning to translate this goal into nursing action.

FURTHER READING

Chinn, P.L., Kramer, M.K. 1995, *Theory and Nursing: A Systematic Approach*, 4th edn, Mosby, St Louis, Chapters 4 and 5.

Emden, C. 1991, 'Ways of knowing in nursing', in *Towards a Discipline of Nursing*, eds G. Gray and R. Pratt, Churchill Livingstone, Melbourne, Chapter 1, pp. 11–31.

Fox, D.J. 1982, *Fundamentals of Research in Nursing*, 4th edn, Appleton-Century-Crofts, Norwalk, Conneticut, Chapter 3.

Lister, P. 1991, 'Approaching models of nursing from a postmodernist perspective,' *Journal of Advanced Nursing*, 16, pp. 206–12 (Forgive this writer's gender bias. He refers, mistakenly, to a number of nursing theorists as male.)

Meleis, A.I. 1991, *Theoretical Nursing: Development and Progress*, 2nd edn, J.B. Lippincott, Philadelphia, Parts 1–3 (Chapters 1–8 inclusive).

Sarantakos, S. 1993, *Social Research*, Macmillan, Melbourne, Chapters 1 and 2.

Sims, S.E.R. 1991, 'The nature and relevance of theory for practice', *Towards a Discipline of Nursing*, eds G. Gray and R. Pratt, Churchill Livingstone, Melbourne, pp. 51–72.

3

WAYS OF KNOWING IN NURSING

BEVERLY O'CONNELL

LEARNING OBJECTIVES

When you have read this chapter you should be able to:

1 List the factors that influence the various ways of knowing in nursing.

2 Describe the sources of knowledge in nursing and evaluate their strengths and limitations.

3 Describe Carper's four patterns of knowing and the five types of nurse knowers.

4 Identify the characteristics of the more artful nurse.

5 Understand the difference between qualitative and quantitative research methods.

Beverly O'Connell, RN, BAppSc, MSc, is a lecturer in the School of Nursing, Curtin University of Technology, Perth. She teaches in the areas of nursing assessment, nursing theory and nursing research. She has an adjunct research appointment with a major Perth teaching hospital and is conducting clinical research.

INTRODUCTION

Nursing is a practice-based discipline that has functioned primarily on knowledge and theories derived from other disciplines—for example, knowledge of cognition from psychology and knowledge of diseases from medicine. More recently, however, much more is being researched and written about nursing itself—that is, 'nursing knowledge'. This knowledge construction is being developed through our ways of knowing in nursing. As our ways of knowing nursing vary, it is important to review this process critically in order to gain an understanding of the factors that affect it, and the strengths and limitations of nursing's knowledge base.

We could hold the view that knowledge that has been developed and accepted by the profession is worthy of recognition and that the need for further review is unnecessary. A simple exercise conducted in a classroom setting illustrates the subjectivity of knowing and shows why a continuous and critical review of the process is necessary. Nine students in an honours seminar class were asked to close their eyes and try to identify the sound they heard. The sound was the ticking of a metronome. Their responses were:

- tapping on a metal box;
- hard plastic against the table;
- lunch box banging on something; and
- tapping against the file.

Finally, one student identified the sound as a metronome. She had heard this sound many times before as her daughters used a metronome to practise playing the piano. This exercise illustrates, in part, that information can be interpreted in different ways, and that this interpretation is influenced by many factors, one of which is experience. Other factors that influence 'knowing' will be discussed later on in this chapter.

As the discipline of nursing moves towards discovering, naming, theorising and knowing nursing, it is important to understand the objectivity and subjectivity of our claims and, more importantly, the context in which these claims are made. Articulating the strengths and limitations of our ways of knowing in nursing and the factors that affect this process, will assist the profession to a deeper understanding and further development of nursing knowledge. We must constantly ask the following questions:

- *How do we know what we know?*
- *Can this knowledge be verified as representing 'the truth'?*

▓   *Does this 'truth' apply across populations and contexts?*

These deep and searching questions have for years challenged the minds of philosophers as they have continued to ask questions about the taken-for-granted ideas and meanings about the world (Hughes 1990). This chapter provides insights into the factors that affect our ways of knowing in nursing and raises issues that need to be considered.

KNOWING

The Macquarie Dictionary (1987, p. 979) defines the word 'know' as 'to perceive or understand as fact or truth or apprehend with clearness and certainty', and 'knowing' as 'having knowledge or information'. Nursing is a practice-based human science where knowing includes knowledge based on observations and research (Meleis 1991). More specifically, nursing knowledge is derived from three main areas—nursing practice, nursing theories and nursing research (Schultz & Meleis 1988). Nursing's focus of concern (i.e. nursing phenomena) is complex and sometimes difficult to describe. Specifically, nursing focuses on the needs of people within the context of their state of health and their environment. How patients respond to their state of health varies considerably from patient to patient. For example, responses to having a mastectomy can range from accepting the loss of a breast to severe grieving that affects the patient's lifestyle. In some instances, the language itself may not exist to capture and explain what is being experienced.

Nursing's knowledge base and its ways of knowing are affected by many different factors. According to the literature (Agan 1987; Carper 1978; Kidd & Morrison 1988; Schultz & Meleis 1988; Vaughan 1992), some of these factors are:

▓   sources of knowledge;

▓   patterns of knowing;

▓   intuitive knowledge;

▓   nurses as knowers; and

▓   research methods used to develop knowledge.

Additionally, in our quest for knowledge we must also ask the right questions, for we will only know and understand when the right questions are asked and answered. One could argue that our knowledge base to date has been shaped by the questions we have asked. The difficulty is actually to recognise when we are asking the right questions. It is necessary, therefore, to reflect constantly on the literature and to raise questions that address our knowledge gaps and advance our professional knowledge base. Furthermore, it is important to recognise the questions that need more urgent answers (Schultz & Meleis 1988). While the literature discusses all these factors about our ways of knowing in nursing, what remains unclear is how they actually relate to one another, or if indeed there is a relationship at all. In light of this, each factor will first be discussed independently, and then any interrelationships will be considered.

SOURCES OF KNOWLEDGE

Vaughan (1992) suggests three prime sources of knowledge that capture some traditional and contemporary ways of knowing in nursing. It is important to examine these sources of knowledge in an attempt to determine their credibility within the contemporary context. Three sources are called tenacity, authority or expert, and a priori.

1 *Tenacity* refers to the traditional way—we know because 'it has always been done like that' (p. 4). More specifically, it is the belief that, because something has always been done in a certain way, then it must be the best way. According to Meleis (1991), people become psychologically comfortable by holding on to **traditional knowledge** and views. Nursing practice abounds with nursing routines and rituals that perpetuate and support the credibility of this source of knowledge (see Walsh & Ford 1989). A simple example is the ritual, performed by night duty staff, of weighing patients before breakfast. This custom continues, although there is very little, if any, empirical evidence to support the belief that weighing patients before breakfast gives a more accurate measurement than weighing them after breakfast or at any other time. Yet patients continue to be disturbed early in the morning because of an entrenched work routine. As the practice of nursing develops from a research base, the legitimacy of this source of knowledge is increasingly being questioned.

2 *Authority or expert* refers to the knowledge that is gained from nurses who have experience or are seen as an authority or role model. Expert opinions are valued and acknowledged as an important source of knowledge. For example, the clinical nurse specialist on the wound care special interest group possesses expert knowledge about wound management. However, Rodgers (1991) states that, in some instances, the endorsement by nurse experts of the 'traditional way' of doing a task poses a danger to the development of nursing knowledge. She defines this type of knowledge as **dogma**—'the unquestioning adherence to authority and tradition' (p. 177)—and argues a need for the profession to recognise and explore instances of dogmatic thinking and to subject these entrenched work practices to critical review. Meleis (1991) acknowledges the value of personal knowledge held and espoused by experts; however, she also cautions its generalisability and its unquestioning transmission from generation to generation. She argues that this practice hinders the growth and development of nursing knowledge. It is necessary to understand, on one hand, the value and worth of this kind of knowledge and, on the other, the potential for it to be misleading. This type of knowledge differs from intuitive knowledge, which is discussed later in this chapter.

3 **A priori knowledge** is derived from a logical deduction process. For example:

Tom has brown hair. He is a boy.

Bradley has blonde hair. He is a boy.

Adam has red hair. He is a boy.

Boys have different coloured hair.

As you can imagine, the validity of this approach depends on the logic of the deductive process. This source of knowledge can have flaws that result in conclusions based on very little information; in some instances, the claims that are made may be difficult to substantiate.

ORAL KNOWING

It is well recognised that nurses function within an **oral culture** (Street 1992). Within this operational mode, knowledge is transferred by word of mouth, from nurse to nurse—it is like an unwritten textbook that is a rich source of nursing knowledge. O'Brien and Pearson (1993) looked at this aspect of knowledge. They conducted a study in a 23-bed professorial nursing unit, using an action research approach, and addressed the question: What do nurses do that makes a difference? Nurses who participated in the study reflected on their actions (within this clinical setting) in order to address the study question. Data were collected from participant and non-participant observation, personal journal keeping and audiotaped semi-structured small group interviews. The results of this study revealed some interesting findings in relation to sources of knowledge. The researchers report that 'how to nurse' is transmitted orally from nurse to nurse and, because society devalues oral knowing, this knowledge remains largely invisible.

> The effect of social devaluation of nursing's orally held knowledge of caring practice has created the situation where understanding and transmission of the knowledge implicit in nursing has only been retained by nurses them-selves and then largely because there has been an implicit understanding of the value of such knowledge derived from the necessity to possess it in order to nurse effectively.
>
> *(p. 121)*

In answering their study question, the researchers report two aspects of care that are common in nursing. First, they note that nurses, due to their continuous contact with patients and familiarity with situations, develop an awareness of each patient's idiosyncratic behaviour. This knowledge assists in their understanding of each situation and influences their actions and the resulting nursing care. Second, as nurses work together they constantly engage in conversations that confirm or refute information and that build on their orally based knowledge.

Although the study also highlighted the uninformative and cryptic nature of the written progress notes (the record of care), the researchers did not discuss the professional ramifications of this factor. Rather, they explained it in terms of the notes being 'unwieldy and time-consuming to compile' (p. 123), thus making excuses for this feature. As nursing care occurs over several shifts involving many staff members, there needs to be a communication system that is more permanent than the spoken word. While the excuse that writing adequate progress notes is time-consuming may be genuine, the failing could be challenged within any professional and legal context. Furthermore, in the present work environment, with short shifts, a reduction in staff overlap time within clinical settings and the introduction of patient care assistants, registered nurses work predominantly in isolation and are therefore unable to build on each other's oral knowledge base. There is, thus, a need for nurse clinicians to develop their writing skills.

The unwritten knowledge held within the oral practice culture needs to be acknowledged and recognised but nursing must learn to surface this knowledge in a written form which can then be discussed and built on.

The findings of O'Brien and Pearson (1993) have some implications for nursing education, because this oral knowledge cannot be taught in a classroom setting—it is specific and occurs within the context of nursing practice. What is specific to this source of knowledge is not only that it exists in an oral form but also that it is *transferred* in the practice setting. Therefore, to tap into this knowledge base it is important for students to be allowed to work side by side with nurses from the practice setting, so that they can listen to the stories that are told and gain information from the oral tradition. In addition, it could be argued that students learn from observing experienced nurses practise and then **modelling** this behaviour. According to Bandura (1977), this modelling is an essential part of professional socialisation. While this situation has merit, it can also be problematic. For example, if student nurses observe something that is in conflict with what they have learnt (theory), it is important for them to discuss and clarify the situation with the experienced registered nurse or the faculty member, and then to discern whether the practice is exemplary and worthy of modelling or is actually an entrenched work practice that has no merit.

PATTERNS OF KNOWING

It is well recognised that nursing is both a science and an art (Johnson 1994). Knowledge of the science component, though developing, is more specific and better defined, while knowledge of the art of nursing is more abstract, complex and difficult to define. Reviewing patterns of knowing in nursing provides some explanation about nursing art and its contribution to patient care.

The seminal work of Barbara Carper (1978) provides information regarding our ways of knowing nursing and emphasises the complexity of nursing practice. She explicated four fundamental **patterns of knowing**—empirics, aesthetics, ethics and personal knowledge. These four patterns of knowing detail how we actually construct our knowledge in nursing, or how we should be constructing our knowledge to enable us to nurse more effectively. While Carper's work has been endorsed and is frequently cited in the literature (Jacobs-Kramer & Chinn 1988; Lumby 1991; Moch 1990; Schultz & Meleis 1988; Smith 1992; Vaughan 1992), she has not continued to publish and further clarify these patterns of knowing. There are some aspects of her work, therefore, that are difficult to explain. More work on these patterns is necessary because, according to Jacobs-Kramer & Chinn (1988) when nurses deliver patient care they use knowledge that is derived from each of these four patterns.

1   Empirics is associated with the science of nursing. This pattern encompasses knowledge that has been derived using an **empirical** approach—in other words, through experiment and observation, using the senses. According to Jacobs-Kramer & Chinn (1988), this type of knowledge is linked to the more traditional sciences.

2   Aesthetics is the pattern of knowing that is primarily associated with the art of nursing. It deals with the more subjective aspects of nursing, those learned within practice settings. Carper (1978) cites **empathy** as an example of this pattern of knowing. More specifically, when nurses understand and feel what a patient is experiencing (i.e.

empathise with the patient), they will develop knowledge over a period of time that helps in understanding the patient's perspective (Carper 1978). With experience, and through the process of representing, interpreting and envisioning past experience, practices of care develop that are unique and individually constructed for each situation (Jacobs-Kramer & Chinn 1988). The concept of caring, which is central to nursing, is grounded in aesthetic qualities (Smith 1992).

3 *Ethics* is the pattern of knowing that is associated with the moral component of care. It is informed not only by an ethical code but also by '. . . the voluntary actions that are deliberate and subject to the judgement of right or wrong—including judgements of moral value in relation to motives, intentions and traits of character' (Carper 1978, p. 20). According to Jacobs-Kramer and Chinn (1988), this pattern of knowing is developed by nurses valuing, clarifying and advocating. They also state that it does not simply mean that nurses use a code of ethics to make a decision but also that they engage in a dialogue that is:

- sensitive to the individual's situation;
- context-specific; and
- accommodates the view that there are multiple realities and what is 'just' in one situation may not be so in another.

To bring this knowledge to the surface nurses must discuss these situations with colleagues and to clarify the different perspectives and actions that are possible.

4 *Personal knowledge* is the pattern of knowing that stems from knowledge about oneself and the use of the 'therapeutic self'. For nurses do not simply implement a nursing intervention—they engage themselves with the patient in a therapeutic way. This pattern focuses on knowing '. . . that promotes wholeness and integrity in the personal encounter, the achievement of engagement rather than detachment; and it denies the manipulative, impersonal orientation' (Carper 1978, p. 20). Personal knowledge transcends objective reality, forms and stereotypes and is not medi-ated by the symbols of language (Jacobs-Kramer & Chinn 1988, p. 131). Carper admits that this is the most difficult pattern of knowing to teach and understand; one could describe it as being 'spiritual' in some ways. Moch (1990) adds that, in a human science that focuses on people and interactions, 'discovery of self' (p. 155) is essential for nursing practice. She further states that discovering, articulating and richly describing instances of personal knowing is essential for the develop-ment of nursing knowledge. It could be argued that this aspect is extremely necessary so that this pattern of knowing becomes more tangible, teachable and transferable.

According to Moch (1990), components of personal knowledge include:

- experiential knowing: becoming aware through participation or by being in the world;
- interpersonal knowing: increased awareness through intense interaction or being with the other person; and
- intuitive knowing: immediately knowing something without use of reason.

All four patterns of knowing are necessary for the understanding and delivery of patient care and should, therefore, be included in nursing curricula (Carper 1978). It is necessary for student nurses to learn how to make the right decisions and deliver nursing care informed by these knowledge patterns. Moreover, this should not be restricted merely to a classroom exercise within the discussion of a case study, but also enacted and discussed in the context of a clinical situation and followed up through reflective debriefing exercises conducted after any clinical practicum. In support, Jacobs-Kramer and Chinn (1988) argue that failure to use these patterns in an integrated way can have a negative effect on patient care; using any one pattern of knowing independently limits the decision-making process and the resulting patient care. An example that highlights this is given in the box on the opposite page.

UNKNOWING

More recently, Munhall (1993) has introduced another pattern of knowing that she calls '**unknowing**'. This pattern is described as 'a condition of openness' (p. 128), where nurses come to terms with and acknowledge what they do and do not know about the patient and the situation. It is based on the premise that individuals are unique and that in any nurse–patient interaction there are two differing perceptions of the situation—the nurse's view of what is happening and the patient's view. These two perceptions are informed by subjective values, beliefs and feelings. Munhall (1993) argues that it is necessary for nurses to acknowledge these subjective views and to keep them in abeyance. It is then necessary for nurses to get in touch with the patient's perceptions and subjective feelings and to act cognisant of the patient's view. Only by knowing the patient's views can the nursing interventions and care be individualised. For this to occur, nurses must approach the nurse–patient relationship without preconceived ideas of individual patients, and try to understand patients' experiences within the context of their own frames of reference.

According to Munhall (1993), the pattern of unknowing can lead to knowledge and understanding that is far deeper and more meaningful for nurses and patients. One could argue that this pattern—unknowing—intertwines and overlaps with Carper's (1978) four patterns of knowing, rather than being a new and separate pattern. Furthermore, it is not clear whether Munhall is simply talking about the nurse being the patient's advocate. **Advocacy** is central to and underpins ethics, personal knowledge and aesthetic knowing. The example on the next page also illustrates this point and highlights Carper's patterns of knowing.

INTUITION AS A WAY OF KNOWING

Intuitive knowing is a way of knowing that develops from experience and it is well recognised that this knowledge makes a difference to patient care and the outcome of that care (Agan 1987; Benner 1984; Benner & Wrubel 1989). One could argue that intuitive knowing is what Polanyi (1967) termed 'tacit knowledge'.

More recently, and within a nursing context, Short et al. (1993) have defined tacit knowledge as 'that knowledge we possess but do not openly express; it involves that part of knowing that we cannot put into words . . . for nurses it refers to the knowledge they can use but do not think about; it is implicit in, and inferred from, their behaviour' (p. 72).

Example

A mother wants her son circumcised for reasons of cleanliness. Informed by contemporary views and knowledge about circumcision (empirical knowing), the nurse is opposed to this procedure. The nurse can act, therefore, in one of two ways: in keeping with his or her own views the nurse can strongly advise the mother against having her son circumcised, thus acting only on one pattern of knowing (i.e. empirical); or he or she can set aside personal opinions and try to see the situation from the mother's point of view (i.e. aesthetic knowing—'making the links', or unknowing—'keeping one's opinions in abeyance'). Realising that the mother's opinion is influenced by her religious beliefs and her husband's view on this subject (i.e. empirical knowing—'knowledge about the patient's cultural background'; ethical knowing—'what is just'; personal knowing, or unknowing: 'keeping one's own opinions in abeyance and seeing it from the mother's perspectives'), the nurse makes a decision. If the nurse were to act only on his or her own knowledge base and beliefs, and advise the mother against circumcision, he or she may cause the mother to be confused and in conflict with her own beliefs. One could argue that the nurse is not acting in the best interest of the mother. In these 'grey' situations, where making a decision is difficult, the combination of the four patterns of knowing provides guidance and is essential for patient-centred care.

It is also easy to see how unknowing intertwines with Carper's four patterns of knowing. Nursing deals with people within the context of vulnerability, where choices and practice options are not clearly defined—for example, the issues of death and dying, or whether patients should be allowed to smoke postoperatively. Such situations offer different options of care that can vary from patient to patient. It is important, therefore, to make decisions based on more than one perspective.

Intuitive knowledge develops with experience. Benner (1984) argues that nurses develop this type of knowledge only after having some years of experience in nursing; she fails to take into account, however, the wealth of experience that nurses bring from their personal lives, their sense of being, which they use in nursing. Intuitive knowledge is what Carper (1978) terms 'personal knowledge'. It is argued that intuitive knowing is a type of knowing not held exclusively by nurse experts and that students (novices) too display intuitive knowing. For example, students who baby sit in order to pay their way through university become very familiar with children, and in some clinical settings they use this knowledge intuitively. While nursing a recovering child (Lisa), a student sought my attention to check Lisa as she knew there was something amiss but did not know what. The student nurse said she had a general feel for children and in this situation things did not seem right. Not being familiar with the setting I handed the situation to the ward staff who confirmed that Lisa was not herself. While the student's action was different from that of an expert nurse, to say it was not intuitive is to underestimate the student's capabilities and the experience she brings to nursing by virtue of her personal experience.

Because intuitive knowledge is silent it remains difficult to teach; however, the model of the reflective practitioner (discussed in Chapter 14) offers a useful means of bringing this type of knowledge to the surface.

NURSES AS KNOWERS

Meleis (1991, p. 138) posed the question: Are nurses' approaches to knowing, understanding and formulating conceptualisations unique? More specifically, does each nurse (the knower) have a different way of knowing? Based on the works of Belenky et al. (1986), who identified five different types of women knowers, Schultz and Meleis (1988) proposed that these types of knowers can be found in nursing. Carper (1978) suggests that part of developing personal knowledge is to understand yourself. It is therefore necessary to understand the characteristics and differences in nurses as knowers, and to review and evaluate the strengths and limitations of these characteristics. These five types of knowers are (Schultz & Meleis 1988):

1   Silent knowers

2   Received knowers

3   Subjective knowers

4   Procedural knowers

5   Constructed knowers.

These knowers are defined in the following way:

1   *Silent knowers* are nurses who remain silent for most of the time because they lack confidence to speak their minds. They accept authority as their legitimate source of knowledge. Their knowledge base remains unarticulated and embedded in silent practice. It may be that these nurses continue to support 'tenacity' as a source of knowledge and give unquestioning adherence to nursing rituals and routines. Students and new nursing graduates who work side by side with this type of knower may find their work experience difficult and sometimes uncomfortable. The challenge in dealing with such situations lies in using Carper's patterns of knowing, trying to see the situation from the knower's perspective, and working through the differences in opinions in a constructive way. However, it must be acknowledged that as this type of nurse operates within a silent mode any discussion and exchange of ideas may be difficult to achieve.

2   *Received knowers* rely on people who are regarded as experts for the source of their knowledge. They use this knowledge unquestioningly. Moreover, received knowers do not create their own knowledge. Perhaps it has been the unquestioning tradition within the nursing profession and nursing practice which has nurtured these types of knowers and the notion that someone else's knowledge has more value and worth than our own. Meleis (1991) states that this practice of unquestioning has led to the wholesale acceptance of ideas and theories in nursing. Jocelyn Lawler (1991) further argues that Australian nurses have, for some time, accepted without question the ideas and knowledge of nursing practice from our North American colleagues. It may be that this acceptance could be explained partly by the theory of the received knowers in nursing and their unquestioning acceptance of other people's knowledge.

3   *Subjective knowers* rely more on their sixth sense—an inner feeling. It is a case of: 'I sense/know what is happening but I don't know why I know that'. These knowers find it difficult to define what they know in more tangible ways because their knowledge comes from their personal experience and from an inner conversation of this experience with the situation in which they are practising. Meleis (1991) states that these types of knowers carry with them a wealth of knowledge that needs to be surfaced and articulated, and thereby contribute to nursing knowledge. According to Meleis (1991), this type of knowledge is what Carper (1978) terms personal knowledge and Benner (1984) calls expert, intuitive knowledge.

4   *Procedural knowers* rely on following procedures step by step, and are careful observers of rules and regulations. They subscribe heavily to the notion of objectivity. Schultz and Meleis (1988) state that these kinds of knowers are especially suited to conducting research because of their objective stance. They further state that researchers and academics are high on the list of members of this group of knowers. While this may have been the case some years ago, more nurse researchers are now using the interpretive and critical approaches to enquiry and it could be argued that contemporary researchers and academics vary along the range of subjective to constructed knowers.

5   *Constructed knowers* rely on a more dynamic approach to knowledge development informed by both subjective and objective stances. They create knowledge and are in themselves part of the knowledge development process. They recognise that knowledge is contextually bound and subject to a number of interpretations that may change over time. According to Schultz and Meleis (1988), this type of nurse believes that knowledge development is an ongoing process that never ends. This belief system would seem to reject tenacity, authority and expert knowledge as being legitimate sources of knowledge.

Nurses as knowers are different, and present with individual ways of behaving that are underpinned by different value and belief systems about what constitutes knowledge and how it is gained. Nurses can also vary as knowers from time to time, from situation to situation; in some instances they may be classified as subjective knowers (intuitive in their response) and in others as constructed knowers. They may not behave consistently as the one type. Given this, it is easy to see why there can be different opinions about knowledge. Our challenge here is to:

■   try to recognise these differences within nurses;

■   put in abeyance our own personal views; and

■   try to work towards and support the approach to knowledge construction that will ultimately assist the nursing profession and its endeavour for optimal patient care.

THE ART OF NURSING

The combination of Carper's (1991) patterns of knowing and Meleis's (1991) description of nurses as knowers has provided some understanding of:

* the art of nursing;

* the knowledge embedded in nursing practice; and

* the knowledge required for nursing practice.

However, the art of nursing remains difficult to conceptualise. According to Johnson (1994), 'nursing art', though central to nursing practice, still remains abstract and difficult to define. She feels it is important to review the way in which nurses practise within a clinical setting and to tease out aspects that will provide an understanding of the phenomenon **nursing art**. Johnson argues that, although several nurse theorists have researched aspects relating to the art of nursing, they have done so in isolation to one another's work. This has resulted in a number of views on what constitutes the art of nursing. In order to consolidate these views, Johnson (1994) conducted a critical examination and systematic analysis of the nursing literature concerning the art of nursing. The study found that there are many differing explanations of what constitutes nursing art. These are explicated in the following ways:

* *Ability to grasp meaning in patient encounters.* The more artful nurses are able to make sense of information and determine what is happening in various situations.

* *Ability to establish a meaningful connection with the patient.* The more artful nurses are able to connect with their patients in a meaningful way. This connection is in some ways expressed in their actions and facial expressions. More artful nurses remain genuine.

* *Ability to perform nursing activities skilfully.* The more artful nurses are skilful in their practice; they are fluent, coordinated and efficient.

* *Ability to determine rationally an appropriate course of nursing action.* More artful nurses act from a sound knowledge base (empirics), using a problem-solving approach.

* *Ability to conduct their nursing practice morally.* The more artful nurses deliver care from a moral base. This includes acting for the 'good of the patient'. These nurses are knowledgeable, competent and caring.

These five explanations of the art of nursing provide further evidence of the complexity of nursing practice and the knowledge required for competent practice. Summarising these conceptualisations of artful nursing, one could say that the more artful nurses actually use all Carper's patterns of knowing in their daily work situations.

RESEARCH METHODS

Research findings are an important source of knowledge development, a way of 'knowing' about nursing. Research focuses on and answers questions about physical and social realities. While we can make sense of the findings and use this information in practice, it is also important to examine critically the method used to derive these results—that is how the findings were determined. As each research method has inherent strengths and limitations, a critical review of the process is necessary. For example, if you wanted to know more about colostomy bags and the effectiveness of each type, you could investigate this in several ways.

- You could conduct clinical research and grade the colostomy bags according to certain criteria, assign scores to each type accordingly and test statistically for significant differences between them.

- You could ask patients and nurses about their experiences of using colostomy bags and which type(s) they found effective under certain circumstances.

- You could speak to the manufacturers, look at the specifications of each bag and grade them accordingly.

Each approach would give you information on your research question, but each set of answers would represent a different perspective or point of view. It is important, therefore, to look more critically at the results in terms of how they were derived (the study method) and evaluate the strengths and limitations of each approach.

For example, it could be said that the first approach, discussed above, was limited as the criteria used to measure effectiveness may not represent the patient's view of what constitutes effectiveness. The second approach neglected manufacturers' specifications and provided only patients' and nurses' perceptions of the effectiveness of colostomy bags. The third approach was limited because it may have illustrated a biased view derived from a manufacturer's specific laboratory testing. This simple concrete example illustrates the strengths and limitations of the study findings in relation to the research method. As nursing phenomena are complex, they are more prone to being misrepresented because of the method of study. The methods used to research nursing phenomena, therefore, require critical review.

As research methods are informed by different philosophies and theoretical perspectives, it is necessary to understand these different perspectives when attempting to determine whether the study method used has adequately and justly answered the research question and dealt with the phenomena of concern in a meaningful way. Wolfer (1993) aptly points out that to say that the method used within a study is driven by the research question only misrepresents the total picture, for the type of method used should also be determined by the phenomena being researched. Hence we must ask the question: What types of phenomena are of interest to nursing? According to Morse (1994), nursing's research endeavour should focus on a few aspects such as human responses to illness and health, the nurse–patient interaction, and aspects of clinical decision making. Keeping this in mind, it is also important to ask the question: Which research method is wholesome enough to answer adequately the questions we are asking about our phenomena of concern?

Broadly, research can be divided into two types—quantitative and qualitative (Burns & Grove 1993; Leininger 1994). The quantitative method is an empirical-analytic approach, while the qualitative method encompasses many research approaches that are different in their philosophical orientation and, to some extent, in the way data are analysed. In addition, some qualitative methods are described as interpretive and others as emancipatory. The four most commonly used qualitative methods are:

- ■ phenomenology
- ■ grounded theory
- ■ ethnography
- ■ critical social theory.

Other less commonly used approaches are philosophical enquiry and historical enquiry (Burns & Grove 1993). Leininger (1994) argues that 'both qualitative and quantitative methods have entirely different philosophic assumptions that need to be acknowledged and observed by researchers'. Table 3.1 summarises the differences between quantitative and qualitative research methods.

TABLE 3.1 A SUMMARY OF THE DIFFERENCES BETWEEN QUANTITATIVE AND QUALITATIVE RESEARCH METHODS

QUANTITATIVE METHOD	QUALITATIVE METHOD
■ Controls settings and variables	■ Studies phenomena in their natural settings
■ Breaks down variables and studies them independently	■ Does not break down variables
■ Uses units of measure	■ Does not use units of measure
■ Measures quantities, uses numbers	■ Uses mainly textual data (words)
■ Outcome predicts (cause and effect) and controls	■ Outcome explains and/or describes and/or emancipates
■ Results are generalisable	■ Results are not generalisable
■ Data must be verified through the senses (must be tangible)	■ All data are valid (i.e. intuition is recognised)

QUANTITATIVE METHOD (EMPIRICAL-ANALYTIC)

The **quantitative research** method is associated with the empirical-analytic perspective, commonly known as the positivistic approach to research (Hughes 1990). It is underpinned by the assumption that the world is structured by law-like regularities that can be controlled (Allen, Benner & Diekelmann 1986, p. 24). Objects and situations can be broken down and studied independently of one another and the outcome of this endeavour is the ability to predict and control situations (Allen et al. 1986). Reality (i.e. knowledge) is constructed through the senses, and information that cannot be verified through the senses is considered not genuine and disregarded (Hughes 1990). Another assumption of this research method is that the findings of the study can be generalised to the wider community—they are not context-specific (Allen et al. 1986).

According to Burns and Grove (1994), the following conditions and controls should be applied to quantitative research.

- ■ Precise instruments with established reliability and validity should be used to measure variables of concern, so that the findings reflect reality.

- Through control of the subjects, the setting and the overall study design, the researcher can reduce the effects of confounding variables.

In addition, Meleis (1991) states that researchers should remain objective and disconnected from their subjects. The critical question here is to discern in what cases or situations these conditions can be applied in nursing.

QUALITATIVE METHODS

The qualitative methods listed previously are all different in their philosophical underpinnings, and it is beyond the scope of this chapter to define these differences. What needs to be noted is what the qualitative methods have in common and how their approach differs from the empirical-analytic approach. **Qualitative research** focuses on understanding the social world of nursing. Qualitative methods, in the main, use textual data that have usually been derived from four main sources: interviews with research participants; field observations; reviews of pertinent documents; and personal journals. This approach usually involves the study of people in their natural settings as opposed to laboratory settings. The findings of the study are context-bound and generalisability is not claimed. As a result of this approach, the information gained from the study arises from the setting itself (Morse 1994). For example, when using a grounded theory approach to study postoperative nursing care in a surgical ward, the researchers would interview nurses and patients as well as observe the postoperative care within the ward. The findings, therefore, reflect what is actually done in practice.

When critically evaluating the findings of studies, and the claims being made, it is necessary to ask certain important questions:

- Can the variables of concern be broken down and studied as single units?
- Do numbers adequately describe the phenomenon, or are words necessary?

If there is a discrepancy or incongruence between what is being studied and the way it is being studied, then the findings of the study (i.e. the knowledge gained) need to be questioned. The complexity of nursing requires it to use many alternative research methods to verify and build its knowledge base. An understanding of the different theoretical perspectives that underpin the various research methods enables a more critical evaluation of research findings, and of the suitability of the method for use in nursing.

Nursing theories have also been developed using different research methods and, therefore, offer diverse perspectives. For example, Roy's adaptation model, a commonly used nursing model, is based partly on Harry Helson's work in psychophysics (Marriner-Tomey 1994), and Parse's human becoming theory has been developed, in part, using an existential phenomenological approach which creates the phenomena from the lived experience of people (Parse 1987). While both models offer nursing a theoretical framework on which to base nursing practice, they have been developed using different research methods informed by different philosophical perspectives. This difference needs to be realised and acknowledged, for when we use these theories to guide practice we will inevitably focus on different aspects of patient care. They also have different ways of interpreting and defining the patient, health, nursing and the environment. Definitions give meaning to things and influence what we purport to know about them.

ARE WE ASKING THE RIGHT QUESTIONS?

After reading the foregoing discussion, it is easy to see that our ways of knowing in nursing are complex and influenced by a multiplicity of factors. More fundamentally, another aspect needs to be considered—are we asking the right questions? It seems logical that we should address issues related to nursing's phenomena of concern, thus adding to our knowledge base. Smith (1992) analysed the type of nursing research being published in three refereed journals and further categorised this research according to the study population. She reported that much of nursing's research focused on nurses themselves—that is, it examined nursing behaviours. If people, health and illness are the focus of nursing, then nurses must ask questions that provide answers and information about people in health and in illness. Furthermore, as nurse researchers are generally not practising nurses, they tend to focus on problems and research questions that are of little concern to nurse clinicians and have limited relevance to practice (Dracup & Weinberg, cited in Weiler & Buckwater 1990). As nursing is a practice-based discipline it is imperative that research questions focus on and address practice-relevant issues, using research methods that do justice to the phenomena of concern.

SUMMARY

Nursing is a practice-based discipline. The knowledge base and ways of knowing are complex, abstract and sometimes difficult to define. They are influenced by many factors. How these factors interrelate is difficult to determine and is not clearly defined in the literature.

Given that the goal of nursing is to achieve a desired outcome that optimises the patient's health—or, where this is not possible, to assist the patient to achieve a peaceful death—certain professional and personal attributes are necessary to nurse. The literature outlines the qualities necessary for competent practice and identifies them as being those held by the more 'artful' nurse.

Artful nursing involves the ability to grasp meaning in patient encounters, thus establishing a meaningful connection with the patient, the skilful performance of nursing activities, the rational selection of an appropriate course of nursing action and the ability to conduct nursing practice in a moral fashion. Collectively, these qualities could be termed 'professional artistry', which results in the careful construction of a tailored plan of nursing care and the delivery of this care in an environment of understanding and activity.

To nurse artfully, nurses must combine the science and art of nursing and use all the patterns of knowing—empirics, aesthetics, ethics and personal knowledge. How aptly nurses use the patterns of knowing is affected by the type of 'knower' they are—silent, received, subjective, procedural or constructed. The characteristics inherent in each particular kind of knower affect the way in which knowledge is acquired, and also the type of knowledge that is recognised (by the nurse) as being legitimate. It is uncertain whether these characteristics are innate, or develop through the socialisation process in nursing, or result from a combination of both.

The various sources of knowledge and the different perspectives of the research methods used to construct nursing knowledge also affect what nurses know and how they use the patterns of knowing (see Figure 3.1). There may be many other factors that are abstract or

FIGURE 3.1 WAYS OF KNOWING IN NURSING

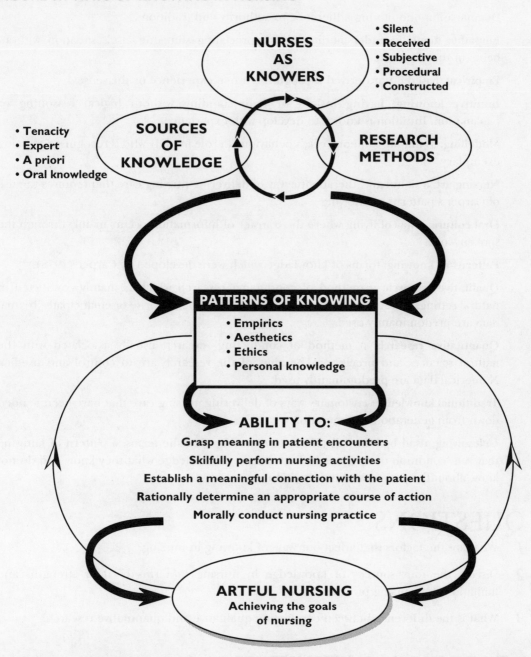

hidden, and remain unarticulated. In order to promote discussion, this chapter has attempted to discuss the more tangible factors and to determine how they relate to each other.

GLOSSARY

A priori knowledge: knowledge that has been derived from a deductive process; this knowledge, however, has not been validated by an empirical study.

Advocacy: the act of pleading for someone else or acting on their behalf.

Dogma: an unquestioning adherence to authority and tradition.

Empathy: mentally understanding and appreciating someone else's situation without being in that situation.

Empirical: based on or derived through the use of experience or the senses.

Intuitive knowing: having insight or understanding without logical reasoning or explanation. Intuition is known to develop with experience.

Modelling: to imitate someone else's behaviour (a role model) who is recognised as being exemplary.

Nursing art: a skilful and therapeutic way of delivering nursing care that requires the use of Carper's patterns of knowing.

Oral culture: a way of living where the transfer of information occurs mainly through the spoken word.

Patterns of knowing: forms of knowledge which were developed by Carper (1978).

Qualitative research: a method of conducting research which is mainly conducted in natural settings. The aims of this research are to describe, theorise or emancipate. Textual data are predominantly used.

Quantitative research: a method of conducting research usually associated with the natural sciences and precision. The aims of the research are to control and predict. Numerical data are predominantly used.

Traditional knowledge: customary ways of delivering nursing care that have been handed down from generation to generation.

Unknowing: used by Munhall (1993) to describe, what she terms, a pattern of knowing that is a 'condition of openness' where nurses acknowledge what they know and do not know about the patient and the situation.

QUESTIONS

1   What are the factors that affect our ways of knowing in nursing?

2   Discuss the four sources of knowledge in nursing in terms of their strengths and limitations for nursing practice.

3   What is the difference between conducting qualitative and quantitative research?

LEARNING ACTIVITIES

1   Within your everyday situation, try to identify people who display characteristics similar to the five types of nurse knowers.

2   Construct a case study where the ethical answers vary because of either different contexts or different people.

4

NURSING PROCESS
A Systematic Approach
to Patient Care

BEVERLY O'CONNELL

LEARNING OBJECTIVES

When you have read this chapter you should be able to:

1 Describe the development of the nursing process and list its stages.

2 State reasons for and against the use of the five-stage nursing process.

3 Undersand the various definitions and types of nursing diagnosis.

4 State the phases of the diagnostic process and the factors that influence it.

5 Understand the factors for and against the use of critical pathways.

INTRODUCTION

Professional nursing practice hinges on the concepts of autonomy and accountability and within this context nurses are required to deliver appropriate care. The effective planning, communicating and documenting of patient care is a vital part of this practice. The problem-solving approach to patient care used in nursing is called the **nursing process**. The nursing process comprises five interconnected though different stages. Collectively, these stages structure how nursing care is determined, delivered, communicated and documented. They are defined in the following way:

1 *Assessment.* Data gathering for the purpose of identifying actual and/or potential health problems.

2 *Diagnosing.* Data analysis and problem identification.

3 *Planning.* Goal setting, and development of a plan of nursing care (nursing intervention).

4 *Implementation.* Application of the nursing care plan.

5 *Evaluation.* Judgements made about the client's progress and the applicability of the nursing care; based on these evaluations, the plan of care is then modified or ceased.

(Alfaro-LeFevre 1994; Iyer, Taptich & Bernocchi-Losey 1991)

The stages of the nursing process are not linear, but dynamic and continuous. The nurse is constantly required to reassess, revise listed problems and alter patient care in order to address the changing needs of the patient. Nursing care is not totally confined to the boundaries of the nursing process, as there are other intuitive aspects to nursing and nurse–patient interactions which in themselves are therapeutic; however, they are difficult to capture within a problem-solving, organised, written framework. The nursing process is illustrated in Figure 4.1.

FIGURE 4.1 PROBLEM-SOLVING APPROACH TO PATIENT CARE

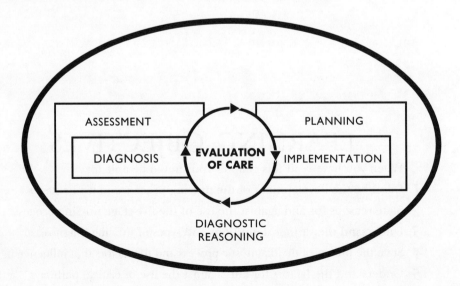

Although most of the stages are action-oriented, they are underpinned by a decision-making process that involves cognitive processes collectively termed 'diagnostic reasoning' (Westfall et al. 1986). The processes involved in diagnostic reasoning resemble generic features of the diagnostic process used by other disciplines, such as medicine (Tanner et al. 1987). There is general agreement that the diagnostic process comprises four phases.

1 Collection of initial data (patient assessment).

2 Generation of initial hypotheses regarding the patient's problem and condition.

3 Collection of more specific information to confirm or eliminate hypotheses.

4 Stating nursing diagnoses/patient problems.

(Thomas, Wearing & Bennett 1991; Gordon 1989).

A substantial body of literature attests to the view that this diagnostic process and patient problem identification is vital to the rest of nursing care (Aspinall 1976; Carpenito 1992; Kim et al. 1984). If patient problems are not identified then appropriate care may not be implemented, thus compromising the quality of nursing care.

This diagnostic process is affected by a multiplicity of factors, some of which are listed below.

■ Attributes of the nurse, such as knowledge base and logical reasoning ability (Woolley 1990).

■ Experience, recency of experience and value systems of the nurse (Benner 1984; Woolley 1990).

■ Contextual factors, such as the patient, the settings in which the assessment interview occurs, and the time allowed to conduct the interview (Woolley 1990).

■ Risk-benefit variables associated with the judgement itself (Tanner 1986). For example, nurses are more inclined to diagnose a patient's psychosocial problems in controlled laboratory settings than in an actual ward setting (Rapley, O'Connell & Tibbett 1995). There are more risks involved in making a judgement in a 'real' setting than in a simulated environment.

More recently, it has been argued that the type of assessment form used may have an important influence on the diagnostic process (Guzzetta et al. 1989; Gordon 1987; O'Connell 1992).

It is important to note all these factors and to try to optimise their effect, in both the delivery of patient care and the teaching/learning process. Also, knowledge of these factors provides insights as to why the decision-making process can vary from person to person and across different contexts and settings.

The nursing process is used widely in Australia; there is, however, some resistance to its wholesale use in some sectors of clinical practice. More specifically, clinicians have criticised the diagnostic language and the prescribed documentation rituals believed to be associated with the nursing process. It is timely, then, that the clinical application of the process is reviewed and modifications made which reflect and suit contemporary nursing practice. However, before any changes are made, it is important to understand why the nursing process was developed and to examine, after three decades of its application, the outcomes of its use in nursing.

This chapter is designed to stimulate students' and educators' thinking about issues related to care planning. It does not provide a prescriptive recipe for nursing practice.

DEVELOPMENT OF THE NURSING PROCESS

Traditionally, nursing care was based primarily on the patient's medical condition and prescriptive medical orders (Johnson & Hales 1989). In the 1960s, the combined effect of a rapidly changing health care system and increasing demands on health care services led to the introduction of defined roles for health care professionals (Yura & Walsh 1988). To establish the professional role of the nurse, and develop nursing as a separate discipline within the health care system, there was a deliberate move to scientise nursing—that is, to make the delivery of nursing care more logical, rational and methodical (Donnolly 1987). As part of this process, in 1967, a group of academics at Catholic University in Washington, USA, explicated an organisational framework called the *nursing process*, which defined systematic stages of nursing practice (Henderson 1987; Yura & Walsh 1988). Given that nursing care was based on prescribed medical orders or instructions from the 'charge nurse', it was necessary to change the practice of nursing and develop it based on a problem-solving framework, where nurses delivered and evaluated care based on their own assessment of patient needs.

The nursing process, as it was originally developed, comprised four stages— assessment, planning, implementation and evaluation. During the first decade of its use, several nurse scholars claimed there was a missing link in the process (Gebbie & Lavin 1974; Aspinall 1976). They argued that, although nurses assessed the patient and then planned care based on this assessment, they did not label the condition/problem that was actually treated. Therefore, it was not clear what the patient's problem actually was and how this problem could be communicated to other nurses involved in delivering patient care. At this stage, the types of problems that nurses treated were rarely communicated in writing, using standard language, and thus remained undefined and unarticulated. To address this deficiency, and to identify and label the common problems that nurses treat, several nurse scholars introduced an additional stage to the nursing process, termed 'nursing diagnosis' (Aspinall 1976; Gebbie & Lavin 1974; Gordon 1976).

THE DIAGNOSIS STAGE AND THE DIAGNOSTIC TAXONOMY

The stage of **nursing diagnosis** follows the assessment stage; it involves the nurse diagnosing patient problems that are of nursing concern and stating these problems using standard labels known as nursing diagnoses. It was thought that the use of standard labels would assist the nursing profession in the identification of nursing phenomena that would enhance nursing discourse (i.e. the discussion and interchange of professional ideas) and research. More specifically, it was argued that standard labels would help in naming, communicating, teaching and researching the health problems that were the focus of nursing care (Gordon 1976). Since nurses work within a multidisciplinary team, where nursing care was traditionally seen as being predominantly medically prescribed, this explication of nursing's unique contribution to health care was also said to be professionally important, as it helped delineate the nursing domain. According to

Carnevali (1983), identifying the nursing domain was crucial for nursing's professional recognition. The two main reasons were as follows:

1 It would assist nurses to gain a clear understanding of the parameters of their practice.

2 It would help to establish nursing as a specific discipline within the health care system and not solely as a supportive adjunct to other disciplines.

To develop the concept of nursing diagnosis and standard diagnostic labels, the first national conference on the classification of nursing diagnosis was held in the United States, in 1973 (Gebbie & Lavin 1974). The North American Nursing Diagnosis Association (NANDA) was formed in 1982. This association's goal is to promote, research and assist with the development of the diagnostic nomenclature and taxonomy. Initially, there was a total of 34 diagnostic categories; currently there are more than 101 diagnostic categories within this taxonomy (Carlson et al. 1991). NANDA organises conferences biennially to provide a forum for professional knowledge exchange and research findings related to the development and refinement of nursing diagnoses and, more peripherally, the nursing process. The NANDA taxonomy list is not exhaustive—as part of the review process, new diagnoses are added to the list and inappropriate diagnoses are removed. This process of review is continuous. NANDA has a set of guidelines for submitting new diagnoses for inclusion in the taxonomy and welcomes submissions from all groups of nurses (see Carpenito 1992).

The nursing **diagnostic taxonomy** developed by NANDA was endorsed by the American Nurses Association and submitted to the World Health Organization (WHO) for inclusion in International Classification of Disease 10 (ICD 10) (Fitzpatrick et al. 1989). It was believed by NANDA that the acceptance of this taxonomy by WHO would assist in the recognition and development of the profession of nursing (Saba 1991). Although the taxonomy was not accepted by WHO authorities for inclusion in ICD 10, this submission is significant for nursing as it demonstrates NANDA's intention of having its taxonomy recognised and endorsed by an international health organisation. At a future date, if the application is successful, the NANDA taxonomy could become the recognised international classification of nursing practice.

In the early 1980s, nursing diagnosis became more widely accepted in Australia. The first Australian National Nursing Diagnosis conference was held on the Gold Coast, Queensland, in December 1991. This conference provided a forum for discussing issues related to nursing diagnosis and, in particular, the use and utility of the NANDA taxonomy within Australia. The papers presented to the conference stimulated lively discussion and information exchange. Conference delegates agreed that, although NANDA's diagnostic taxonomy had some limitations for Australian nurses (some nursing diagnoses were perceived as being difficult to understand), it was a worthwhile concept for nursing practice and should be further developed and refined. Although no formal national nursing diagnosis group was formed, it was agreed that the next conference would be held in Perth.

Entitled 'Clinical Application of Nursing Diagnosis: Nexus or Nonsense', the Second National Nursing Diagnosis conference was held in Perth, in November 1994. Many papers were presented, both for and against the use of nursing diagnosis, and these generated discussion and lively debate. Conference delegates presented arguments from various schools of thought (e.g. the feminist and caring perspectives), offering different views of the use and utility of this concept. Papers presented at the conference addressed numerous and diverse patient problems that are of nursing concern—for example, the experience and discomfort of postoperative flatulence, patients' sexual concerns in relation to their state of health, and the role strain experienced by caregivers (family members) of the frail and elderly. It would seem that the labelling of patient problems has encouraged nurses to research different types of phenomena that are of nursing concern, thus building up nursing knowledge. At the end of the second conference there was overwhelming support by conference delegates for the further development of nursing diagnosis and its use in Australia.

THE INTERVENTION AND OUTCOMES TAXONOMY

Further to the development of a nursing diagnostic taxonomy, considerable research and work has been done on the development of both a nursing interventions classification system and an outcome classification system (McClosky & Bulechek 1993). It was believed that this would assist in the development and articulation of commonly used nursing interventions. A Nursing Interventions Classification (NIC) system has been developed in accordance with this idea; however, the use and utility of this taxonomy within the Australian context needs to be further explored and validated.

USE OF THE NURSING PROCESS

Since its inception, the nursing process has been used increasingly by nurse academics, administrators, clinicians and staff development nurses. In 1980, the American Nurses Association endorsed the diagnosis stage of the nursing process by defining nursing as '. . . the diagnosis and treatment of human responses to actual or potential health problems' (Carlson et al. 1991, p. 4). More recently, the Australian Nursing Council Incorporated (ANCI) has listed nursing competencies for national registration which are classified under domains of practice. One domain, Problem Framing and Solving, has been developed, based on the nursing process (ANCI 1994). Factors affecting the first two stages of the nursing process will be discussed. A schematic representation of these factors is given in Figure 4.2.

NURSING DOCUMENTATION

Nursing documentation usually comprises an assessment form, a master problem list, a nursing care plan or an interventions list, and a record of patient progress. This documentation is essential for continuity and communication of nursing care. It also serves as a legal record of the patient's care.

TYPES OF ASSESSMENT FORMS

Nursing assessment is the foundation of the nursing process. These assessments are conducted using an assessment form. In general, nursing assessment forms have evolved, with each clinical setting constructing its own forms based on senior nurses' perceptions of what constitutes pertinent information. Some assessment forms have been developed using a more structured approach, such as assessing patients' activities of daily living.

FIGURE 4.2 SCHEMATIC REPRESENTATION OF THE FACTORS THAT AFFECT CARE PLANNING

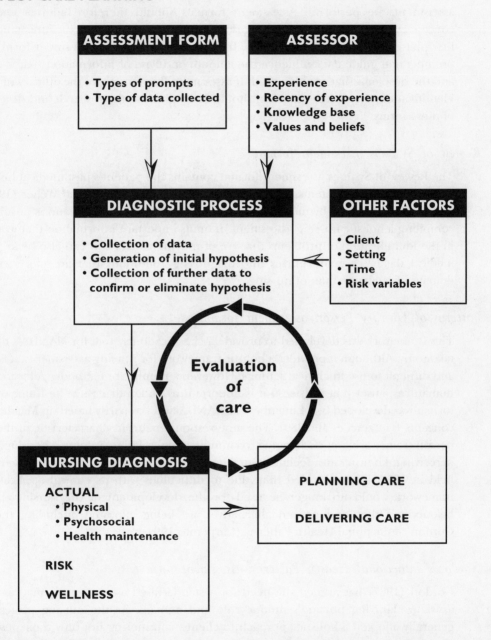

General information such as the patient's next of kin, prosthesis used, and whether the patient wears dentures is also included. Assessment forms contain both subjective and objective physical assessment information. These forms usually address and comply with both legal and medical record standards.

More recently, two structured assessment formats have been developed—the Gordon's Functional Health Patterns and the Patterns of Unitary Person Framework. Another commonly used assessment format is the Review of Systems approach; however, this is more commonly used by the medical profession. The features of these formats are discussed below. Guzzetta (1990, p. 303) states that 'the tapestry of holism is woven by the assessments we perform'. Assessment formats should therefore address and reflect concepts within this holistic framework. As the collection of patient information is the first phase of the diagnostic process, the terms listed on the assessment form serve as prompts that guide and influence the amount and type of information that is collected and the problems that are identified. If assessment forms improve the efficacy of problem identification, then some attention should to be given to the research and development of these forms.

Review of Systems assessment format

The Review of Systems assessment format contains the patient's past medical history and a review of all body systems. According to Guzzetta et al. (1989) and Weber (1988), this type of format is used by medical practitioners to diagnose disease and is unsuitable for compiling a holistic nursing assessment. It omits important information that would assist in the identification of problems that are of nursing concern. It can also be argued that medical databases guide nurses into diagnosing conditions that are more within the domain of medicine than of nursing.

Patterns of Unitary Person assessment format

This framework was developed to provide a classification system for NANDA's diagnostic taxonomy. Although it provides a holistic framework for nursing assessments, it is abstract and difficult to use in clinical settings. However, a number of textbooks refer to the nine human responses that it lists, so it is important to be familiar with the framework. This format was developed by 14 members of NANDA and was partly based on Martha Roger's concepts (Guzzetta et al. 1989). The nine response patterns characteristic of the unitary person framework are: exchanging, communicating, relating, valuing, choosing, moving, perceiving, knowing and feeling (Guzzetta et al. 1989, p. 7). At the NANDA conference held in 1994, it was decided that, due to difficulties with its clinical application, this framework would no longer be used for the development of the nursing diagnostic taxonomy. Other options and alternatives are being explored, including the use of Gordon's Functional Health Patterns (Carpenito 1994).

Gordon's Functional Health Patterns assessment format

Gordon (1987) has argued the need for a standardised assessment format, as it would assist in clarifying nursing's unique role and domain. As the nursing profession has generally adopted a holistic approach to clients, considering not only their physical but also their psychosocial and spiritual dimensions, an assessment form that encompasses these dimensions would seem more appropriate. Gordon (1987) developed an assessment format for this purpose, based on the belief that all human beings have in common 11 **functional health patterns** that contribute to their health, quality of life and achievement of human potential. These eleven functional health patterns are:

1   health-perception–health-management pattern;

2   nutritional–metabolic pattern;

3 elimination pattern;

4 activity–exercise pattern;

5 cognitive–perceptual pattern;

6 sleep–rest pattern;

7 self-perception–self-concept pattern;

8 role–relationship pattern;

9 sexuality–reproductive pattern;

10 coping–stress-tolerance pattern; and

11 value–belief pattern (for further information see Gordon 1987).

INFLUENCE OF ASSESSMENT FORMS ON THE DIAGNOSTIC PROCESS

Nurse scholars argue that the Gordon's Functional Health Patterns framework provides a format for holistic assessment that guides nurses to identify patient problems and plan appropriate care (Field & Winslow 1985; Carpenito 1992). The following studies support this view.

Padrick et al. (1987) conducted a study on the diagnostic process, using a convenience sample of 43 subjects. The subjects' diagnostic reasoning strategies were elicited in response to nine videotaped patient situations. The researchers found that, in general, subjects correctly accepted hypotheses if they collected the appropriate data and that they seldom made incorrect decisions if they had the necessary information. However, in cases where subjects had not collected appropriate data, they were much more willing to accept incorrect hypotheses than to reject them. The researchers emphasised a need for clinicians to focus on obtaining relevant cues, as definitive information assists the problem-solving process.

Thiele et al. (1986) investigated the effects on diagnostic accuracy of teaching **cue recognition** (a cognitive process used in diagnosing) to a group of 80 student nurses. The study's results revealed that teaching cue recognition, using computer-assisted instruction, improved the accuracy of clinical decision making. The researchers reported, however, that students frequently leapt to incorrect conclusions based on inadequate assessment information.

These studies strongly emphasise the importance of obtaining relevant client information. If relevant cues and definitive information assist problem identification, then nursing assessment forms must contain appropriate prompts to elicit germane data to facilitate the accuracy of the problem-solving phase. It is also important that the forms help clinicians to obtain information that is of direct relevance to nursing practice.

Studies that have evaluated assessment formats support Gordon's arguments about the efficacy of the GFHP assessment format. These studies found that the use of a modified Gordon's Functional Health Patterns assessment format generated a significantly greater frequency of nursing diagnoses and more diverse types of diagnostic categories than did other routine assessment formats (Dowd et al. 1987; Soares-O'Hearn 1987; Henning 1991).

More recently, and within an Australian setting, O'Connell (1992) conducted a study to determine the effect the assessment format had on the efficacy of the diagnostic process. Analysis of the data revealed that, when student and registered nurses used the Gordon's Functional Health Patterns (GFHP) assessment format, they stated significantly more correct diagnoses and significantly fewer incorrect and medical diagnoses than when they use the Review of Biological Systems (ROBS) assessment format. In addition, when both student and registered nurses used the GFHP assessment format, they stated significantly more diagnoses in the psychosocial and health maintenance categories than when they used the ROBS assessment format.

The findings of this study also support the views of Guzzetta et al. (1989) and Weber (1988), who argue that the Review of Biological Systems assessment format is unsuitable for compiling a nursing assessment as it is medically focused. The results of the O'Connell study provide empirical support for the argument by illustrating that, when both student and registered nurses used a ROBS assessment format, they stated significantly more diagnoses that were classified as being medical than when they used a GFHP assessment format.

In addition, the GFHP assessment format guided nurses into eliciting and documenting significantly more assessment data that also correlated with the recommended criteria outlined within the Standards for Nursing Care (ANF 1989). In the light of these findings, the use of the GFHP framework in educational institutes and clinical agencies is worthy of consideration. These findings emphasise the need for clinical and educational agencies to review the cues (headings) on commonly used assessment forms, because they influence not only the information that is collected but also the way in which this information is synthesised. Furthermore, it is important that the forms comply with recommended Australian nursing standards.

NURSING DIAGNOSIS/PROBLEM IDENTIFICATION

The outcome of performing an assessment is problem identification. Most health care professions diagnose patient problems—what varies is the knowledge base of the profession, the focus of concern and the labels used. Unlike medicine, which focuses on pathological biological phenomena, conceptualised as disease states, and the identification of illness, nursing focuses on human responses (of a person, group or community) to their general state of health and/or illness (Bennett 1986; Iyer, Taptich & Bernocchi-Losey 1991). Nursing diagnoses therefore differ from medical diagnoses as they focus on human responses to a state of health or illness, rather than on disease states themselves.

Nursing diagnosis, or problem identification, is the most controversial stage of the nursing process. Most of the critique has been directed at NANDA's nursing diagnostic taxonomy. The diagnostic labels devised by this group comprise the first component of a nursing diagnosis and are sometimes referred to as a diagnostic category. NANDA has continued to research, devise and revise diagnostic categories and has organised them within a framework. Although NANDA has done a considerable amount of work developing nursing diagnosis, nurses in all countries should test the applicability of each diagnosis within their work settings. It is important to select and use only those nursing diagnoses which seem appropriate and have meaning for nurse clinicians in Australian settings.

DEFINITIONS OF A NURSING DIAGNOSIS

The introduction of the diagnosis stage into nursing and the use of nursing diagnoses to describe client problems identified by nurses resulted in a need to define the concept, and also to standardise the language used to describe similar problems across health care settings. Nurse scholars have developed a number of conceptual and structural definitions of a nursing diagnosis.

- The *conceptual definition* of a nursing diagnosis defines the concept of nursing diagnosis and specifies how it differs from other types of diagnoses, such as medical diagnoses.

- The *structural definition* of a nursing diagnosis refers to how you write a nursing diagnosis, commonly termed the 'nursing diagnostic statement'.

There are several conceptual definitions of a nursing diagnosis. The challenge for Australian nurses is to review these definitions and determine whether they are useful and have the potential to reflect the types of patient problems encountered in Australian practice settings. Although these definitions share a common idea, they emphasise different aspects. As the concept of nursing diagnosis is less than 20 years old, it is likely that this definition will be reviewed and updated as the research and knowledge base of the discipline develops. NANDA's definition of a nursing diagnosis is as follows:

> A nursing diagnosis is a clinical judgement about individual, family, or community response to actual and potential health problems and life processes. Nursing diagnoses provide the basis for selection of nursing interventions to achieve outcomes for which the nurse is accountable.
>
> *(Carroll-Johnson 1991, p. 368)*

There is agreement that a nursing diagnosis consists of a number of components (i.e. has a defined structure); however, the actual number and nature of the components recommended differ among theorists. Some suggest the use of two-part statements, while others prefer a three-part statement. A typical two-part statement recommended by a number of eminent nurse scholars is shown here (Shoemaker 1984; Ziegler et al. 1986; Iyer et al. 1991).

Example

Activity intolerance related to difficulty breathing on exertion

This statement contains two phrases (shown in italics) joined by the words 'related to'. The first describes the client's actual or potential problem, or response to the condition, and the second defines the cause or aetiology of the problem or response and directs nursing interventions.

In contrast, Gordon (1987) advocates the use of a three-part statement where the first component is the client's actual or potential problem, or response to the condition; the second is the aetiology (when known) or factors that relate to the client's condition; and the third outlines the defining characteristics or cluster of signs and symptoms.

Example

Altered nutrition: More than body requirements, related to *dysfunctional eating patterns* (Carlson et al. 1991, p. 66).

The first part of the statement discusses the client's problem, and the second and third parts of the statement direct nursing intervention and substantiate the existence of the problem.

Though useful in the classroom, three-part statements are lengthy and cumbersome in clinical practice.

While there are different methods of writing nursing diagnostic statements, it is important to expose students to all definitions and to remain flexible until concepts have been more clearly refined and defined. Lengthy nursing diagnostic statements, using words that are not culturally explicit or easily understood, should be avoided. Clinical and educational agencies should discuss and decide on agreed conceptual and structural definitions, so that the confusion and ambiguity surrounding the use of nursing diagnosis can be minimised.

Types of nursing diagnosis

Nursing diagnosis includes not only diagnosing actual problems, but also making risk diagnoses and wellness diagnoses. These types of diagnoses are defined in the following way:

- *Risk diagnosis* is a clinical judgement that an individual, family or community is more vulnerable to developing the problem than others in the same or a similar situation. Risk diagnoses are supported by risk factors that guide nursing interventions intended to reduce or prevent the occurrence of the problem (Carroll-Johnson 1991, p. 374). Risk diagnoses are written using a two-part statement, where the first part states what the patient is at risk for and the second part directs nursing intervention. For example: 'High risk for injury related to impaired vision'.

- *Wellness diagnosis* is a clinical judgement about an individual, family or community in transition from a specific level of wellness to a higher level of wellness (Carroll-Johnson 1991, p. 375). This diagnosis is written using the phrase 'Potential for enhanced'... followed by the process which can be improved. For example: 'Potential for enhanced health maintenance'. This type of diagnosis is used mainly by community health nurses, where prevention of diseases and health promotion is important. However, its use must not be confined to these settings as it is important for all nurses to focus on these aspects of care and include them in the discharge plan.

Errors in writing nursing diagnostic statements

The research literature has identified some common errors made in writing nursing diagnostic statements. Specifically, some diagnostic statements do not observe the structural and conceptual definitions of a nursing diagnosis (Ziegler 1984; Castles 1984;

McLane, Lancour & Gotch 1986; Thomas 1987; Myers & Spiers 1987; Serrell 1987). Ziegler (1984) evaluated 168 nursing diagnoses generated by 90 masters level graduate nurses for adherence to the structural and conceptual definition of a nursing diagnosis. A self-designed instrument was used, comprising 12 criteria derived from the structural and conceptual definitions of a nursing diagnosis (stated in the literature). The findings revealed that only 10 diagnostic statements met all the criteria.

In addition, some nursing diagnoses could be identified as being medical diagnoses (O'Connell 1995). Looking at the legal aspect, Fortin and Rabinow (1979) state that medical and nursing diagnoses focus on different aspects: medicine on disease states and nursing on patient responses to their state of health. This excludes, therefore, from the realm of nursing diagnosis, health problems for which the accepted treatment is legally defined as being under the practice of medicine. This is an important point—a study conducted within the Australian context reports that when nurses state nursing diagnoses using any descriptive terminology, they inadvertently use medical terminology and medical diagnoses (O'Connell 1995). This practice can leave nurses open to litigation as they are diagnosing beyond the scope of nursing practice.

Another inconsistency in identifying nursing diagnoses is the lack of documented data to support the existence of a particular nursing diagnosis. It is professionally and legally important that nursing diagnoses listed in the patient problem list are substantiated by subjective and objective information contained in the patient's assessment form. According to Carpenito (1992), each nursing diagnosis has many cues (defining characteristics) and aetiologies; it is important, therefore, to list as many pertinent cues in the patient's assessment form as possible, so that the listed problems are substantiated by the assessment data. A recent study (Rapley, O'Connell & Tibbett 1995) revealed that 20 per cent of diagnoses listed were not supported by information contained in the patient's assessment form. This lack of documented evidence substantiating the existence of the recorded nursing diagnoses is unprofessional and needs to be addressed. Quite often, quality assurance audits of patient records examine compliance with medico–legal standards; however, little emphasis is placed on auditing the assessment form for the quality of the content and substantiation of the nursing diagnosis by the information contained in the assessment form (Rapley et al. 1995). This review is necessary to evaluate adherence to professional standards.

Finally, some studies have also questioned the issue of **interrater reliability** in relation to the diagnostic concept. Specifically, do nurses who diagnose patients at approximately the same time state the same nursing diagnosis? A study conducted by Castles (1984) examined whether nurses who evaluated the same client, within a period when the client's condition remained stable, recorded the same nursing diagnoses. The subjects (n=21) participating in the study were primarily degree nurses familiar with the concept of a nursing diagnosis and who worked in an intensive care unit that had a high reputation for nursing care. The results revealed that practising nurses making assessments of the same client at approximately the same time do not arrive at the same conclusion. In addition, they reported different signs and symptoms as the basis for their conclusions.

COLLABORATIVE PROBLEMS

Carpenito (1992) introduced the Bifocal Clinical Practice Model, which extends the parameters of nursing judgements. Guzzetta and Dossey (1983) argue that in areas of critical care, where the practices of nursing and medicine are entwined, nursing diagnoses do not adequately reflect the interdependent role of the nurse. Hence, there is a need to establish specific labels for these interdependent problems. Carpenito developed this concept further and labelled problems that fall into this interdependent zone as 'collaborative problems'. These problems have different conceptual and structural definitions to nursing diagnoses (which fall into the independent zone).

Collaborative problems are conceptually defined as:

> certain physiological complications that nurses monitor to detect onset or changes in status. Nurses manage collaborative problems utilising physician-prescribed and nursing-prescribed interventions to minimise the complications of the events.
>
> *(Carpenito 1992, p. 38)*

Collaborative problems are written using a different structure to a nursing diagnosis. They are written using a two-part statement, where the first part is the phrase 'potential complication'; the second part states the actual pathophysiologic state or medical condition that the nurse is attempting to monitor or prevent. The words 'potential complication' can be abbreviated, using the letters 'PC' followed by a colon. An example of a collaborative problem presented by Carpenito (1992) is: 'Potential complication: Pulmonary embolism' or 'PC: Pulmonary embolism'.

Carpenito also emphasises the importance of including the first part of the statement ('potential complication'), as its omission may lead to the problem being interpreted as a medical diagnosis.

There appear to be some inconsistencies associated with collaborative problems. According to Alfaro (1990), collaborative problems are not usually documented in the nursing care plan, because nursing interventions for collaborative problems are usually determined by hospital policies, procedures and standards, or by medical orders. Collaborative problems are only documented on the nursing care plan when such conditions do not exist.

Some nursing scholars present an opposing view to the use of collaborative problems in nursing. Iyer et al. (1991) and Gordon (1987) acknowledge the independent and interdependent roles of the nurse, but they query the need actually to label the interdependent problems in any specific way. This theoretical debate continues and remains unresolved. Although derived to assist nurses in labelling client conditions that require both medical and nursing intervention, the concept of collaborative problems adds to the confusion surrounding the nursing diagnostic language.

OUTCOME STATEMENTS

As part of the patient care planning process, each nursing diagnosis statement should have an accompanying **outcome statement** that clearly states the goal and outcome of the treatment; it should be stated in terms that are measurable so that the progress of care can be easily determined. According to Alfaro LeFevre (1994), it is important to classify outcome statements into cognitive, psychomotor or effective domains and to use appropriate words to describe the goals of care. The outcome statement should clearly state a specific level of improvement that can be achieved within a set time frame. The inclusion of a time frame is important, to enable the success of the treatment to be reviewed and evaluated accordingly. All outcome statements must be realistic so that both the patient and the nurse are able to achieve the goal.

Example

Nursing diagnosis

Self-care deficit (feeding); related to decreased strength and ability to cut food.

Outcome statement

Patient will:

- maintain hydration as evidenced by a good urine colour and output, evaluated daily;

- maintain current weight till discharge; and

- increase level of independence and be able to eat independently by discharge.

In the present economic climate there is increasing emphasis on the outcomes of patient care and the effectiveness of the nursing interventions to achieve these outcomes. Therefore, it is vital that the outcome statements observe the specified conventions and—through an evaluation process—are able to illustrate goal achievement or a need for the plan of care to be changed.

NURSING INTERVENTIONS

To achieve treatment goals, nursing interventions are determined in collaboration with the nurse, the patient, the medical officer and the allied health team. Hospital policies and procedures also influence the type of care that is given, as there are set standards and care for certain procedures. For example, patients who have patient-controlled analgesia are monitored in a specific way according to hospital standards. During clinical experience it is wise to refer to the policy and procedure manuals within the health care settings for specific information. It is important that the plan of care is reviewed periodically and updated to reflect actual care. Very often, care is changed and this change recorded in the progress notes, but no alteration is made to the care plan.

PROGRESS NOTES

Patient care within any clinical agency is continuous from admission to discharge. A record of the ongoing care and patient progress is essential, not only to facilitate the communication process but also to provide a legal record of patient care. The primary focus of the written narrative should be the patient's responses to the nursing care (outcomes of care), and any changes in the patient's condition. In other words, documentation should focus on *outcomes of care* rather than the actual care itself, as the plan of care is clearly detailed in the nursing care plan. Several acronyms are used to assist the documentation process by providing structure to what is written. Commonly used acronyms include SOAP, SOAPE (which are discussed below) and **D**ata **A**nalysis **P**lan (DAP).

Example

Subjective information: Patient states, 'I don't feel well and my leg hurts'.
Objective information: Temperature 39°C, swollen red lesion 2 x 2 cm.
Analysis of this information: Inflamed abrasion to right calf.
Plan: Dress daily according to the wound management plan.
Evaluation: *Record the outcome/effectiveness of the care.*

One of the criticisms of the SOAP documentation format is that it does not contain a cue for documenting the evaluation of care and, although the SOAPE version addresses this weakness, it is cumbersome and lengthy for clinical use. Lampe and Hitchcock (1987) introduced a more focused documentation format that concentrated on reporting three main aspects of care and, more importantly, placed greater emphasis on the patient's response to the care. This format is known as focus charting and uses the acronym DAR.

- **D**ata/Diagnosis: signs and symptoms, nursing diagnosis

- **A**ction: nursing actions/interventions

- **R**esponse: patient's response to care

This method of charting was clinically evaluated and the researchers reported that its use improved the content in nursing notes (Lampe & Hitchcock 1987).

Whatever system is used to document care, it is important that it follows a few rules: the handwriting must be legible; the narrative should be accurate and brief, and cover the substantive issues; patient care and critical events should be documented in the sequence in which they occurred (Staunton 1991). In some clinical settings, documentation is prepared at the end of a shift; this practice is unsafe as it relies heavily on the nurses' memory. Also, if the patient is transferred to another area before the end of a shift, the notes may not reflect actual patient care and outcomes.

THE CASE FOR AND AGAINST USE OF THE NURSING PROCESS

Currently, although the nursing process has been generally accepted and is used in most countries where nursing is regarded as a profession, some groups still argue against its use and question its utility. These arguments for and against are discussed below.

ARGUMENTS IN FAVOUR OF USING THE NURSING PROCESS

Several features have been discussed in support of the nursing process. It potentially provides:

A problem-solving approach to patient care that enhances accountability

One of the outcomes of achieving professional autonomy is greater professional accountability. Accountability for patient care requires that care is given based on a problem-solving approach. Within this framework, it is important that the discipline of nursing develops its body of knowledge through research. This research should address the types of problems that are of nursing concern, the interventions that nurses perform and the outcomes of these interventions. The nursing process framework supports and facilitates this process—it is a problem-solving process, and the assessment, diagnosis and intervention stages are developed using an empirical approach.

A common language for nursing practice

Using a standard language enhances nursing discussion worldwide. Nurse scholars have argued that the development of standard labels and language within a diagnostic taxonomy would provide the foundation for developing nursing knowledge and communicating this knowledge, thus developing a clearer understanding of nursing practice (Hinshaw 1989). It has also provided the impetus to think about the types of patient problems that require nursing interventions. Further, within today's health care system, with the increasing use of automatic computer clinical information systems, Hovenga (1991) emphasises the need for the use of standard nursing labels and language to assist in articulating nursing care within automated computerised information systems. This is important because it increases the visibility of nursing's contribution to patient care.

Increased visibility of nursing

Reflecting on her experiences, Hockey (1981) states that as nurses were—and still are—the largest group in the health care sector, it was easy for administrators to establish the large labour cost of the nursing service; but in the absence of prescribed nursing care and a formal system for documenting this care, administrators were unable to identify the actual services that nursing provided for this cost. Therefore, it was easy for them to absorb and justify budget reductions within this sector. This was due to the *invisibility* of the nursing service. Before the introduction of the nursing process in Australia, and a formal system of documenting care, it was usual practice in some hospitals to discard the nursing notes when the patient was discharged. The nursing process has helped to formalise the way in which nursing care is delivered and documented, and thereby has increased the visibility of nursing care.

Enhanced patient care and evaluation

Nurse administrators argue, from a legal and audit standpoint, that the documentation accompanying the nursing process is necessary because it provides the basis for evaluating patient care through quality assurance audits (McCourt 1986). It is also suggested that it provides a framework for increasing the quality of nursing care, by ensuring that patient care is based on assessment and diagnosis, and thereby specifically and scientifically addressing the unique needs of each patient (Mallick 1981). Failure to assess patients individually can result in an overemphasis on the patients' medical condition and the mechanisation of care, with little attention paid to patients' overall well-being and their responses to their state of health. This could have a detrimental effect on the quality of the overall care.

A framework for teaching

It is well documented that students and novice nurses need structure (Thomas, Wearing & Bennett 1991). The nursing process provides a structured framework and a language that facilitates the teaching and learning of some aspects of nursing.

ARGUMENTS AGAINST USING THE NURSING PROCESS

The nursing process, particularly the diagnosis stage, has been widely debated in the nursing literature. Nurse academics have argued, from a philosophical stance, about whether articulating nursing care within a mechanistic framework, which uses discretely defined labels to detail patient problems, adequately captures the complexities of patient problems and whether it can, therefore, act to facilitate the delivery of nursing care. This philosophical discussion raises several issues:

- Barnum (1987) questions the congruency between the reductionist approach used in nursing process and the assumptions of nursing's holistic philosophy.

- Several authors (Pearson 1988; Lawler 1991; Cooney & Watts 1992) point out the similarities between the nursing process (in particular the diagnosis stage) and the biomedical model, and emphasise that the latter is reductionistic and has a narrower focus than that espoused by nursing.

- Henderson (1982) argues that the nursing process confines nursing practice to a narrowly focused regime, ignoring the intuitive approach to care.

- Masso (1990) states that, as other members within the health care team do not understand the nursing process, it acts as a barrier and limits communication within the health care team.

- From an ethical perspective, Mitchell (1991) emphasises that the lived experience of illness is multidimensional and unique to the person experiencing it. The issue of the nurse diagnosing and labelling the responses of another human being raises certain ethical questions.

CLINICIANS' RESISTANCE TO THE NURSING PROCESS

Though the nursing process is used widely in clinical areas, some clinicians resist its use and question its utility. While clinicians acknowledge the usefulness of the problem-solving approach to patient care, they emphatically argue that the nursing diagnosis language is difficult to understand, and the prescribed documentation within this framework is time consuming and unreflective of actual nursing care (McHugh 1991; Prideaux 1991). This negative attitude towards use of the nursing process has resulted in poor and inconsistent usage within the clinical setting. The clinicians' arguments have been, and still are, contested by some nurse academics, administrators and staff development nurses, who argue that it enhances accountability and communication among nurses. Some clinicians' resistance to the use of the nursing process has been explained by certain academics and staff development nurses in terms of a lack of knowledge of the nursing process and a need for further in-service education (Cunning & Pflederer 1986).

Although there is no cited empirical literature that offers an explanation for these differences in opinion, it may be that the lack of consensus among nurse academics, administrators, clinicians and staff development nurses is due to the different objectives of these groups. Clinicians are involved in the direct delivery of patient care rather than focusing on administrative and theoretical aspects; although these aspects are acknowledged, they may seem removed from actual care and, therefore, unimportant.

The argument that lack of knowledge of the nursing process is an important factor is supported by a study conducted by Bowman, Thompson and Sutton (1983). This study indicated that the use of a structured educational program about the nursing process created positive attitudes towards its use among nursing staff. However, other studies have produced results that conflict with this finding. These studies reviewed the effect of an educational program that focused on the nursing diagnosis stage of the nursing process, as it is believed that this stage is the most difficult to understand and use. A study conducted by Meade and Kim (1984) demonstrated that an education program on the documentation of nursing diagnoses had no effect on the overall standards of such documentation in clinical practice. These findings are supported by Carstens (1984), who found that an in-service program on nursing process had no effect on registered nurses' ability to identify and label valid nursing diagnoses. Fredette and O'Neil (1987), in the first part of their study, examined the relationship between increased didactic theory on nursing diagnosis and the efficacy of diagnosing in clinical practice. The findings revealed no significant differences between the two groups. In addition, Smeltzer and McCreary Juhasz (1990) found no significant relationship between nurses' educational preparation and planning patient care. The results of these studies raise the question as to whether the argument of a lack of knowledge of the nursing process is valid, or whether there are other reasons for the resistance of clinicians.

Street (1992) offers another explanation; she claims that within clinical nursing there exists an oral culture which is effective, though disconnected from the highly organised written culture. This oral culture is inherent in the type of interactions in which nurses engage in their day-to-day dealings with patients, relatives and the interdisciplinary team. She states that the organised written culture has been driven by the need to mirror the more recognised medical culture. As the nursing process is an example of this written culture, it may be unsuitable for nurse clinicians, whose professional culture is purported to be different. Within a clinical setting it is well recognised that the verbal and tape-recorded handovers are an important mechanism in the discussion and communication of patient care. Although useful, this verbal handover does not comply with legal standards and may expose nurses to litigation. It must be recognised that the verbal handover is an adjunct to the formal documentation system—it does not replace it.

OUTCOMES OF THE NURSING PROCESS

The literature has identified both positive and negative outcomes of the use of the nursing process. These are summarised below.

POSITIVE OUTCOMES

The nursing process is seen to have several positive outcomes.

- It provides an organisational framework for the delivery and documentation of nursing care.

- It provides a framework that increases the quality of care, because it is based on individual patient assessment and not merely on the patient's medical diagnosis.

- The documentation that underpins the nursing process provides the basis for evaluating patient care through quality assurance programs.

- It assists in the explication of nursing's unique contribution to patient care within the health care team.

- It provides an impetus for discussion about the nursing domain within and across countries.

- It provides a framework by which nursing services can be accounted for within computerised systems.

- It provides a structured approach which can be used to teach nursing.

NEGATIVE OUTCOMES

Several negative outcomes of the nursing process have also been identified.

- It takes a reductionistic approach to care.

- It is incongruent with nursing's oral professional culture.

- It is seen to undermine the value of intuitive care.

- The language is esoteric and unreflective of actual nursing care.

- It acts as a barrier and limits communication within the health care team.

- It involves too much documentation.

PRAGMATIC OUTCOMES

The discussion surrounding the use and utility of the nursing process is necessary and professionally important. Nursing is, after all, a young discipline with a developing knowledge base; critical review of its developing knowledge base is necessary to help shape its future and reshape the nursing process as deemed necessary. Also, as professional nursing agencies demand the use of a problem-solving approach to patient care (ANCI 1994), in the absence of a better alternative the nursing process provides this problem-solving framework for patient care. Its use enhances nursing's accountability for care and provides a framework and language for communicating and researching patient problems that are of nursing concern. This is necessary if nursing is to develop its practice, based on a platform of research. In addition, certain other methods being used to plan and mechanise care, such as care checklists, are problematic; although they streamline documentation, they confine nursing to a series of tasks that do not truly reflect nursing's contribution to patient care.

LINKING THE NURSING PROCESS AND NURSING THEORY

Nursing theories provide a perspective or a view of nursing. Based on this perspective, the individual, the environment, health and nursing are defined. Within any clinical setting, nursing theories are operationalised using the nursing process. For example, Orem's theory of nursing combines the theories of self-care, self-care deficit, and nursing systems (George 1990). A simple description of how this theory is operationalised, using the nursing process, is given below.

Using Orem's model, patients are assessed and information elicited about the three self-care requisites—universal, developmental and health-deviation. Patients are also assessed in terms of their adequacy, knowledge, skills and capability or capacity to perform self-care operations to meet each component of the therapeutic self-care demand (Orem 1991). Self-care deficits are diagnosed and listed. A plan of care is developed where the nurse helps the patients by:

- acting or doing;
- guiding;
- supporting (physically or psychologically);
- providing an environment that enhances personal development; and
- teaching.

(George 1990)

The determined goals are achieved, guided by the theory of nursing systems. The nurse does everything for the patient (defined as the *wholly compensatory system*), the nurse does some activities for the patient (defined as the *partially compensatory system*) or the nurse supports and teaches the patient to be independent (defined as the *supportive educative system*) (Meleis 1991). Finally, progress is evaluated and the care modified. All stages of the nursing process have been used; however, they are guided by a theoretical perspective. Some of the criticisms regarding the nursing process might be addressed if more clinical settings used a nursing theory and model to deliver patient care.

CRITICAL PATHWAYS

Another newly developed method of delivering patient care is **critical pathways**. Health care services are funded on the types of medical cases they treat. More specifically, each medical diagnosis and treatment procedure has been classified under a Diagnosis Related Group, which attracts a predetermined sum of money. Hospitals are trying to match the cost of patient care to the amount of assigned funds. To do this they have developed critical pathways for common medical diagnoses.

Critical pathways are specifically designed patient care plans which are developed in collaboration with the health care team—that is, nurses, doctors and the allied health team. The plans contain the critical and key stages of treatment and a time frame for achieving each stage. The aim of the care is to achieve a desired patient outcome within a particular time frame by the discharge date. Plans are developed based on the most cost-effective pattern of care for a particular diagnosis or treatment procedure (Bowers 1994; Nelson 1993; Metcalf 1991). The plan of care is prescribed before the patient is admitted, and the tasks of each health care team member are listed. The plan anticipates that the patient's recovery will occur in a sequential and uninterrupted manner—if the patient does not achieve the goals as prescribed, this is documented on a variance chart and further investigated to determine the reason for it. The rationale for this investigation is to improve the quality of care by understanding the pitfalls and changing practices of care accordingly. An example of a critical pathway is shown in Figure 4.3.

While the concept of critical pathways has economic merit, its actual use presents a number of problems.

■   It is based on the biomedical model and locks nursing into this framework.

■   It is task oriented and mechanises care.

■   It is not sensitive to individual needs and recovery rates.

■   It is insensitive to patients' feelings and may be upsetting for patients who are unable to achieve the prescribed goals.

■   It replaces the problem-solving approach to care with a more prescriptive approach.

The problematic aspects of critical pathways are endorsed by the findings of a recent Australian study, which reviewed novice and expert nurses' clinical judgements in a ward setting where critical pathways were used (Greenwood & King 1995). Based on the interpretations of the textual data, the researchers cautioned the wholesale use of critical pathways in its present form, as its use constrained and stifled the thinking of expert nurses. The findings of this study demonstrated that the use of critical pathways hindered the delivery of quality care: the care prescribed within the critical pathway formed the basis for physically oriented patient care, with very little emphasis on other aspects of care (e.g. psychosocial needs) or further addressing the individual needs of each patient. Another point of concern raised by the researchers was that the prescriptive care plan relies on the assumption that the nurses understand the reasons for the interventions. They questioned whether nurses really know why they are giving this care, and whether they are able to determine cases where the prescribed care is inappropriate. There was also evidence to suggest that the use of critical pathways in its present form has the potential to automate care, rather than grounding it within a problem-solving approach (Greenwood & King 1995).

It should also be noted that the development of critical pathways has been driven by economic rationalism. The critical pathway outlines the most cost-effective method of delivering patient care for various medical conditions and procedures. Departing from the critical pathway increases the costs of delivering patient care and may not be viewed favourably by management. If departing from the critical pathway is viewed negatively, nurses may feel reluctant to do so. A case study from the field illustrates this point (see box on p. 72).

It is important to recognise that changes in work practices create changes in behaviour. The long-term effects of these changes and their ramifications for both patient care and the nursing profession are unknown. Critical pathways have only recently been used in Australian settings; their value and worth need to be further evaluated before they are implemented in clinical settings.

FIGURE 4.3 CRITICAL PATHWAY FOR ROUTINE SURGICAL CONDITIONS

Patient's name: _____

Admission date: _____

DRG number: _____

	DAY 1 (date) Admission	DAY 2 (date) Operation	DAY 3 (date) Post-op (Day 1)	DAY 4 (date) Discharge
Diagnostic tests	Full blood picture U's and E's			
Medications	Pre-medication	Intravenous analgesia		Discharge drugs
Treatments	Admission Assessment Observations	Post-op observation regime	BD observations Wound care	Wound care
Diet	Fast at midnight	Light diet as tolerated	Light diet	
Elimination	Routine urine test	Check urinary output postsurgery		
Activity		As tolerated with assistance	Ambulant	
Patient education	Leg and deep-breathing exercises Plan discharge needs			Care of the suture line Explanation of the discharge drugs
Follow-up appointments				Surgical outpatients
Variation	☐ Yes ☐ No *State reason*	☐ Yes ☐ No *State reason*	☐ Yes ☐ No *State reason*	☐ Yes ☐ No *State reason*

Note: The procedures listed on this critical pathway are not conclusive. Individual hospitals develop their own critical pathways which reflect patient care in their respective agency. Some critical pathways also specify the heath care professional responsible for each particular task.

> ### Case study from the field
>
> I was working in a small, 100–200 bed hospital. I was tape-recording my report for the oncoming shift, when another registered nurse entered the room and asked if Mr Smith could have oxygen. I told her that there would be no problem in giving him up to 2 litres without a medical officer's order (nursing discretion). She stated that she did not feel comfortable with that because at another hospital she had been disciplined for using her clinical judgement and departing from the critical pathway. She left to look for the nurse in charge of the patient. I passed the patient's room five minutes later. The patient was clearly in respiratory distress and although he was attended by the cardiac arrest team the patient died. The question remains: would this patient have died if the nurse had not been reprimanded previously for not following the script? (Mahan 1994)

SUMMARY

The five-stage nursing process was developed to provide a problem-solving framework for nursing practice and a structured way of documenting patient care. Currently, this process underpins professional nursing standards, competencies and the practice of nursing in many settings. Though widely used in both clinical and educational settings, some nurses are opposed to its use as it is seen to be reductionist and incongruent with nursing's philosophy. However, in the absence of a better alternative, and with competing interests in the workplace, it provides a structure for the delivery and articulation of nursing care that is patient centred and outcome focused.

GLOSSARY

Collaborative problems: Certain physiologic complications that nurses monitor to detect onset or changes in status. Nurses manage collaborative problems using both nurse and medical officer prescribed interventions.

Critical pathways: specifically designed patient care plans (addressing particular patient conditions) which are developed by the health care team—that is, nurses, doctors and the allied health team. These plans outline the critical stages of treatment and a time frame for achieving each stage. The aim of the critical pathway is to outline patient outcomes within a desired time frame and predictable cost structure

Cue recognition: a stage in the assessment/diagnostic process where the nurse recognises relevant signs and defining characteristics (cues) as being an important indicator of the patient's overall problem.

Diagnostic taxonomy: a classification system for nursing diagnosis development. Nursing diagnoses are categorised and listed in an order (groups and connected subgroups of nursing diagnoses) according to the order in which they were received by NANDA and their level of observation and relationship with other nursing diagnoses.

Functional health patterns: a format for conducting a nursing assessment developed by Dr Marjory Gordon. There are 11 functional health patterns common to all human beings which address both physical and psychosocial aspects.

Interrater reliability: 'the degree of consistency between two raters who are independently assigning ratings to a variable or attribute being investigated' (Burns & Grove 1993).

Outcome statements: goal-directed statements that objectively describe the goals and expected outcomes of nursing interventions.

Nursing diagnosis: the second stage of the nursing process where nurses diagnose patients' problems that are of nursing concern and record these problems using standard labels called nursing diagnostic statements.

Nursing process: a problem-solving approach to nursing care that is comprised of five stages: assessing the patient, diagnosing the patient's problems, planning patient care, implementing patient care and evaluating the effectiveness of patient care.

Risk diagnosis: a type of diagnosis that specifically relates to a situation where the patient is more vulnerable and at risk of developing further illness or injury.

Wellness diagnosis: a type of nursing diagnosis that specifically relates to a situation where the patient is capable of enhancing or promoting their state of health and wellness.

QUESTIONS

1 Define each stage of the nursing process.

2 What are the reasons for and against the use of the nursing process?

3 What are the problems associated with the use of critical pathways?

4 Discuss some ways in which the nursing process could be modified to suit contemporary nursing practice.

LEARNING ACTIVITIES

1 In a group, discuss the factors that influence the diagnostic process, listing examples.

2 Write three nursing diagnoses and accompanying outcome statements. Critique the outcome statements, stating whether they are realistic, unambiguous, measurable, behavioural and/or achievable.

FURTHER READING

Alfaro-LeFevre, R. 1994, *Applying Nursing Diagnosis and Nursing Process: A Step-by-Step Guide*, 3rd edn, J.B. Lippincott, Philadelphia.

Nursing Diagnosis, published by the North American Nursing Diagnosis Association, Nurse Com, Philadelphia, is a journal which is also very useful. The email address is 73764.123@compuserve.com.

5

NURSING THEORISING IN THE UNITED STATES AND AUSTRALIA

Social and Professional Contexts

JUDITH CONDON

LEARNING OBJECTIVES

When you have read this chapter you should be able to:

1. Demonstrate an understanding of the conditions that led to the emergence of nursing theorising in the United States in the 1950s.

2. Explain the context of the major changes that occurred in nursing theorising over the four decades from the 1950s to the 1990s.

3. Describe similarities and differences in the influences on nursing theorising in the United States and Australia.

Judith Condon, RN, DipNursEd (NSW College Paramedical Studies), BA (Hons), MEd Stud (FUSA) has been a lecturer in the School of Nursing at the Flinders University of South Australia (and its predecessors: the South Australian College of Advanced Education and the Sturt College of Advanced Education) for many years. Her interest has been chiefly in the improvement of educational practice in nursing, and in curriculum development and evaluation. More recently, Judith has been working in the area of nursing theory development, concentrating on the social, intellectual and professional contexts that have impacted on its development. She is also very interested in the potential of critical reflection for the improvement of practice.

INTRODUCTION

Why did nurses in the United States begin to theorise about nursing practice in the 1950s? In order to find some answers to this question, it is essential to understand the social and professional contexts that nurses found themselves in at this time. The view of theory development taken in this chapter is that theory in the human sciences cannot capture cause and effect relationships in some external reality about which all are agreed, as is possible by and large in the physical sciences. Rather, theory in the human sciences emerges as a result of what it is possible to think, write or say within specific historical periods, influenced by ideology, sociocultural factors such as institutions and the economy, and political factors.

To appreciate the nature of theory development in nursing, therefore, it is important to understand the social, intellectual and political contexts in which it emerged, developed and changed. An understanding of the social context of theory development is important for the critique of theory. Knowledge of the conditions under which a theory was developed will allow more intelligent assessment of that theory and a more informed judgement of its appropriateness for particular situations in nursing in a different time and place.

Before going further it is important to clarify how theory is being defined for this chapter. As you will have found from your reading of the second chapter in this text, the term 'nursing theory' has a number of possible meanings. In the past it generally meant 'that which was learnt from texts or in the classroom'. In this meaning it was often set in opposition to 'practice' or 'the real world' or 'clinical'. Today it is more likely to mean 'grand theory'—that which attempts, in a global way, to explain everything in nursing. Examples are: adaptation in Roy; self-care in Orem; a health care system in Neuman (Fitzpatrick & Whall 1983).

In some of these 'grand theories', which are also described as conceptual models or conceptual frameworks (Fawcett 1980; Fitzpatrick & Whall 1983), theoretical statements are often not clearly defined and may not have been tested empirically or explored by other research paradigms.

Theories of the mid-range are theoretical statements about more circumscribed phenomena in nursing which have usually arisen out of research or have been tested by research. Micro theories deal with unidimensional concepts and also have a clear relationship with research.

Another form of theory that has been of interest since 1988 to nursing academics and clinicians in Australia is personal theory. No practice is atheoretical. Even nurses who have never heard of nursing theory will have personal theories (which may be tacit), by which they organise and interpret nursing. Exploration of your personal theory, particularly if accompanied by an uncovering of its history and the social, ideological and political constraints shaping and constraining it, can lead to insights about practice and illuminate possible changes for the better, in practice (Street 1991).

In this chapter some consideration will be given to these different forms of theory and the conditions surrounding their adoption.

In order to explore the social context of theory development in nursing, we will be seeking the answers to two central questions.

1 (a) What were the conditions that led to the emergence of formal theorising in nursing in the 1950s in the United States and its development over the next 30 years?

(b) What was the Australian experience during the same period, and what were the similarities and differences?

2 (a) What influenced the form and substance of nursing theories in the United States?

(b) What influenced the form and substance of Australian nursing theories?

The experience in the United States will be considered first, because the move to theory there predated and influenced the Australian experience. It will be argued that in both countries education has had perhaps the greatest influence in motivating nurses to theorise about nursing and nursing practice. As nursing education and registration became more closely regulated in the early part of the twentieth century, and gradually moved into the higher education sector in the second half of the century, nursing academics developing curricula for preregistration, and postgraduate students were forced to state clearly their conceptualisations of nursing. These conceptualisations were, as Bruni (1991) argues, profoundly influenced by the increasing desire of nurses for professional status. This argument will be explored further below.

THEORY DEVELOPMENT IN THE UNITED STATES

Afaf Meleis (1991), in her excellent book *Theoretical Nursing: Development and Progress,* has carefully and clearly set out the key milestones and stages in theory development in the United States; these will be only briefly canvassed here before a more lengthy examination of the context in which these changes occurred. Meleis dates the birth of nursing theory to the period between 1955 and 1960, with Columbia Teachers College, New York, as the first centre of theorising (1991, p. 33.) As Meleis shows, of the theorists who offered conceptions of nursing during this period, Peplau, Henderson, Hall, Abdellah, King, Wiedenbach and Rogers were educated at Teachers College (1991, p. 33). From there, the influence of these nurses spread widely. For example, Peplau went on to Rutgers and also held senior positions in the American Nurses Association (Marriner 1986). Henderson became associated with Yale University, and Wiedenbach joined the staff at Yale where Orlando was working as a research associate and later as a faculty member. Yale became another important centre for theory development (Meleis 1991).

The key event isolated by Meleis in the period 1961–65 was the 1965 position paper of the American Nurses Association, 'in which nursing was defined as care, cure and coordination and in which theory development was identified as a most significant goal for the profession of nursing' (1991, p. 37).

Between 1966 and 1970, several significant theory conferences were held at Case Western Reserve University, the University of Colorado and the University of Kansas, with key papers being published in *Nursing Research* and other journals, recently founded, such as *Nursing Science* and *Image*. These conferences and subsequent publications were important in widening the debate about theory in nursing and for the first time focused attention on the value of theory for practice (through the work of Dickoff, James & Wiedenbach 1968a, 1968b). Until this time, theory had only been used in education or as a framework for research by Columbia Teachers College or Yale students (Meleis 1991). **Metatheoretical** concerns raised in this period concerned 'whether theories should be basic or borrowed, pure or applied, descriptive or prescriptive' (Meleis 1991, p. 38).

Between 1971 and 1975, nursing academics, having accepted that nursing was a field about which theory might be generated, became preoccupied with further metatheoretical issues, such as the structural components of theory and analysis of theory (Meleis 1991). In 1972, an initiative with far-reaching effects was enacted by the National League for Nursing's Council for the Accreditation of Baccalaureate and Higher Degree programs. A criterion for accreditation of programs by the League was that the nursing curriculum be taught within a conceptual framework. This often led to the adoption of one of the 'grand' theories as a conceptual framework (Meleis 1991).

The period 1976–80 saw a continuation of metatheoretical debates with a dawning recognition that knowledge development in nursing had been overly constrained by the **empiric–analytic paradigm**. Carper's (1978) paper proposing four patterns of knowing in nursing was seminal in enlarging nurses' vision of the sources of nursing knowledge (Meleis 1991). As discussed in Chapter 3, Carper identified 'four fundamental patterns of knowing' in nursing, '(a) empirics, the science of nursing; (b) aesthetics, the art of nursing; (c) the component of personal knowledge in nursing; and (d) ethics, the component of moral knowledge in nursing' (1978, p. 13).

In 1978, the Nursing Theory Think Tank was formed with the aims of utilising existing theory and developing new theories 'to describe and explain nursing phenomena to predict relationships, and to guide nursing care' (Meleis 1991, p. 42).

In 1980, two papers were published which summarised the concepts central to nursing as nurse, person, health and environment (Flaskerud & Halloran 1980; Fawcett 1980). These had first been named by Walker in 1971, and refined by Yura and Torres in 1975. It was not until after 1980, however, that these 'domain concepts' (Meleis 1991, p. 43) in nursing gained general acceptance, becoming the standard against which other concepts such as caring were argued for.

As Meleis (1991) documents, by 1981–85 the theory literature was showing an acceptance of theory for nursing. The focus shifted to the relationship of theory to different research and practice problems, and analysis and comparison of theories. The period 1986–90 saw continuation of some of the earlier debates about nursing's scientific and disciplinary status, but from a more confident, less exploratory standpoint. The focus of theorising had shifted by this period from broad questions, such as 'what is nursing?', to issues within single domains (Meleis 1991). This represented a move from grand theorising to mid-range or micro theorising.

A much broader view of knowledge development and research became evident, with publications by Allen (1985) and Allen, Benner and Diekelmann (1986), for example, advocating that nursing researchers use a range of methodologies appropriate to the problem or phenomenon under investigation. This was more helpful than much of the literature of the early 1980s, which had tended to polarise discussions on methodology into *either* **quantitative** *or* **qualitative** methods as being most appropriate for nursing.

In a 1992 paper, Meleis commented that nursing theorising appeared to have entered a period of philosophical debate which in part revisited some earlier questions on the role and future of nursing. Meleis (1992) had predicted that the testing of propositions arising out of nursing theories would become a top priority, with special focus on improving practice. That this has not eventuated is perhaps not so surprising. While most of the 'grand' theorists have attracted disciples who have been conducting their nursing research and practice from particular theoretical frameworks, many other nursing researchers are 'non-aligned', pursuing their particular research interests and generating mid-range or micro theories pertinent to their own interests.

This, then, is the situation today, with some ongoing heart-searching about the status of nursing as a science (Packard & Polifroni 1991) and a discipline (Newman, Sime & Corcoran-Perry 1991), and much diversity in research methodology and knowledge generation in nursing.

The foregoing is clearly a very brief and simplified survey of some of the key events and stages of theory development in nursing in the United States. Meleis (1991), among others, is an excellent source for the detail of these events. It is more important for our purposes to try to answer the question about the conditions that led to nursing theorising taking the forms it did. As mentioned in the Introduction to this chapter, education is held to be a key influence on the development of nursing theory.

NURSING EDUCATION IN THE UNITED STATES

University courses for graduate nurses in education and administration were developed as early as 1898 at Columbia University Teachers College (Bevis & Watson 1989). The first undergraduate baccalaureate nursing program was created in 1909 at the University of Minnesota, when the School of Nursing associated with the university hospital was transferred to the university (Bevis & Watson 1989). It was not until after World War II that there was any substantial move into the tertiary sector but, by 1951, 9184 women were enrolled in baccalaureate programs in 195 schools of nursing in universities or colleges (Gilkey 1953, in Thibodeau 1983), with 350 schools in operation by 1959 (Bevis & Watson 1989).

In 1951, associate degree programs for 'technical nurses' were developed as two-year college programs, gradually taking over from hospital diploma programs and bringing most, but not all, nurse education into institutions of higher learning (Bevis 1988). The move to the higher education sector influenced nursing theory development in at least six important ways:

1   The requirement of nursing academics for graduate education.

2   The development of higher degrees in nursing.

3   The development of nursing research.

4   The influence of the National League for Nursing (NLN) on curriculum development—behavioural objectives.

5   The influences of the NLN on curriculum development—conceptual framework.

6   The influence of other disciplines.

These factors will now be considered in some detail.

Requirement for graduate education

Nurses teaching in the higher education sector required graduate education. Teachers College, Columbia University, as mentioned above, provided graduate courses for nurses in education and administration based on the theories of those disciplines (Meleis 1991). Other nurses gained their graduate education in disciplines such as sociology, psychology, physiology, anthropology, history and philosophy, with most doing their higher degree work in education (Bevis & Watson 1989). At that time, educational and psychological theory was dominated by **positivist behavioural** theory, and other disciplines such as sociology were strongly **empiricist**. These disciplines were an important influence on the development of the thinking of many nursing theorists—for example, Leininger's doctoral studies were in anthropology, King's in education, Barnard's in psychology and Roy's in sociology (Marriner 1986). It should be noted, however, that other theorists were influenced by non-empiricist thinkers, such as Carl Rogers in the case of Lydia Hall, and Harry Stack Sullivan, in the case of Hildegard Peplau (Marriner 1986).

Development of higher degrees in nursing

Some of the nurses with baccalaureate degrees in nursing lobbied for masters and doctoral degrees in nursing. The development of higher degrees in nursing (very few before the 1960s) provided the impetus for nursing academics trained in disciplines other than nursing to attempt to articulate the theoretical base of nursing. Subsequently, with higher degrees in nursing, the amount of nursing research being conducted expanded dramatically, with an inevitable increase in theorising about nursing.

Development of nursing research

Nursing academics in universities, in common with other academics, were required to research and publish and, by 1952, there were sufficient nursing researchers seeking publication, and nurses interested in reading nursing research, to see the launch of the journal *Nursing Research*. A number of federally funded initiatives in the 1950s and 1960s also helped to establish nursing research. In 1955 the Special Nurse Research Fellowship Program was commenced in the Division of Nursing of the National Institute of Health, and in 1962 the Nurse Scientist Graduate Training Grants Program was established, providing support for nurses to pursue doctoral studies in one of the basic sciences (Meleis 1991).

As Ellis (1985, p. xiii in Nicoll 1992) notes, the development of nursing research gave rise to a number of questions that are essentially theoretical questions: 'What is nursing research? What is nursing? What should be researched? How should nursing research be done?' As early as 1960, Schlotfeldt claimed that: '[t]he primary task of nursing research is to develop theories that serve as a guide to practice' (Meleis 1991, p. 39). Because this was written in 1960, it may be assumed that Schlotfeldt meant empirical research.

Curriculum development—behavioural objectives

By the late 1950s and early 1960s both State boards of nursing and the National League for Nursing had based their criteria for the accreditation of hospital, college and university undergraduate programs on the rational, linear Tyler curriculum model. If a school of nursing could not demonstrate that it followed the model, with clearly delineated objectives and measurable outcomes, then students were not eligible to sit for State board licensure examinations and, until 1988, schools would not be accredited by the National League for Nursing (Bevis & Watson 1989). During the early 1960s, following the publication of Mager's book, *Preparing Instructional Objectives* (1962), many nurse educators attended workshops on writing behavioural objectives (Bevis 1988). By 1972, with the publication of Bevis's book on curriculum development in nursing, which was to become a standard text for nurse education, Tyler's model was inextricably tied to behaviourism (Bevis 1988). Since 1988 there have been moves to deinstitutionalise the Tyler model (Bevis & Watson 1989).

The Tyler model is a behavioural, empirical model which adheres to the dictum of Thorndike, an early behavioural psychologist, that 'whatever exists, exists in some amount: and therefore can be measured' (Bevis & Watson 1989, p. 26). In this model, objectives are to be stated in a manner that guides not only teaching and the selection of learning experiences, but also the changes required in the students' behaviour, to be measured by assessment procedures (Bevis & Watson 1989). This is a technical model of curriculum development and professional education, and has been subjected to severe criticism (Schön 1983; Carr & Kemmis 1986; Grundy 1987). In such an approach to education, only the measurable is valued; the immeasurable or difficult to measure are reduced to components in which the parts may not add up to the desired whole. For example, empathy may be reduced to a formula consisting of paying attention (leaning forward, open body position and eye contact) and reflection of the other's content and feelings, with no room on the checklist for the evaluator's professional judgement as to the appropriateness and effect of the communication.

This approach to curriculum is also premised on the belief that there are right or wrong answers to all questions in nursing, and that there is no student-generated question which cannot be predetermined by the teacher.

This was to take a technical–rational approach to professional education in which the practitioner's role was to apply scientifically determined solutions to problems that could be anticipated and clearly defined. The clinician's role was to assess the problem and apply the correct scientific solution (Schön 1987). In this, nursing modelled itself on other professional schools, such as medicine, architecture, engineering and education, all of which had been similarly seduced by the promise of the application of science to solve human problems. By the 1980s, disenchantment with this promise was being experienced in many professional schools, which had found that practitioners do not tend to solve human problems as the model implied they should, and that human problems were infinitely more complex and 'messy' than those that could be isolated in a scientific experiment (Schön 1983).

Curriculum development—conceptual framework

In 1972, the National League for Nursing's Council of Baccalaureate and Higher Degree Programs approved its 'Criteria for the Appraisal of Baccalaureate and Higher Degree Programs in Nursing', including the criterion that nursing curricula should be based on a conceptual framework (Meleis, 1991, p. 41). This criterion was not revoked until 1983, when it was changed to the more flexible statement: 'the curriculum is logically organised and internally consistent' (NLN 1983, in Diekelmann, Allen & Tanner 1989).

The work of a number of theorists was developed in large part as a conceptual framework for curriculum development—for example, that of Sr Callista Roy, Betty Neuman, Martha Rogers, Imogene King and Myra Levine (Fitzpatrick & Whall 1983).

The 1972 decision to have nursing curricula based on a conceptual framework reflects the excitement about the potential of theory in academic nursing in particular and the commitment to establish nursing as a science.

However, the decision was met with confusion by the staff in many schools of nursing, with a solution being found in the adoption of one of the published, though usually untested, theories of nursing as the curriculum framework (Diekelmann, Allen & Tanner 1989). The requirement at least had the effect of making known the work of nursing theorists to a large number of nurses; but it may well have contributed to the fruitless search that pervaded the thinking of many in the 1960s and 70s for *the* grand theory of nursing, which would explain everything in nursing. It may also have diverted attention away from the development of theories for practice (Meleis 1991). This desire for 'a theory of everything' can of course be understood in the light of the view of science and knowledge development held by nurses at that time, based on the science of the physical sciences. This will be considered further later in this chapter.

Influence of other disciplines

The wholesale adoption of the behavioural model of education by schools of nursing in the United States reflected the widespread belief in empiricism in the scientific community of the country. The dominance of psychology and education by behaviourism, and sociology by empiricism, reflected a belief that the methods of the natural sciences could be used in the human sciences to solve the problems of humanity. During World War II, enormous advances had been made in science and technology, which in the post-war period were applied to civilian use. By the late 1950s, the launching of Sputnik by the then United Socialist Soviet Republic, and the resultant scientific race in the atmosphere of the Cold War, created a strong focus on science. Great scientific advances were also made in medicine and other domains, adding to the belief, perhaps most clearly exemplified by the 1969 US moon landing, that science would find the answer to all human problems.

Paradoxically, these certainties were being expressed during a period of great cultural upheaval, with the black rights movement gaining momentum in the 1950s and early 1960s, student rights and women's rights groups challenging the status quo by the late 1960s, and the upheaval of the Vietnam war in the late 1960s and early 1970s. The challenge offered by these human rights movements was also a challenge to the myth of science as a panacea. Clearly, science had not been able to find solutions to all human problems (or even articulate what these problems might be). Empirical science had been on the ascendancy in the physical sciences since the time of Francis Bacon (1561–1626) and Isaac Newton (1642–1727); it was adopted for the human sciences in the mid nineteenth century by Comte who, using the natural sciences as his model, 'proposed to advance the study of society to the scientific level of thought which natural science had already reached' (Jones 1975, p. 176). Comte envisioned a scientific sociology comprising 'social statics concerned with describing the laws of order, and social dynamics concerned with describing the laws of progress' (Jones 1975, p. 176). For Comte, and for many of the scientists in the emerging social sciences, the function of science was to be able to generalise about how things happen in order to be able to control events, thus providing the knowledge with which administrators and bureaucrats might bring about an orderly society (Jones 1975).

VIEWS OF KNOWLEDGE

The view of knowledge inherent in these beliefs, which have so dominated twentieth century social/human science and nursing, is 'that valid knowledge can only be established by reference to that which is manifested in experience' (Kolakowski 1972, in Carr & Kemmis 1986, p. 61); that is, knowledge has its foundation in external reality, to be discovered by sensory observation. The method of discovery is the scientific method, most usually equated with the **hypothetico-deductive** method (Carr & Kemmis 1986), in which hypotheses with observable consequences are generated; objective measurements are made under controlled conditions that ensure the validity of the measures; and measurements repeated to ensure their reliability. The aim is to be able to generalise from the observations and generate laws.

Because this view of science dominated the disciplines in which nurses were gaining their higher degrees and conducting postgraduate research, it is the view which rapidly came to dominate nursing theorising and research. This approach was reinforced by the criteria adopted for evaluating research proposals, by agencies funding nursing research; these criteria were those of empiricism (Meleis 1991), as by and large they continue to be to the present day.

Nursing academics, theoreticians and researchers strove to establish nursing as an empirical science because, for the most part, they knew no other legitimate approach to knowledge development. Jacox and Webster (1986), in arguing against an earlier paper on theory development written in purely empiricist terms by Jacox in 1974, explain the problem.

By the late 1960s, the theories of Hildegard Peplau, Dorothy Johnson, Ida Orlando and Dorothea Orem, among others, had been in circulation for some time.

When 40 nurses met at Western Case University in 1969 and the University of Kansas in 1970 to discuss theory and its implications for nursing, eight had recently completed doctoral degrees in sociology or education, bringing to the conference the empiricist views of science held by those disciplines, which were as yet largely uninfluenced by the changes in conceptions of science taking place in philosophy and at least some of sociology. As Jacox and Webster (1986, p. 364) describe, the views of those at these conferences were to be highly influential and yet were based on 'pre-1960 notions of science'. It was, by and large, not until the 1980s that there was a shift from the 'overly rigid and narrow accounts [based on empiricism] of what theories are and how they are developed' (Jacox & Webster 1986, p. 365). By then, nurses were recognising that a purely scientific view of theory development was often incompatible with their beliefs about nursing, and that empirical research was not suitable for the investigation of many of the phenomena nurses were interested in (Jacox & Webster 1986).

Before moving on to explore the Australian experience, consider the extent to which the questions posed in the Introduction have been answered.

It has been argued here that education has, in a variety of ways, been the dominant factor motivating nurses to theorise about nursing: in designing curricula for undergraduate and postgraduate programs; by providing a framework for an outcome of the research done by academics and students; by influencing the view of knowledge development and approach to theorising adopted by nursing. These educational goals are inextricably linked to the professional goals of nurses and are exemplified in the promotion of nursing theory by the American Nurses Association and the National League for Nursing.

While the goal of finding the 'grand' theory of nursing has been abandoned, the goal of establishing prescriptive theory for nursing has not (Meleis 1991). This goal reflects the empirical origins of nursing theory, even though it is tempered these days by the recognition that nursing knowledge has many sources other than empirical sources, and that descriptive theory may be as fruitful in illuminating nursing as prescriptive theory.

THE AUSTRALIAN EXPERIENCE

As yet there is no chronicler of the Australian experience of nursing theory development such as Meleis (1991) has been for North American nursing. In the Gray and Pratt book, *Towards a Discipline of Nursing*, a number of authors explore the state of the discipline including its 'theoretical base, its research approaches and its knowledge development' (1991, p. 2). There have also been several conferences which have considered nursing theory. A brief though necessarily incomplete survey will be undertaken here (incomplete because the sources of theory exist in many places, such as unpublished higher degree theses and curriculum documents which, although they are public documents, have not been widely published). Because there are few published theories in Australia as yet, a variety of role statements (e.g. from the National Health and Medical Research Council and the Australian Nursing Federation) will be examined in some detail along with the social context of the changes.

Until the early 1970s, the dominant influence on the thinking of Australian nurses was British nursing in the traditions of Nightingale. The Royal Victorian College of Nursing was established in 1934 to offer postgraduate courses for nurses, with the NSW College of Nursing and the College of Nursing Australia in Melbourne, being established in 1949 (Russell 1990). Before these colleges were established, nurses who wished to obtain postgraduate qualifications in education or management had been required to go to Britain. The influence of the British tradition continued, even when postgraduate courses became available in Australia. For example, one of the founders of the NSW College of Nursing, Muriel Doherty, who had been sister-tutor at Royal Prince Alfred Hospital, Sydney, and co-author of an influential nursing text (which will be considered below), received her Sister Tutor Certificate from the University of London (Russell 1990; Doherty, Sirl & Ring 1963).

Before considering the few examples of published Australian nursing theory, major role statements spanning the three decades 1960–90 will be examined, to establish the shifts in thinking about nursing which occurred in that time.

The 1963 publication of the tenth edition of Doherty, Sirl and Ring's *Modern Practical Nursing Procedures* (revised by Smith, Lew & Tomlinson) provides a convenient starting point for a survey of role statements in Australia. The role of the nurse is defined in the first chapter, entitled 'Ethics and hospital etiquette', and is taken from the *First International Code of Nursing Ethics*, presented in 1953 by the 10th Quadrennial Congress of the International Council of Nurses (ICN).

> Professional nurses minister to the sick. They assume responsibility for creating a physical, social and spiritual environment which will be conducive to recovery; they stress the prevention of illness and promotion of health by teaching and example. They render health service to the individual, the family and the community and co-ordinate their services with members of other health professionals. Service to mankind is the primary function of nurses.
>
> *(Doherty et al. 1963, p. 1)*

While the language is dated, much of this statement when taken at face value might be accepted by nurses today. However, given the changes, since 1963, in institutional, societal and theoretical contexts of care, and in the perceptions of nurses and their clients of nursing and health care, the connotations implicit in the statement make this conception of nursing very different in spirit from that of the 1990s. For example, the language of vocation is implied in 'minister to the sick' and 'service to mankind'; in keeping with this ethos is the passivity—indeed, near invisibility—of the patient/client, who is present only as the recipient of care in this definition. The patient is also defined as ignorant, being satisfied to base his or her relationship with the nurse on trust alone: 'The patient comes to you in simple faith—offer him sympathy, respect his confidence, inspire him with courage, hope and a feeling of security' (Doherty et al. 1963, p. 4).

The ICN Code (1953), cited by Doherty et al. (1963), lists 14 statements which are a mixture of the responsibilities and personal attributes of the nurse, beginning with: 'the fundamental responsibility of the nurse is threefold; to conserve life, to alleviate suffering and to promote health', and including: 'The nurse is under an obligation to carry out the physician's orders intelligently and loyally and to refuse to participate in unethical procedures; the nurse sustains confidence in the physician and other members of the health team; incompetence or unethical conduct of associates should be exposed but only to the proper authority' (in Doherty et al. 1963, p. 2).

The first statement, which establishes 'the fundamental responsibility of the nurse', can be read as a mirror image to that of medicine, with the nurse's role being clearly defined by its relation to medicine (Doherty et al. 1963, p. 2).

The vocational element of this 1963 definition of nursing, and nursing's subservient and dependent role, is emphasised by Doherty et al. in the following section on hospital etiquette.

> The spirit which makes one observe hospital etiquette is ethical. It demands loyalty and a cheerful co-operation with all those with whom the nurse comes in contact—the patients and their relatives, medical officers, matron, sisters, fellow nurses and other members of the hospital staff and the general public.
>
> *(Doherty et al. 1963, p. 3)*

Clearly, a nurse is to judge 'the right thing to do' in terms of the orders of those who are his or her superiors.

Nursing is defined as hospital nursing and in this text has clear links back to Florence Nightingale in its reference to 'the harmonious and restful atmosphere of the wards, and the quality of the care and attention received therein' (Doherty et al., 1963, p. 4) and in its 'Advice to Student Nurses':

> Have no regrets—you are on the threshold of your career, with unlimited opportunities for a full and satisfying life of service—a life in which you can give of your best in the knowledge that you are privileged to carry on the great example set by 'The Lady with the Lamp'.
>
> *(Doherty et al. 1963, p. 4)*

The advice continues with a note on the importance of education as a means of understanding the patient, controlling the nurse's own instincts and emotions, performing nursing skills with intelligence and finding ways to improve nursing care (1963).

The following caveat is then offered:

> Hours are regulated, but this should not prevent the nurse from doing good work, and the spirit that has imbued nurses from earliest times can still be hers, the spirit of willing and cheerful service. A nurse's first obligation is to care for and tend the sick, and in a modern training school, this must not be sacrificed by non-technical duties and academic work. She must have sufficient knowledge and understanding to enable her to take part in the prevention of disease, in the great fight against it and in the rehabilitation of the patient.
>
> *(Doherty et al. 1963, p. 5)*

Nightingale's vocational view of nursing is reflected in this 1963 text. She also held education to be very important and in earlier writings explicitly defined nursing knowledge as different from that of medicine (Nightingale 1859/1970, pp. 74–5). In later statements there is a contradiction which is reflected in the 1953 *First International Code of Nursing Ethics*. Nightingale described nursing as the 'skilled servant of medicine, surgery and hygiene' (1882/1954, p. 335, in Fitzpatrick & Whall 1983, p. 22) and compared nurses with 'the building staff' and physicians with the 'architect' (Cook 1942, p. 270, in Fitzpatrick & Whall 1983, p. 22). As Fitzpatrick and Whall comment, 'these remarks were likely aimed at appeasing the physicians who complained that Nightingale's nurses were over-educated' (1983, p. 22).

Clearly, Nightingale's earlier vision was lost to nursing over the next century, with medical **discourse** dominating the emergent nursing discourse (Meleis 1991).

In Doherty et al. (1963), as has been shown, the biomedical model dominates thinking about the role of the nurse, with disease conceptualised as the enemy to be defeated.

The subservience of education to service is also made quite clear, even in a 'modern training school' (Doherty et al. 1963, p. 5). It is ironic that this claim on the 'first obligation' of the nurse, with the sacrifice of education if necessary, was hollow. As White (1972) reports, 39 per cent of nursing duties in 1971 involved non-nursing work.

The remainder of this 1963 text, in keeping with its conception of the role of the nurse, and the dominance of service over education, is presented as a 'procedure manual': that is, as sets of explicit instructions on the setting up for, performance of and cleaning up after a wide range of nursing tasks.

It is noteworthy that the text's revisers, while citing the 1953 ICN Code of Ethics (from a British publication), seem unaware of the ICN's 1961 *Basic Principles of Nursing Care* written by Henderson, or of Henderson's 1955 text, *Principles and Practices of Nursing*, both of which are organised around basic needs and symptoms, rather than the tasks that characterised the Australian text.

As mentioned above, Doherty and also Ring, two of the original authors of the text, had Sister Tutor Certificates from Kings College of Household and Social Science, University of London. Smith, Lew and Tomlinson, the text's revisers, had all been awarded the Sister Tutor Diploma from the NSW College of Nursing.

Australian nursing was founded in the Nightingale tradition and continued to be influenced by British nursing traditions through those Australian nurses who had completed their tertiary education in the United Kingdom. It was to be another decade before Australian nursing took note of the changes occurring in the United States. However, this 1963 definition marks the end of a long period of certainty about the role of the nurse. The next 30 years saw profound changes in the ways in which nurses conceptualised their role. The changing definitions can be read as a marker for the ferment of political activity that nurses were engaged in over this period to improve their educational, professional and industrial status.

When White (1972) wrote her report, *The Role of the Nurse in Australia*, for the National Health and Medical Research Council (NHMRC), she included an annotated bibliography of 100 published and unpublished papers written in the five years between 1966 and 1971, on the present or future role of the nurse. The purpose of the report was to define and identify 'the present and future roles of the nurse in relation to the needs of the Australian community' (1972, p. 2). In defining the 'present role of the nurse', White concludes:

> There would be little disagreement among nurses, doctors and patients that the basic role of the registered nurse in primary, acute and long-term care involves those functions relating to the personal care of the patient. The word 'patient' is taken to mean any person well or sick, in any health care setting, who is receiving the services of a professional provider of health care for the purposes of promoting, maintaining or restoring health or minimising the consequences of illness.

> *(White 1972, p. 6)*

This statement marks a clear shift in emphasis from that of Doherty et al. (1963). Nursing is defined in terms of 'the personal care of the patient' rather than the biomedically influenced conservation of life, alleviation of suffering and promotion of health. The word 'patient' is also expanded to include 'the well' as a recipient of health care and marks a return to Nightingale's definition of a nurse as a person who had the 'charge of the personal health of somebody', whether sick or well (1859/1970, p. 6).

It is likely that White's reclaiming of 'the well' was influenced by Virginia Henderson. When she was commissioned to write this report, White had recently returned from Columbia University Teachers College where she had obtained her education doctorate. Henderson had been one of the group of nursing academics at Columbia during the 1950s and 1960s. Henderson states in the preface to her revision of the fifth edition of *Textbook of the Principles and Practices of Nursing* (Harmer & Henderson 1955): 'Throughout the text I have proceeded on the premise that nursing is a service to both well and sick' (in Henderson & Nite 1978, p. vii).

In the same text in 1955, Henderson had defined nursing. The following statement, written for the ICN in 1961, was an adaptation of her 1955 definition.

> The unique function of the nurse is to assist the individual, sick or well, in the performance of those activities contributing to health or its recovery (or to a peaceful death) that he would perform unaided if he had the necessary strength, will or knowledge. And to do this in such a way as to help him to gain independence as rapidly as possible.
>
> *(in Henderson 1966, p. 15)*

Nursing care is defined as assisting the patient to fulfil 14 fundamental human needs, ranging from the physiological, psychological and spiritual to activities of daily living. White's 'elements of clinical practice' reflect Henderson's thinking on the functions of the nurse:

> Many elements of clinical practice are common to primary, acute and long-term care and form the fundamentals upon which specialist expertise is later built. These elements include: maintenance or restoration of basic functions (respiration, elimination, nutrition, circulation, rest and sleep, locomotion and communication); observing and reporting signs of actual or potential change in a patient's condition; assessing his physical and emotional state and immediate environment; giving instruction, information, support and advice to patients and relatives.
>
> *(White 1972, p. 6)*

Among the conclusions of the report, White notes:

> The idea is perpetuated among nurses, other professionals and members of the community that nursing is predominantly concerned with disease and disease processes, rather than individuals and their particular needs.
>
> *(White 1972, p. 34)*

White looks forward to a time when 'a larger proportion of nurses are educated in institutions of higher education [and] traditional nursing roles will be examined and reassessed for their relevance and adequacy in meeting the health needs of the community' (1972, p. 13). She foresees an expanded role for the nurse within hospitals and in the community. White's document provided evidence for the industrial struggles of the mid 1970s to remove non-nursing duties such as food distribution and cleaning from nurses' work. It was also timely in relation to the changes to health care, especially in community health, initiated by the Whitlam Labor government which came to office in 1972.

In 1973, the Nursing Committee of the National Health and Medical Research Council presented a brief report entitled *The Role of the Nurse in Australia* to the 76th Session of the Council, which was published in 1974. In this statement, the nurse's role is accepted as 'complementary to that of the doctor' and as being 'general and comprehensive' in comparison with 'the special, more closely defined, roles of other health professionals such as physiotherapists . . . '.

The report goes on:

> For the individual patient, doctor and nurse together provide care for the whole person within particular areas and levels of expertise. In addition to providing basic physical care, the nurse is healer, adviser, comforter, confidante, and technician. Of these, the functions of healer or treater have been predominant.
>
> *(1974, unnumbered page)*

This is an early reference to nursing as care of the 'whole' person and, unlike later definitions, includes the doctor with the nurse in partnership providing care for the whole person. Also, in this statement, healing and treating are emphasised in contrast to later statements which emphasise care.

The report has a somewhat defeatist and negative flavour, noting that 'the nurse performs, and has been expected to perform tasks ranging from the frankly domestic to the highly technical', including the specialist duties of allied health professions such as physiotherapy, when the physiotherapist is unavailable (1974, unnumbered page).

Thus the impression is conveyed that nursing has little control over its own work and no clear sense of the potential of its role, justifying White's conclusion:

> Many nurses are not practising at their highest capacity, and the potential for the nurse in a clinical specialist role, complementary to that of other health professionals has not been realised.
>
> *(1972, p. 34)*

These role statements became part of the ammunition in the battle to improve work and education conditions for nurses.

In 1973, as a response by nurses to indicate their concern about the inadequacy of preregistration nursing programs to prepare nurses to work across the range of practice arenas listed in the 1973 NHMRC document mentioned above, a working party was formed to develop goals for the provision of nurse education in Australia (Wood 1990). The committee consisted of representatives of the Royal Australian Nursing Federation (RANF), now the Australian Nursing Federation (ANF); the Royal College of Nursing Australia; the NSW College of Nursing; and the National Florence Nightingale Committee of Australia. The reports, Parts I and II, *Goals in Nursing Education*, were published in 1975 and signalled the beginning of a unified, national approach to the transfer of all preregistration nursing education to the higher education sector. Prior to this, attempts at reform had been hampered by: 'a lack of national unity, insufficient and inefficient communication between state leaders, no broad framework or development of national leadership, a lack of decision-making ability and a lack of national cohesion' (Manock 1973, pp. 30–1).

In the meantime, nursing organisations in individual states had been negotiating with state governments for preregistration nursing education to be conducted in colleges of advanced education. In 1974, the first tertiary nursing students entered the Diploma of Applied Science (Nursing) conducted by the Royal College of Nursing Australia, Melbourne (transferred to the Lincoln Institute of Health Sciences in 1977, now part of La Trobe University). In 1975, diploma nursing courses commenced in Western Australia, South Australia and New South Wales, and a second began in Victoria. In 1976, a second course commenced in New South Wales. Thus, when the *Goals in Nursing Education* working party compiled its report, it was able to adopt as its 'Philosophy of Nursing' a statement taken from the proposed nursing curriculum of the Western Australian Institute of Technology (now Curtin University), 1974.

This is a very different statement from those seen previously and remarkable in that it was written in 1974, only a year after the 1973 NHMRC role statement. It is quoted in full opposite, as it appears in the *Goals in Nursing Education, Part II: Report of the Working Party* (1975), because it introduces themes which were to be influential over the next two decades.

As in the United States (Meleis 1991), the requirement of nursing academics in Australia to develop curriculum documents, which became, in part, a defence of nursing's place in the academy, led to descriptions of nursing that were broadly based. This 'Philosophy of Nursing' takes a position on nursing's role and demonstrates the need for a broadly based tertiary education.

It is clearly, among other things, a political statement in which nursing claims its 'special role' in relation to other members of the health care team—a belief it had been unable to articulate in 1973. The nurse's care of 'the whole person' reflects the 1973 NHMRC statement; however, this nurse provides whole care in his or her nursing capacity, not as 'doctor and nurse together' in which the nurse's role is seen as complementary to that of the doctor (NHMRC, 1973). In this document, the language has shifted so that the nurse is represented as working 'interdependently' with doctors and other health care workers, and as actively participating in decision making and assuming responsibility and accountability for his or her own decisions.

Decision making is conceived of in terms of the nursing process. This is the first appearance in a national nursing document in Australia of a concept introduced in the United States by Orlando in 1961 (Hargreaves 1981) as part of the movement to establish nursing as 'scientific' and to justify nursing care on the basis of objective data and verifiable, replicable results. This statement, however, is careful to talk about the nursing process in relation to the 'unique health requirements of the recipient'. This is unlike some other uses of the term, which imply a greater ability to generalise care.

Other themes which were to persist are those of nursing over the life span and the recognition of humans as physical, psychological and social beings in interaction with their environment. While this had been recognised in earlier definitions, the notion had not previously been articulated quite so clearly. Less clearly articulated is the indication of the recognition that the health of the society and the environment can influence an individual's health. It is, however, a long way from the notion of the individual as the battleground on which the war against disease was fought (Doherty et al. 1963).

Philosophy of Nursing

Nursing as an occupation is as old as humanity itself. Mothers gave origin to nursing; it has always been associated with care and remains the most personal and vital service one human being can perform for another.

Nursing provides a service to society. In providing this service it becomes a social system within the larger system of health care. It affects, and is affected by other systems, such as medicine and social work, as well as society itself. As the medical, social and nursing participants in health care have developed, and other participants, such as physiotherapists, have been introduced, it has become important that each practitioner identified his or her special role and activities in the delivery of health services.

The role of the nurse is health care, which she [sic] performs in a variety of settings. It includes health education, prevention of illness, early detection of disease, care of the acutely and chronically ill, and rehabilitation. She must assume responsibility for making constructive contributions for the improvement of nursing, and of society through teaching, administration and research.

The nurse is concerned with the whole person, in health, or in illness, from conception to death. This implies care throughout the entire life cycle, beginning with the pre-natal period and extending to senescence. The nurse is concerned with the nature of man [sic] as a physical, psychological and social being and his interaction with his environment. She supports man's right to develop his maximum potential in order to realise his individuality and to participate as a fully functioning person in his society.

However, the nurse recognises that man's realisation of his maximum potential is influenced by his state of health and the health of his society.

Health implies a quality of living, a process by which the individual adapts to his physical and social environment. It can be measured by the ability of the individual to adjust to and cope with the variable conditions, demands and stresses of life.

The goal of modern nursing is to assist individuals or groups to achieve optimal health by minimising or eliminating those factors which cause disruption in health, and to deal effectively with or adjust to health problems where the individuals or groups cannot meet these situations themselves.

To function effectively in this extended role the nurse uses an analytical process to assess the health status of individuals or groups, formulates, implements and evaluates a plan of nursing action based on the unique health requirements of the recipient. In this capacity the nurse actively participates in decision making and assumes responsibility and accountability for her own decisions. In performing this service she works interdependently with medical practitioners, social workers and other members of the health care team whose purpose it is to help people achieve, maintain and regain optimal health.

(Goals in Nursing Education, Part II: Report of the Working Party, 1975, pp. 10–11)

Claiming as a human right the development of one's maximum potential in order to realise one's individuality, and recognising that achievement of this right will be influenced by the state of health are also new concepts in Australian nursing. They reflect the community-wide social and attitude changes occurring in Australia and internationally in response to the human rights movements in the early 1970s. This statement marks a remarkable shift in the conceptualisation of nursing in the 11 years since Doherty et al.'s 1963 chapter on ethics and hospital etiquette.

In 1983, the NHMRC commissioned another analysis of the role of the nurse in Australia. The report (published in 1984) adopts Virginia Henderson's definition of the function of the nurse, quoted above, citing the 1969 *Basic Principles of Nursing Care* version, first developed in 1955 as previously shown. Some of the inclusions in *Goals in Nursing Education, Part II* (1975) appear here with the recognition of the need to take account of the diverse backgrounds of clients, given the multicultural nature of Australian society.

Also appearing specifically for the first time in such a document is the goal of providing 'a personal service and a family centred approach' (1984, p. 85) as an antidote to the 'rapid changes in society' and increased 'social stress and dislocation' (1984, p. 85). This is a clear example of theory generation within a role statement written with other purposes in mind. Although not meant as theory, or generally seen as such, statements like these eventually became part of nurses' beliefs about their role, irrespective of how possible they may be to enact.

The statement also reflects the new emphasis in the community on personal responsibility for health care, noting the nurse's role in promoting health maintenance and self-help and assisting 'individuals in making informed choices about their lifestyle' (1984, p. 85). This reflects the individualism and economic rationality which dominated the consciousness of the Western world in the 1980s.

The nurse's role continues to be defined in terms of the nursing process, with its scientific underpinning.

By 1983, nurses had taken their place in the community health movement, initiated by the Whitlam government in 1972. This statement predicted a primary health care role for nurses in a health care system in which 'the dividing line between hospital and community based nursing service is becoming less well defined' (NHMRC 1984, p. 87). The Alma-Ata World Health Organization (WHO) Declaration on primary health care had been published in 1978 (Wood 1990). This is altogether a more confident and assertive statement than that of the NHMRC in 1973. Nursing education had been in the higher education sector for 10 years, albeit for less than 10 per cent of students, Australia-wide (Russell 1990).

As noted above, the requirement of nursing academics to articulate nursing clearly for curriculum documents had raised the level of thinking and debate about nursing in Australia. Also contributing to the debate was the fact that nursing was being organised nationally in its crusade to achieve its nursing education targets (of tertiary education for all preregistration nurse students and technical college (TAFE) education for enrolled nurses).

The RANF (1984) statement of the same period carefully uses the language of health:

The primary responsibility of the nursing profession is to provide direct health care and education for people in relation to the prevention of illness,

the promotion, restoration and maintenance of optimal health, and the
achievement of a dignified death.

(RANF 1984, unnumbered page)

The language of 'health' can be seen as an attempt to free nursing of the dominance
of medicine and to claim its own and different territory. This is articulated clearly in
the following:

In circumstances of ill-health, rather than focussing on the diagnosis and
treatment of disease, nurses are concerned with the response of the person
and the fulfilment of needs within that context.

(RANF 1984, unnumbered page)

Needs are then defined in terms of Henderson's list of 14 human needs, found in the
ICN *Basic Principles of Nursing Care* (1969). The influence of Henderson is also seen in her
citing of an unknown Canadian physician who said there are two essentials: care (by the
nurse) and cure (by the physician). However, Henderson goes on to claim a therapeutic
function for nursing as well as the caring function (1966, p. 17). Care is often claimed now
for nursing without any sense of the curative nature of nursing. An example will be seen
in the Australian Nursing Federation (ANF) 1989 role statement below.

Not surprisingly, in this RANF (1984) statement 'the process of nursing' is defined as
the *nursing process*. Two years earlier, nursing process had been directly linked to nursing
accountability and the 'measurement' of nursing in the RANF's National Quality
Assurance program, launched in 1982, and in the *Standards for Nursing Practice* (RANF
1983). These are clear examples of the political nature of such statements with their
professional claims, in this case still couched in the language of prediction and control,
that is, in the language of empiricism.

While earlier documents have referred to care of the whole person, this is the first
statement of its kind in Australia to use the term 'holistic care' although the term had had
currency in the United States for some years (e.g. Jean Watson's 1979 work on caring):

Nursing differs from most other health professions in that the nurse
provides holistic care by simultaneously attending to the biological,
psychological, social and spiritual needs of people.

(RANF 1984, unnumbered page)

Also appearing for the first time, although without definition or elaboration, is the
idea of nursing as an 'enabling relationship'. This will reappear in the Australian Nurse
Registering Authorities Conference (ANRAC) competencies (1990).

Finally, it is noteworthy that this RANF statement (1984) also includes the first national
claim that nursing is 'a discrete health care discipline'. The claim is made here in relation
to nursing's responsibility for the education of practitioners, and research into and
evaluation of practice. Nursing's legitimate control over these functions had only recently
been won. For example, in South Australia, nurses had only gained a majority on the
Nurses' Board in 1970 and a nurse chairperson in 1978 (Durdin 1991, p. 240).

In 1989, the ANF published *Nursing in Australia: A National Statement* in conjunction
with other national nursing organisations. It notes, clarifying the perspective taken in
the statement:

> The focus of nursing is *caring* and in broad terms nursing is the *relationship* which occurs between the nurse and the consumer within whatever context the relationship exists. The ultimate goal of this relationship is a state of health appropriate to the individual's needs and desires.
>
> *(1989, unnumbered page; emphasis added)*

This constitutes another considerable shift in the conceptualisation of nursing, from the performing of tasks in 1963 (Doherty et al.), delivering personal care based on fundamental needs (White 1972), comprehensive care (NHMRC 1984) which is holistic (RANF 1983) to nursing as a relationship whose **existential** goal is the 'state of health appropriate to the individual's needs and desires' (ANF 1989). The statement goes on to define health, context, consumer and nurse, with clear parallels to the North American nursing domains.

Until 1989, the North American influence on Australian nursing had, at least explicitly, been confined to that of Henderson, in these national statements on nursing, although higher education nursing curriculum documents showed the influence of many other theorists (Dunlop 1992).

The ANF publication (1989) was the first time to call the patient/client the 'consumer', using language that reflects the growth of consumerism as a social and political movement (McMurray 1995). While the language leads to a conceptualisation of the role in terms of a provider (nurse), and a recipient (consumer), there is also, in the language of empowerment, a focus on the relational aspects of the role. The 'consumer' is now a partner in health and health care and the nurse an 'enabler' (McMurray 1995). This can be seen as an indication of the adoption by Australian nurses of the principles and premises of primary health care, which had been largely ignored by nurses in the United States (McMurray 1995).

The definition of nursing focuses on caring and relationship, as cited above. The definition goes on:

> Nursing encompasses processes and activities by which the nurse establishes an empowering relationship and gives direct care designed to promote a health state which is optimal for the individual. In circumstances of ill-health, rather than focusing on the diagnosis and treatment of disease, the nurse is concerned with the response of the person and the fulfilment of needs within that context.
>
> Nursing differs from other health professions in that the nurse provides holistic care by simultaneously attending to the biological, psychological, sociocultural and spiritual needs of people.
>
> The essence of nursing is caring. Nursing care is manifested by the creation of an environment which empowers the individual to:
>
> - maintain personal integrity, identity, autonomy and self esteem;
>
> - contribute to the process of nursing care as an equal partner by collaborating in and expressing satisfaction with the planning, implementation and evaluation of the program of care;

- assume progressive responsibility for self-care to maximum potential;

- express satisfaction with the extent to which significant others have been identified and supported;

- communicate personal health status, strengths, resources, feelings and concerns;

- be . . . free from injury;

- experience maximum comfort;

- maintain optimum physiological function;

- engage in optimum activity;

- increase and apply knowledge related to health, and actual and potential health problems.

In circumstances where because of age, illness or disability an individual is unable to participate effectively in the process of care, the word 'individual' is intended to include 'significant other(s)' or other person(s) representing the individual's interests.

(ANF 1989, unnumbered pages)

The first paragraph of this section of the ANF's (1989) definition can be seen as a continuation of the Henderson tradition. In the first two paragraphs, the notion of 'an empowering relationship' is new, while the remainder has not changed since the 1983 RANF statement. This 1989 statement shows strong evidence of other North American influences, too—for example, Orem's concept of self-care (1971, 1980), Watson's (1979, 1985) human caring; and Gadow's existential advocacy (1980). The naming of the recipient of nursing care as an equal partner in care, and the use of the language of empowerment, indicates the influence of **critical social theory** on nursing. These ideas had entered the North American literature, with regard to research, with Allen, Benner and Diekelmann in 1986 and Thompson in 1987. However, the publication in 1988 of the Diploma of Nursing curriculum of the School of Nursing at Deakin University (which had been influenced by the critical theorists Kemmis and Smyth, both of whom were in the School of Education at Deakin at the time) probably had a far greater influence in Australia on the dissemination of the ideas of critical social theory and their potential for improving nursing practice. Certainly, after this time, the rhetoric of empowerment entered nursing discourse.

In 1990, the Australasian Nurse Registering Authorities Conference published national competencies for the registration and enrolment of nurses. These are known as the ANRAC competencies and, from 1993, as the Australian Nurse Council Inc. (ANCI) competencies. The development of competencies occurred in the context of the Federal government's industrial legislation on enterprise bargaining and the need to be able to judge the competency of immigrants with overseas qualifications. While many trades, in particular, reduced competencies to a checklist of skills, nursing developed a more global set of competencies to be assessed by the professional judgement of competent clinicians.

As part of the documentation a statement of 'philosophy' was offered, which reflects much of the content of the 1989 ANF statement:

(a) Nursing is a service which is authorised and valued by society.

(b) The focus of nursing care is health. Nurses are concerned with enabling people to remain healthy, return to a state of optimum function, behaviour or state of mind, and with assisting the dying to achieve a dignified death.

(c) Nursing addresses the complexity and uniqueness of the whole person in the environmental context.

(d) Nurses provide care, simultaneously attending to the biological, psychological, social and spiritual needs of the person, and by being acutely aware of the interrelationships between these needs.

(e) The effect of nursing care should be positive and should result in benefit, physically, emotionally and/or spiritually, to an individual or group.

(f) In circumstances of ill health, nurses focus on the response of individuals and groups to health problems, and their ability to contend with these responses.

(g) Nursing is an art and a science. The essence of nursing lies in a unique interplay of knowledge, intuitive and logical thought and compassion for others.

(h) The interaction of cognitive, affective and psychomotor skills is essential for nursing practice.

(i) Nursing knowledge is derived from qualitative and quantitative research and from the experience of nurses.

(ANRAC May 1990, p. 64)

Notable in this statement is the consideration of the origins of nursing knowledge and the claim that nursing is both art and science, depending not only on knowledge and logic but also on intuitive thought and compassion. There are echoes of the influential North American nurse Barbara Carper's 1978 'patterns of knowing' here, as well as Benner's (1984) work on intuition and experience.

The domains of practice of registered nurses are defined as:

(i) Professional/ethical practice

(ii) Reflective practice

(iii) Enabling

(iv) Problem framing and solving

(v) Teamwork.

(ANRAC 1990, pp. 26–7)

The descriptions of the domains demonstrate strong North American influences, mostly from the nursing literature but also from education and general professional education literature (e.g. Schön 1983, 1987). The domains of reflective practice and problem framing and solving probably owe more to the literature on expertise from Benner (1984) than to critical social theory. However, that influence is also present in the consideration of the potential for improving nursing arising out of the reflective practice and personal theorising of experienced nurses.

Wood (1990) has a chapter defining nursing in her book on the role of the Commonwealth Government in nursing from 1921–91. She cites the North American nurses Henderson (in Henderson & Nite 1978), Watson (1979) and Diers (1986) in order to define nursing and part of the ANF (1989) statement on the nurse's role in empowering clients. Wood goes on to provide a long 'wish-list' of attributes which she sees as 'essential' to the nurse. This may be read in the 1990 version of the chapter, 'Ethics and hospital etiquette' (Doherty et al. 1963), considered to be the first in this survey of definitions of nursing. Where Doherty et al. (1963, p. 3) write of the need for 'loyalty and a cheerful co-operation', Wood believes that nurses must:

- have a healthy self-respect and conduct themselves with dignity;

- treat each other with tolerance, patience, honesty and respect;

- choose positive relationships and avoid becoming enmeshed in negative thinking and behaviours;

and 30 others in similar vein, canvassing continuing education, patient advocacy, nursing process, working conditions, improvement of nursing, health care and team work.

(1990, p. 15)

Perhaps the point with the strongest echo to the vocational past of nursing is the statement that nurses 'are prepared to show mercy to those who oppress them and to live with their scars with dignity' (Wood 1990, p. 15).

Finally, in this chapter from Wood, is a reference to nursing theory. 'The delivery of care becomes the process of theory building. In other words, in care, theory attempts to reflect practice' (Wood 1990, p. 14).

This assertion follows a statement on the range of functions of the nurse, among which are embedded the phases of the nursing process. It is not clear what is intended by this statement other than that theory should arise out of practice. Wood (1990) cites Benner (1984) as the source of her thinking here, but the juxtaposition of theory-building with the nursing process makes it unclear whether Wood means hypothesis generation and testing, phenomenological theory development or even the uncovering of personal theory through reflective practice with the intent to transform practice. This is, however, the first time theory-building has been included in a national statement on nursing.

The most recent report on the role of the nurse in Australia was prepared in 1991 by Robinson for the NHMRC. This statement makes the claim that '[t]he role of the nurse in

Australia over the past century has remained relatively stable' (NHMRC 1991, p. 1) with the caring aspect of nursing remaining constant but the context in which care has been carried out being one of continuous change. The persistence of Virginia Henderson's 1955 definition of the unique function of the nurse gives weight to Robinson's claim. However, if the role has remained fundamentally the same, the ways in which nurses have conceptualised the role and implicitly theorised about nursing have changed enormously in the last 30 years.

Robinson (1991, p. 1) lists the changes that have affected the role performance of the nurse as follows:

- the changing role of women in society;

- advances in science and technology and the resulting increased ethico-legal dilemmas and a changing demand for the nursing workforce;

- the changed nature of nursing education;

- the changing direction of health care towards promotion, maintenance and self-help;

- increased consumer awareness and demands for easy access to health care;

- increasing economic constraints;

- spiralling health care costs;

- an increasing number of aged persons, many of whom will have chronic disabilities; and

- the emergence of a more multicultural population.

The nurse is defined in terms of a 'complementary caring relationship' with the patient, similar to the ANF statement (1989), and there are also allusions to Henderson's needs and Orem's self-care. The definition of nursing also demonstrates the influence of the caring theorists, holism and the nursing process and makes the political claims that nursing is 'a discrete health care discipline' and that nurses have professional status.

In describing the role components, Robinson alludes, somewhat ambiguously, to the nurse's role in theory development: '[to] refine theoretical and practical knowledge in clinical situations' (NHMRC 1991, p. 7). It is not clear how theory is conceived of here, but there is a possibility that it is in purely empirical terms, where theory is separate from and directs practical knowledge—that is, that practice is atheoretical. This conjecture is supported to some extent by the following statement, from the final section of the report, on the future role of the nurse:

> [Nurses] are increasingly active in undertaking nursing research, and the development of conceptual frameworks of nursing, enabling the nurse to predict and prescribe nursing practice.
>
> *(Robinson 1991, p. 11)*

It cannot be said that nurses in Australia are 'active in the development of conceptual frameworks of nursing' which might enable them to predict and prescribe nursing practice. Certainly, nurses are engaged in many forms of research and are developing micro and mid-range theories which are helping them to understand, transform and/or predict the outcomes of practice more effectively. However, the notion of the development of conceptual frameworks (or nursing models or 'grand' theory) can be seen as an outdated empiricist ideal stemming from the work of the nurse theorists in North America from the 1950s to the early 1980s.

The changes in the way Australian nurses have conceptualised their role in the past 30 years have been immense, even if, as Robinson claims, the role in its caring aspect has remained relatively constant (1991).

The following changes have been described:

1 from nursing as subservient, the servant of medicine, to nursing as complementary to medicine, to nursing as interdependent with medicine;

2 from vocation to profession and health care discipline;

3 from task orientation, to comprehensive care, to holistic care;

4 from task assignment, to personal care, to nursing as an enabling relationship;

5 from art to science (nursing process), to art and science;

6 from patient as passive to patient as actively involved in decision making;

7 from hospital nursing to primary health care and nursing across the life span;

8 from received knowledge to knowledge creation.

It should be re-emphasised that this survey of role statements is not a survey of nursing theory in Australia. Nevertheless, these role statements contain, at least implicitly, theoretical statements which have been influenced by:

- nursing's political struggle to establish itself as an independent health profession with control over its work and education;

- the desire to establish nursing as a legitimate 'discrete health care discipline' (RANF, 1984, p. 5);

- developments in nursing in the United States;

- the recognition of the multicultural nature of Australian society;

- better educated recipients of health care; and

- the 'rights' movements, including women's rights and patients' rights.

Such a chronological cataloguing of role statements demonstrates the cumulative and dependent nature of such changes. The shifts from the 1963 textbook statement to that for the NHMRC in 1991 would be inconceivable without an understanding of what came in between.

AUSTRALIAN NURSING THEORY

There is only one example of grand theorising in the tradition of the United States by an Australian nurse, that of Betty Andersen (1991). Andersen has been developing her theory over the past 20 years, with the earlier versions developed in response to nursing curricula evaluations and the later versions (in common with a number of her North

American counterparts, as has been described above) to provide a conceptual framework for curriculum development for undergraduate nursing programs in the higher education sector (see Andersen in Gray & Pratt (1991) for details).

Lawler (1991) has developed a theory of the mid-range from her doctoral research, based in sociology, in which she observed nursing and interviewed nurses about their practice of basic nursing care. In particular, she focused on how nurses deal with the problem of the body. Lawler argues that 'nurses practice in a somological way' (1991, p. 215); that is, 'nurses help a patient/client to live in a body which will not work properly' (1991, p. 225); that nurses' care for bodies violates normal social rules and nurses need to find ways to manage their own and patients' embarrassment or misconstruing of the event.

Lawler illuminates the way in which nurses manage basic body care and in so doing argues that the trend towards holism, which has dominated nursing rhetoric in Australia since the 1983 RANF role statement, has not been grounded in research on nursing. Rather, Lawler argues, the trend towards holism 'has grown out of a perceived need to enhance nursing practice, to raise its status, to make it more humanistically [sic] oriented, and to professionalise and scientise the occupation' (1991, p. 216). This is similar to the arguments of Bruni (1991) noted above.

From her doctoral studies in nursing, Taylor (1994) has also developed a theory of the mid-range. She argues that nurses are therapeutic because of 'the sense of shared affinity that nurses and patients have for one another as humans'. This 'ordinariness in nursing . . . potentiates nursing as a caring and curing force in people's lives and makes their stay in health care contexts manageable and familiar for them' (1994, p. 230).

More theory at this mid-range level can be expected, given the increasing number of nurses engaged in higher degree and other research.

CHANGES IN NURSING EDUCATION IN AUSTRALIA

As was the case in the United States, changes in nursing education had a profound effect on nursing theory development in Australia.

Australian State and Federal governments had been concerned about nursing since the late 1940s, with 15 expert committees reporting between the 1960s and 1970s (Russell 1990). Concern related primarily to issues of recruitment and wastage of student nurses (in excess of 50 per cent in New South Wales between 1962 and 1968; 36 per cent in Victoria and 44 per cent in Tasmania in the same period (Russell 1990, p. 57)) and the numbers of registered nurses leaving nursing.

Typical of the findings were those of Chittock (1968). Chittock, a nurse educated in the United States, who had taught nursing in Canadian universities, was commissioned as a short-term World Health Organization consultant to advise on public health courses at both the NSW College of Nursing and the College of Nursing Australia (Russell 1990). To fulfil her commission, Chittock found it necessary to examine preregistration nursing education in New South Wales and was scathing in her criticism:

Although there has been enormous growth of opportunities, nursing has not shared in these advancements. At the age of seventeen, the entrance age to schools of nursing, students are cut off from any educational program that would enlarge their vision, develop their potential resources and make them aware of the social, political and cultural problems they must face as citizens. Nursing education at the basic level remains a trade which students learn over a period of three or four years in a very limited environment. Perhaps no other group of young people in modern society receives such a narrow, restricted and unimaginative type of education.

(Chittock 1968, in Wood 1990, p. 6)

By 1974, a series of expert committees—for example, Noble (1974), Livingstone (1976), Sax (1978) and Russell (1990, p. 103)—were supporting the change from the apprenticeship system to tertiary-based education for at least some nursing students.

There was also strong consensus on the need for curriculum change but little agreement on the direction of change. As Russell (1990) reports, most supported the inclusion of behavioural science, more biological science and medical subjects and also administration and teaching. Closer integration between theoretical and clinical components of the curriculum was generally endorsed. In discussions of the so-called 'theory-practice gap', theory was equated with classroom teaching and 'the gap' used in arguments to justify the transfer of nursing to the tertiary sector, with teachers having control over both theoretical and clinical components of the course (Yuen 1984).

It wasn't until the late 1980s that theory began to mean the specific relationship between nursing theory and nursing practice (Speedy 1989) although, as has been shown above, the work of the North American nursing theorists had been influencing thinking about nursing in Australia since the early 1970s.

As described above, nurses had for the first time become united nationally with the publication in 1975 of the *Goals in Nursing Education Part I* and *Part II* documents. Achieving the goals was to take another 10 years in New South Wales, with the transfer of nursing education to the tertiary sector occurring in 1985, and another 8 years in the rest of Australia, with the transfer completed in 1993.

The arguments accepted by the Interdepartmental Committee of the Commonwealth ministers for Education and Youth Affairs, and Health, in 1984 to support the transfer were as follows (Wood 1990, p. 210):

- the trend to shorten hospital stays, focusing hospital care on the acutely ill;
- increased emphasis on technology which is constantly changing;
- increased complexity of drugs and treatments;
- a rapid increase in scientific knowledge;
- the recognition that existing hospital-based nursing programs no longer adequately meet the needs for an appropriately skilled nursing workforce; and
- increased demand for community nursing.

It is noteworthy that these reasons are largely in the domain of scientific and technological knowledge. The reasons given by nurse leaders from the *Goals in Nursing Education, Part II* (1975) document, onward, were considerably more wide-ranging as has been shown.

The shift to tertiary education made demands on nurse educators that reflect the experiences of nurse educators in the United States. Most had Diplomas of Teaching from one of the Colleges of Nursing. Nurse educators upgraded their qualifications to bachelor level and looked around for masters and doctoral degrees; until the second half of the 1980s, they found none in nursing in Australia. A few completed their formal education in the United States or Britain, but most undertook their higher degree work in other disciplines such as education, psychology or sociology.

It was probably the introduction of masters degrees in nursing, with coursework topics in nursing theory and the requirement for nursing research which, as in the United States, most raised the profile of theory in nursing in Australia, and alerted nurses to the potential of theory for improving practice. Once higher degrees in nursing were available in Australia, more clinicians had access to study and research at this level. In the late 1980s, with the introduction of the career structure, there were direct links between educational preparation and career level at least in some states (Silver, 1989). This provision was later to be removed.

SUMMARY

As it was argued in the first section of this chapter, understanding of the rise of theorising in nursing in the United States in the 1950s, and its subsequent developments over the next 30 years, can be enhanced by an understanding of the intellectual, social, professional, political and ideological contexts nurses were part of.

As was the case in the United States, changes in nursing education and the seeking of professional status have been the key influences in changing the way in which Australian nurses conceptualise nursing.

Because theorising in Australia has lagged behind that in the United States, Australian nurses have had the benefit of learning from and selectively using the work of their North American colleagues. Although there has been some metatheorising on 'grand' theory in the tradition of the United States (see, for example, Gray & Pratt 1991) and some theorising in the context of curriculum development, Australian nursing theory appears to be emerging from the results of research into the practice of nursing.

The changes to the ways in which nursing has been conceptualised in Australia in the last 30 years can only be understood in the context of the times in which they occurred and as part of the struggle of nurses to achieve professional status and educational and industrial justice over that period.

GLOSSARY

Behaviourism: an influential approach in psychology and education which, in an endeavour to establish a science of behaviour or learning, confines itself to the study of observable behaviour.

Critical social theory: an approach in sociology which developed as a critique of Marxism. Critical theorists are motivated by a desire to create a more socially just world and, therefore, have an interest in relating theory to politics and to the critique of ideologies and domination.

Discourse: a way of referring to written or spoken language which takes account of the extent to which the particular words used, structure what it is possible to think about something, and thus gives rise to particular social practices.

Empiricism: belief that knowledge is based on observation of experience, sensations and concrete situations in the real world; based on a correspondence theory of truth, in which such observations are assumed to correspond to the real world. In research, the *empiric–analytic paradigm* has been equated to the scientific method, or *hypothetico-deductive method*, in which a hypothesis is generated about a cause/effect relationship and observations made in controlled experiments. The goal of empiricism is prediction. Also loosely termed *quantitative* research, because of the measurement (of observations) component.

Existential: from existential philosophy, the belief that individuals create themselves through choosing and acting responsibly.

Metatheory: 'in most cases *meta* may be translated as *the study of the characteristics of*' (Angeles 1992, p. 183). Thus, metatheory is the study of the characteristics of theory.

Positivism: an extreme form of empiricism which, when applied to the social sciences, claims that scientific method is the only source of knowledge about reality; that such science is value free and that the goal of science is prediction and control.

Qualitative methods: approaches to knowledge development which have as their goal the understanding of the qualities of something.

QUESTIONS

1 Discuss the relationship between the desire of nurses for professional status and theory development in nursing.

2 Isolate the theoretical statements implicit or explicit in the Australian role statements and discuss the social context of their appearance.

3 Discuss the ways in which Robinson's (NHMRC 1991) list of changes affecting nurses' role performance may have had their effect.

LEARNING ACTIVITIES

1 Ask to see a copy of the statement of 'philosophy' or rationale section of the curriculum document that is framing your learning. Discuss the theoretical statements implicitly or explicitly stated in it. To what extent do these guide your clinical practice and the way you conceptualise nursing?

2 Ask to see the 'philosophy' statement of the nursing department in an agency where you are engaged in clinical practice. Does it, either implicitly or explicitly, have theoretical statements within it? If there are currently no parallels between the philosophy and practice, what changes would need to be made for the philosophical statements to be enacted in practice?

FURTHER READING

Deakin Institute of Nursing Research 1988, *Bridging the Gap! Between Nursing Theory and Nursing Practice*, conference proceedings, Deakin University, Geelong, Victoria.

Dunlop, M. 1992, *Shaping Nursing Knowledge: An Interpretive Analysis of Curriculum Documents from NSW Australia*, Royal College of Nursing, Australia, Melbourne, for an interpretive analysis of the development of nursing theory in the United States and its influence on Australian nursing.

Guba, E.G. (ed.) 1990, *The Paradigm Dialog*, Sage, Newbury Park, for differences in approaches to research and theory development.

Kaluchi, J.F. & Simmons, H. (eds) 1992, *Philosophic Inquiry in Nursing*, Sage, Newbury Park, for philosophical debate in nursing (United States).

Lincoln Centre for Research Nursing Practice 1988, 'Shaping nursing theory and practice: The Australian context', in *Proceedings from 3rd Nursing Research Forum*, La Trobe University, Melbourne.

Meleis, A. 1991, *Theoretical Nursing: Development and Progress,* 2nd edn, Lippincott, New York and Nicoll, L. 1992, *Perspectives on Nursing Theory*, 2nd edn, Lippincott, New York, for theory development in the United States.

Quality Health Forums 1991, *Science, Reflectivity and Nursing Care: Exploring the Dialectic*, proceedings of the National Nursing Conference, Melbourne. This conference focused on the contribution of critical social science to nursing knowledge development in Australia.

Quality Health Forums, in association with the Faculty of Nursing and Health Sciences, Griffith University 1993, *Critical Theory, Feminism and Nursing: Empowering Nursing's Future*, proceedings of the National Nursing Conference, Melbourne. This is another example of a conference that was focused on the contribution of critical social science to nursing development.

South Australian College of Advanced Education 1989, *Theory and Practice: An Evolving Relationship*, proceedings of the National Nursing Theory Conference, Sturt Campus, Adelaide.

6

CONSIDERATIONS OF CONTEXT
The Crucial Moderator

ROSALIE PRATT

LEARNING OBJECTIVES

When you have read this chapter you should be able to:

1 Explain the concept of 'context' and provide examples of context from the perspectives of place, time and individual.

2 Consider the context within which you are applying any theory to clinical practice.

3 Include context as a matter of routine as one of the elements that influence the process of your practice.

Rosalie Pratt, RN, CM, DNE, BA, MHPEd, FCN(NSW), FRCNA, is Associate Professor in the Faculty of Nursing, University of Sydney. She was Pro-Dean of the Faculty of Nursing from 1992–95, and has held teaching and administrative positions in the higher education sector and the New South Wales College of Nursing since 1977. Her clinical specialty was in the field of spinal injuries nursing.

Rosalie has been active in nursing organisations since 1960. She is currently Censor-in-Chief of Royal College of Nursing, Australia (RCNA) and has served on the six-member Professional Services Committee of International Council of Nurses, Geneva, 1989–93. Rosalie is honoured by being the only person invited to deliver the three Orations: the Patricia Chomley Oration, RCNA (1980), the Florence Nightingale Oration (1983) and the Annual Oration of NSW College of Nursing (1995). Rosalie has been writing and editing nursing publications since 1970.

INTRODUCTION

In common with all people, nurses do not live and work in a vacuum. Nurses' practice, whatever its focus, is always situated within a particular context—a context which is multifaceted and which critically influences many aspects of nursing practice. The first part of this chapter addresses the concept of context in terms of place, time and people as individuals. *Place* can be considered from at least local, national and international perspectives. Associated issues include those of culture, ethnicity, society, **demographic** trends, politics, the economy and the natural and built environments. These issues link to a consideration of the concept of context from the perspective of *time*. There are three considerations here. The first is the prevailing nature in a particular place of, for example, cultural and social **mores**, politics, the economy and the environment. The second is the **currency** of the ideas and the philosophy behind any particular nursing theory or model. The third is time in the sense of your work time, the way in which you organise it and the demands made on it. Both place and time are linked in the formation of the unique context of every person as an *individual*.

Invariably, the context within which any activity occurs acts as a significant moderator on that activity. It is crucial, therefore, always to consider the nature and influence of the context in which nursing practice is occurring, in which theory is being applied to the process of practice, and in which theory (and knowledge) are being derived from practice.

The second part of this chapter is based on the suggestion that, given these considerations of context, theories and models of nursing should be addressed at two different levels, if they are to be useful for application in nursing practice (whatever the focus of the practice: clinical, educational, administrative, research) and if they are to be informed usefully by practice.

The first level might be described as **superordinate**. This is an abstract, general and inclusive level at which a theory might be developed initially. At this level, nursing and its associated **phenomena** can be considered as concepts, essentially without reference to the context of practice.

The suggested second level is **subordinate** to this, and is that of the *application* of a theory to, or the *generation* of a theory from, a specific nursing context, with its multi-faceted nuances of place, time and individual patient being.

THE CONCEPT OF CONTEXT

Hinds and Chaves (1992) have asserted that health professionals' ability 'to understand humans, their health, and other related phenomena and to use this understanding to promote meaningful life experiences ... depends on knowledge of the multiple *contexts* in which these phenomena exist' (emphasis added). One of the definitions given by *The Macquarie Encyclopedic Dictionary* (1990) for context is 'the circumstances or facts that surround a particular situation, event, etc.'. The *Australian Pocket Oxford Dictionary* (1976) adds the phrase 'general setting'. The word comes via late Middle English from the Latin *contextus* meaning 'connection'. For the purposes of this chapter, context will be considered in terms of *settings* and *circumstances*, and the connections between them. From a slightly different perspective, in relation to people as individuals, context has been defined as 'a lens from which persons view their world' (Dunn, Brown & McGuigan 1994).

CONTEXT FROM THE PERSPECTIVE OF PLACE

Broadly, local, national and international *settings* in relation to the practice of nursing are the first issue for consideration. Each then provides a frame within which to view other issues or *circumstances* of place. The circumstances addressed for each will include culture, ethnicity, society, demographic trends, politics, the economy, and the built and natural environments.

THE LOCAL SETTING

The local setting refers to the place where you live and practise nursing. Clearly, the size of that setting will vary depending on whether you practise in a tertiary referral hospital in a capital city and live in one of the city's suburbs; or practise in a remote area encompassing many thousands of square kilometres and live in an isolated settlement within that area; or practise and live in any number of different settings between these two extremes. Even if you live in a city but work as a community or district nurse, or as a nurse practitioner within the community, the circumstances of your local setting may be markedly different from those of a colleague who works in an institution such as a hospital or nursing home in the same city.

Local circumstances

It is unlikely that there will be much variation in terms of culture, *very broadly defined*, whatever your local setting within Australia. Subcultures, however, and culture defined in relation to particular ethnic groups, may manifest quite distinctly within particular local settings. Similarly, Australian society, *broadly defined*, may not vary greatly in relation to local setting, but in terms of social status and groupings, for example, distinctive local characteristics are likely to be apparent. Such characteristics will invariably include ethnicity and features such as the age spread of a population demonstrated through demographic studies. Likewise, the organisation of systems such as the health care system and of institutions such as hospitals will be broadly similar across Australia. There may, however, be local variations as, for instance, with the management of the organisational context within which you work. This *may* impose constraints on the way you practise nursing.

Thus, if you work and live in a city, your local circumstances may include:

■ a subculture of homeless men;

■ a population which is predominantly 'working class';

■ various ethnic groups, members of which may be recent immigrants or refugees; and

■ a large proportion of young to middle-aged people and their children.

If you practise in a hospital within this setting, you will be able to define additional distinctive features. These will include the way the hospital is managed and its relationship with the local community, as well as the **case mix** of patients, and their age and gender characteristics. At the other end of the spectrum, if you practise as a remote area nurse, the major proportion of those you work with may be Aboriginal people with completely different circumstances of culture, society, demographic trends and case mix. In addition, the way in which the delivery of health care is organised and managed in such a context will be completely different from the organisation and management of health care delivery in a metropolitan hospital.

Other issues relevant to local circumstances include politics, the economy and the natural and built environments. The first two—politics and the economy—are, of course, closely connected. Indeed, the term 'politics' is used to encompass a number of elements. These include, but are not necessarily limited to, the political system of a country, and hence government (and the ideological complexion of the government of the day), legislation, public policy and bureaucracy at all levels—national, State and local. Also included are the way in which systems such as the health care system, and institutions such as hospitals within that system, are organised and managed.

Clearly, all sociopolitical systems are inextricably related, but one other of particular significance for you as a nurse is the industrial relations system and associated legislation, because of its impact on your income and working conditions, which constitute a part of your context—see, for example, the special workplace issue of *The Australian Nurses Journal* (1993).

'Politics' also refers to the power relationships which pervade society (again at all levels), and the 'games' in which people engage to achieve and maintain relative positions of power.

In a local Australian setting, both politics and the economy will reflect to some extent State/Territory and national circumstances. For example, similar political ideologies (if not parties) are likely to be represented at local government level. Funding at this level depends in part on funding from, and the relevant legislation of, a particular State, which in turn depends largely on funding from, and the relevant legislation of, the Australian Government. There may also, however, be purely local considerations, such as:

- the complexion, organisation and policies of your local government entity;

- whether the institution where you practise is funded publicly or privately (or whether, indeed, you practise privately); and

- what local politics, in terms of power relationships and games, are in operation both inside and outside the institution.

In another sense, economics is linked with social status in terms of income, assets and associated lifestyles. Clearly, socioeconomic status and resources may vary considerably between, and within, local settings.

Pause for a moment and think about how the variables mentioned so far in this section might affect your nursing practice. For example, in relation to culture, your patients' religious and health-related beliefs and practices may necessitate modifications in the way you nurse them if the outcomes are to be favourable. If English is your patients' second language, your ability to communicate effectively with them may be compromised, perhaps gravely. There may be a 'generation gap' between you and some of your patients. Their socioeconomic status and lifestyle may make it difficult for you to implement desirable nursing interventions.

This chapter is not designed to elaborate details of the concepts of, or Australian issues associated with, culture, society, ethnicity, demographic trends, politics or the economy. It is anticipated that such matters will be addressed elsewhere in your undergraduate program. It is important, however, that you *apply* the knowledge you gain from those studies to your considerations of context. Useful reading to enable you to pursue the issues further, in relation to the national or particular local contexts, could include Gardner (1989), Commonwealth Department of Community Services and Health (1989), Bates and Linder-Pelz (1990), Sax (1990), Reid and Trompf (1991), Saggers and Gray (1991), Davis and George (1993), McCoppin and Gardner (1994), Palmer and Short (1994) and Stanley (1994).

It is evident that both the local built and natural environments will influence health and illness, and therefore nursing practice, to a significant extent. The built environment includes the buildings in which you live and work. The natural environment refers to the geography and geophysics of an area, and in your local setting *may* be associated with politics and the economy. Useful reading could include Ewan, Bryant and Calvert (1991), Pratt (1992) and Ewan et al. (1994).

THE NATIONAL SETTING

The national setting refers to Australia as a whole, incorporating six States and two territories. Clearly, it is possible to consider the particular State or territory where you live and work as an *intermediate* context between your local setting and the national Australian setting. A fruitful exercise could be for you to identify State/territory issues which distinguish this setting as a context from both local and national contexts. How, for example, does your State's *average* unemployment rate vary from the country's *average* rate and from your particular local context's *actual* rate? (Be aware that unemployment is likely to have adverse consequences for people's health.) Are the demographic trends in your State different from those of the country as a whole *and* from those of your local context? Does your State's ethnic mix vary from the overall Australian mix and from that of your work setting? (New South Wales, for instance, has a significantly different mix from other States—see Millett 1995 and Byrne 1995—but a remote area in New South Wales such as Wilcannia has a different mix from metropolitan Sydney, and many areas within Sydney also differ from each other—see Phelan 1995.)

National circumstances

As was implied in the previous section on the local context, from the national Australian perspective the concepts of culture, society, ethnicity, demographic trends, politics, the economy and environment **subsume** related concepts and issues at local levels. They vary significantly, however, from the same concepts and associated issues in other countries, even in those countries with which Australians share a common heritage. A distinctive characteristic of our national context, for example, is the diversity of its natural environment. Likewise, one of the most striking features of contemporary Australian society is its inclusion of such a diverse range of ethnic groups (and therefore of cultural mores), whether of immigrant/refugee or original Australian (including Torres Strait Islands) derivation. It is obvious that this ethnic mix changes over time, and in doing so changes both national and local contexts. Similarly, all the other national circumstances will vary over time, some much more rapidly than others.

Pause again, and consider how each of the variables of circumstance might affect policy and legislation at a national level. For instance, large numbers of immigrants, particularly refugees, might affect immunisation policy. Policy in relation to illegal refugees might have implications for health care and nursing in certain local contexts. Demographic trends might affect policy and legislation in relation to the age pension, and consequently the socioeconomic status of this particular group of people. Despite the diversity of its natural environment, large tracts of Australia are prone to cyclical drought, for a variety of reasons. When drought is widespread, it is likely to have serious consequences for national output and income, and hence for national spending. In these circumstances, the funding available to the States and Territories for such enterprises as health services is likely to be diminished. It is evident that this is likely to impose constraints on funding in local contexts and may therefore have implications for the way nurses practise in these contexts.

THE INTERNATIONAL SETTING AND CIRCUMSTANCES

The world has become a global village and in so doing has made it imperative to consider contexts beyond those of national boundaries. All the circumstances considered in relation to local and national settings are influenced to a greater or lesser extent by related circumstances in other parts of the world—that is, by the international context. This context includes international organisations such as the World Health Organization, the International Labour Organization and various United Nations' instrumentalities, with many of which Australia has formal relationships. It follows that the policies and conventions of such global organisations may well impact on public policy in Australia and thus on the working context of nurses. Other pertinent organisations in this regard include the International Council of Nurses and international specialty nursing associations, such as the International Society of Nurses in Cancer Care. Moreover, lessons can be learnt (and applied) from experiences in other countries, particularly those with contexts similar to our own.

Again, there are intermediate contexts between those of Australia and those of the world as a whole. For example, Australia is a part of the South Pacific region and is geographically closer to the countries of Asia than to those of Europe. Another fruitful exercise could be for you to consider distinctive circumstances within the Pacific or Asian regions which might impact on the Australian (and your local) context. By way of illustration, think of features of the natural environment, such as the Pacific 'ring of fire', and the effects which the associated earthquakes and volcanoes in the region might have on the creation of refugees and on their subsequent migration, or on the regional economy.

CONTEXT FROM THE PERSPECTIVE OF TIME

As suggested earlier, circumstances will vary over time, whatever the setting. In defining the circumstances of your context, therefore, whether local or national, you should also query whether the characteristics of culture, society, ethnicity, politics, environment and so on, which you are taking into consideration, are *contemporary*—that is, applicable to the present time and not just historical features gathered from your reading. Certainly, your nursing practice is influenced in part by its history, and the current context of your practice is always historically situated—that is to say, it has been created by all the many circumstances which have impacted on it, or influenced it, in the past. Nevertheless, it is important to distinguish between the past and the present, because the circumstances of the 'here and now' will inevitably have the more profound impact on your practice and on the way in which you apply any theory or model to the process of that practice.

This suggests that you should keep yourself informed about current circumstances, at least in your local and national settings, and preferably in the international setting as well. Additionally, you should be knowledgeable about current as well as historical circumstances in relation to the health care and industrial relations systems within which you work. How do you become (and remain) thus informed and knowledgeable?

Books may help you with historical background and also, provided they are of recent publication date, with the contemporary scene. Examples (only) for your reading could include Donahue (1985), Morse (1988), Gray and Pratt (1992a), Nutbeam et al. (1993), Fry (1994) and Gray and Pratt (1995a). Recent reports such as that of the National Review of Nurse Education in the Higher Education Sector (Reid 1994); of the Advisory Committee to the Multicultural Nursing Workforce Project (1991); or of the National Aboriginal Health Strategy Working Party (1989) may also be helpful. More 'up-to-the-minute' sources, however, are journals, newsletters and the various daily or weekly news media.

Relevant nursing journals in the mid 1990s, for example, include *The Australian Nursing Journal, The Lamp, Contemporary Nurse, Collegian, The Australian Journal of Advanced Nursing* and *International Nursing Review*. The Australian Nursing Council Inc. (ANCI) publishes an informative quarterly newsletter and a number of the specialist nursing organisations in the country publish regular journals or newsletters. Some specialist organisations publish internationally—for example, *International Cancer Nursing News*, the quarterly newsletter of the International Society of Nurses in Cancer Care. Examples from the print media would include *The Sydney Morning Herald's* series of articles entitled 'Sydney's Asian shift' (see Mellor & Mills 1995; Mellor 1995a; Mellor 1995b; Lague 1995; Coultan & Mellor 1995; Scott 1995); and that newspaper's *Good Weekend* articles, 'The last gasp' (Maslen 1995) and 'Made in Japan' (Drew 1995).

THE CURRENCY OF IDEAS

There is another sense in which the concept of currency is applicable to context from the perspective of time. Are the ideas that underpin a particular nursing theory or model still the most up to date? Is the thinking on which the theory is based at the 'cutting edge' of nursing knowledge and research? Does the philosophy (i.e. the set of beliefs and principles) that imbues the theory 'fit' comfortably—with your national (and local) setting if it originates in another country, with your local setting if it originates elsewhere in Australia? And how will you judge the currency of ideas and the cutting-edge status of knowledge?

Again, your best source is likely to be national nursing journals. In the mid 1990s, these would include, but not necessarily be limited to, *Nursing Inquiry, Contemporary Nurse, Collegian, The Australian Journal of Advanced Nursing* and *The Australian Journal of Holistic Nursing*. The published proceedings of conferences held in Australia may also be useful. Be avid in your curiosity, your enquiry, your reading. There is nothing more exciting than an idea that engages your attention with its potential; and nothing more challenging intellectually than such an idea which needs adaptation to your own context because it has originated elsewhere. Be vigorous in seeking out contemporary Australian nursing literature apart from journals—you may be fortunate in terms of your timing. Current cutting-edge texts, for instance, include Lawler (1991), Gray and Pratt (1992b), Taylor (1994), Gray and Pratt (1995b) and Gray and Pratt (1995c).

WORK TIME

Another sense in which time is of the essence, in relation to context, is time defined as daily work time. Think about it and you will realise that this has two aspects—the way in which you organise your time at work and the demands made upon that time. Clearly, the first is influenced to a considerable extent by the second. A graphic illustration of this came to light in an article about oncology nurses:

> There is no typical day for oncology nurses . . . the atypical becomes typical . . . Time was a central metaphor used in the descriptions [of a typical day for nurses who work with patients with cancer]. The amount of time available influenced nurses' abilities to perform a certain quality and quantity of work. Demands on time, whether legitimate or illegitimate, were *the context* for the day-to-day work (emphasis added).
>
> *(Deatrick & Fischer 1994, p. 35)*

CONTEXT FROM THE PERSPECTIVE OF PEOPLE AS INDIVIDUALS

All human beings are unique in terms of the individual amalgam and background configuration which they bring to an encounter with a health care system and the nurses who practise within that system, in a particular context of place and time. Regardless of the reasons that bring people to such encounters, they also bring totally distinctive configurations of gender, age, attributes, capacity and background—configurations which define their own personal context, the 'lens from which [they] view their world' (Dunn, Brown & McGuigan 1994), including their health/ill-health experiences.

Pause and consider the various elements that can be included in a definition of attributes, capacity and background. Attributes include physical, physiological and psychological dimensions, as well as attitudes and attitudinal determinants such as beliefs, values, interests and needs. Capacity includes the ability (or potential ability) to perform on physical, intellectual, emotional and spiritual planes. Background refers to a combination of factors including culture, ethnicity, socioeconomic status, upbringing, lifestyle, the individual history of health and ill-health (and previous encounters with the health care system and nurses), and all other unique experiences related to a person's living and being. It is always within the context of the complexity of unique configurations of age, gender, attributes, capacity and background that nurses engage in clinical practice with individual people.

CHANGE

Perhaps the most compelling common feature of contexts across all settings within the global village in the last years of the twentieth century is that of *change*. Wherever you live and work, you will face change—constant, often rapid, seemingly relentless change. This variable affects all the circumstances that have been mentioned so far in this chapter in relation to context from the perspectives of place, time and person. Change occurs locally, nationally and internationally. Although written more than 25 years ago, Toffler's *Future Shock* (1970) remains a seminal reference in this regard, as indeed does his *The Third Wave* (1981). Change cannot be avoided and must be taken into account in any consideration of context. It is the crucial connection between context from the perspective of place and context from the perspective of time, since it is the quintessential determinant of the currency of circumstances and ideas.

It seems to me that this notion of change represents one of the most telling arguments for studying and/or developing (and deriving) theories of nursing at one level, and utilising (i.e. applying) them at another level.

THEORIES AND MODELS OF NURSING IN CONTEXT

In the first part of this chapter it has been suggested that the concept of context is multifaceted and can be considered from the perspectives of place, time and person. The pervasive feature of change in all contexts has been drawn to your attention. The second part of the chapter is based on the contention that it is important not to apply theories and models of nursing to your practice (or generate them from your practice) in an arbitrary fashion without due consideration of context. Hence, it will be suggested that, in order to take considerations of context into account, theories and models of nursing need to be addressed on two different levels if they are to be applied effectively in practice. (Practice can be defined as clinical practice, education, administration, research or scholarship. At this stage in your career you will be focusing on clinical practice.)

The first, or superordinate, level is abstract, general and inclusive; it is applicable universally—that is, regardless of the (local) practice context. At the second, or subordinate, level nurses must fashion details for application in particular contexts of place, time and individual patient being.

A Canadian nurse (Gendron 1994) very effectively uses the analogy of a tapestry to illustrate the concept of the art of clinical nursing practice. A similar analogy can be used in relation to context. A tapestry (or indeed any other piece woven on a loom or frame, such as a carpet) is comprised of two elements, the warp and the weft. The warp is the standard, basic component. For the present purpose, imagine it as a series of bare, closely aligned threads set vertically across the frame. The weft comprises threads woven across the warp. The particular texture and colour of the weft threads, and the technique of weaving used, determines the individual pattern that results.

> The weft of nursing care for each person is unique, based on a foundational warp of generalized knowledge and skill. As the tapestry of care develops, the weft displays an ever changing matching of nursing approaches to the person's needs, interests and values; a sensitive awareness of the *total context* of care . . .
>
> *(Gendron 1994, p. 29, emphasis added)*

Thus, in a very similar vein, the superordinate level of theory development can be equated with the warp (which in another place Gendron refers to as '**acontextual** knowledge . . . and conceptual ideas'—emphasis added); while the weft is equated with the subordinate level, with nurses weaving individual patterns of practice in accordance with particular contexts.

THEORY DEVELOPMENT AT A SUPERORDINATE LEVEL

What are the variables—the bare warp threads—usually addressed in nursing theories at the superordinate level? It seems to me they are as follows:

- people who are nurses;
- people who are (traditionally called) patients (but may now, depending on the context, be called clients or consumers or customers);
- the health of people who are patients (and nurses); and
- the relationships between the above three variables, particularly the interaction between people who are nurses and people who are patients with the express purpose of achieving healthy outcomes.

I have stated these variables very broadly and apparently simply but they contain the possibility of a number of differing assumptions in regard to definitions, beliefs and ideas. Such possibilities would include, for instance, definitions of 'nurse', 'nursing' and 'health'; beliefs about the nature of nursing work, and thus about the relationship of nurses both with their patients and with, for example, other members of the health care team; and ideas about what constitutes appropriate 'health outcomes'.

I believe that these variables, treated as elements within a nursing theory, will only have universal applicability (and continue to act as standard, basic warp threads) if they are considered as concepts in an abstract, general and inclusive way. As soon as concrete examples, particular instances and 'exceptions to the rule' (i.e. exclusions) start to be introduced into the theory, it begins to lose its universal applicability and a weft pattern begins to emerge. Pause and consider this proposition and you will understand how it is so. By definition, a 'variable' is apt to vary or change, or liable or capable of being varied or changed (*The Macquarie Dictionary 1981*). As we have seen, one of the likely determinants of such change is specific context.

THEORY APPLICATION AT THE SUBORDINATE LEVEL OF SPECIFIC CONTEXTS

One of the variables often addressed at an abstract or general level in nursing theories is 'environment'. Certainly, environment can be defined in conceptual terms but inherent in this concept is the *inevitability* that, in terms of practical application, environment depends on context. In previous discussion in this chapter, environment as a contextual variable was rather narrowly defined in terms of the built or natural environment. Clearly, however, it is a concept that can be applied equally to all the other variables of context that have been addressed. Indeed, the word 'environment' can be (and often is) used interchangeably with the word 'context'. This appears to be the way it is used by a number of nursing theorists (see, for example, Fawcett 1984, p. 5; Meleis 1985, pp. 27, 29–30). I would argue that an abstract and general consideration of environment thus broadly defined will not facilitate the application of a theory to nursing practice in a particular context.

To enable such applicability, nurses must weave onto the warp of an acontextual theory a weft pattern of clinical practice which incorporates their own particular contextual elements. As Gendron (1994) suggests: 'The warp structure includes nursing interventions for particular symptoms and disease states . . . A holistic view of Person is another warp string, and this perspective might be integrated within a variety of possible nursing theories or conceptual frameworks'. The origin of any theory will determine the extent to which consideration has to be given to national (and State/territory) settings as well as the local setting. For example, if the theory originates overseas, it will be sensible to consider details of applicability in the Australian context in the first instance before focusing on your local setting.

What follows are suggestions for a systematic approach, or framework, which it might be useful for you to adopt in your pursuit of applying any theory to *your* context—its setting and its circumstances of place, time, change and individual patient being.

Philosophical assumptions

Particularly when a theory originates overseas, you should begin by querying whether the ideas that inform it at the superordinate level are in tune with current thinking in your local context. For example, in the framework of what definitions of 'nurse', 'nursing' and 'health' has the theory been developed? What ideas about appropriate 'health outcomes' are evident in the theory? If such definitions and ideas do not appear to be in tune with the current context of your nursing practice, are they so at variance that to try to adapt the theory is likely to be an exercise in industrious futility?

Are there philosophical assumptions (i.e. assumptions about beliefs and principles) underlying the theory in relation to the variables that comprise its substance at the superordinate level? If so, do these fit comfortably with the nursing philosophy current in your local context? For instance, what beliefs about the nature of nursing work and of the relationships between nurses and their patients, and nurses and their co-workers are inherent in the theory? It may be that a difference in philosophical assumptions, in relation to the nature of the relationship between nurse and patient, is so glaring that the theory is fundamentally incompatible with practice in that context. Consider, for example, the difference between a philosophy of nursing that views the patient as an essentially passive recipient of nursing 'care' (and care which is concerned with the current ill-health problem only), and one that sees the patient as an active and equal partner with the nurse in focusing on resolution of the current ill-health problem in relation to the person's health as a whole.

This is a suitable juncture to pause and consider the feature of change, which was mentioned earlier. If your intention is to embrace a particular theory as a framework for your clinical practice in anything other than the short term, you should think carefully about whether the theory in question has been developed at a sufficiently abstract, general and inclusive level to accommodate with relative ease the (rapid) change that is likely to occur in many of your local contextual circumstances. If it appears to you that this is *not* the case, then it may be prudent to consider adopting another theory that does fit this criterion.

Political assumptions

In relation to a theory that originates overseas, you should next query whether there are political assumptions underlying the theory. If you believe there are, ask yourself whether these assumptions remain valid in the Australian context. Is the political system (and the range of political ideologies within that system) the same as in Australia? Ask the same question in relation to these issues: public policy concerning health; the legislation which governs practice as a nurse (professionally and industrially); and the funding and organisation of the health care system, including the way in which nursing service is organised and nursing care delivered. Even among the so-called Western 'democracies', there may be significant differences of emphasis in relation to, for example, conservatism and social reform, free market and government-controlled economies, and centralisation or devolution of political power. Such differences will inevitably affect public philosophy, policy, funding and organisation in regard to a country's health care system. (Compare and contrast, for example, the funding and organisation of health services in Australia, the United States and Britain.)

In relation to the delivery of nursing care, are hospitals staffed with a skill mix of registered nurses, enrolled nurses and undergraduate students of nursing (however these categories are titled) or by registered nurses only? What type of delivery system is used— patient assignment, team nursing, primary nursing? Are (independent) nurse practitioners an established part of the system? If you find significant differences emerging as you answer such questions, you should then ask whether these differences are likely to affect the application of the theory to the Australian context.

As we have seen, the term 'politics' (and hence political assumptions) incorporates a number of elements. Some of these may vary *within* Australia. Thus, you need to weave weft threads of State/territory (and local government) politics into the warp of the theory, even if it originates in Australia but in another setting. Finally, the political and (socio)-economic context of your particular place of work may influence the way in which you apply the theory to practice. A privately funded hospital may be a radically different proposition from one that is publicly funded (particularly in times of economic constraints). Consider, for example, potential differences in relation to the following: the socioeconomic backgrounds and therefore (possibly) the case mix of the patients; the sophistication and currency of the technology used in regard to diagnostics, therapeutics and information systems; management systems and styles; nursing delivery systems; nurse:patient ratios; and the pace of practice.

Sociocultural considerations

You should follow a similar questioning approach (for both overseas and Australian theories) when considering your circumstances in relation to culture and society. Remember from the previous discussion that you will be querying the local context in relation to a number of aspects, including ethnic groups and the associated variables of culture and length of residence in Australia, subcultures, social strata and demographic patterns. In essence, in this exercise, you will be identifying the *backgrounds* of the patients you are nursing, and then weaving these as weft threads through the warp of the theory in question.

To which ethnic groups do your patients belong? What are the implications of their ethnicity in terms of, for example, cultural mores, religious beliefs, philosophy of health and illness, diet? Are they recent immigrants (and refugees)? Are they indigenous? To which socioeconomic stratum do they belong? Are they members of a particular subculture, of a minority group, of a group which attracts stigma or discriminatory practices or disadvantage? What is their age range? Is one gender predominant? What circumstances of ill-health have brought them into a nurse–patient relationship with you—that is, what is the case mix of your patients? If the application of theory to practice is to be effective in terms of healthy outcomes for your patients, it is crucial that such details of your patients' sociocultural contexts are taken into consideration.

Listen to a highly respected Aboriginal nurse (Joan Winch AM) talking about nurses acting as change agents in the context of Aboriginal health care: 'Be aware of what you are doing. Do not set out to change a culture. Weave a programme around this so that traditional concepts can be kept with safe practices included' (Winch 1989).

Environmental considerations

You should give some thought to the possibility of either the built or natural environments (or both) in which you work affecting the way in which you utilise a theory in your practice. For instance, the physical structure of a hospital unit may influence the relationship you are able to develop with your patients. Think, for example, about the implications, from at least two different points of view, of having patients situated in four- or eight-bed 'wards' as compared with single- or two-bed wards—how might each configuration affect the privacy with which you are able to conduct conversations with, and carry out assessments of, a patient; and how might each affect the amount of time you have available to spend on direct nursing care?

Likewise, the circumstances of your local natural environment may influence a number of practice variables. Consider, for example, the effect that a polluted natural environment may have on people's health and therefore on the patient case mix where you work. Consider the effect that extremes of temperature may have on the way you practise your nursing. Consider the presence of any conservation versus employment issues which may be affecting your local politicoeconomic context.

Considerations of individual patients and their being

Finally, with the focus on your patients as individuals, you should weave your weft threads of unique attributes and capacity. Together with details of your patients' backgrounds, you must seek to discover the complexities of their being, at least in so far as these are pertinent to your encounter. In a sense, the total time span of your relationship with patients is a voyage of discovery about those patients as people, and the ways in which their attributes and capacity may be harnessed for the purpose of resolving their present problem(s) and also in pursuit of their longer-term health and well-being. It is clear that these considerations of personal being demand nursing skills of observation, 'tuning in' and sensitivity.

> One needs to attune to and synchronize with the person being cared for
> . . . . To do this, a keen awareness of the total context of the person and
> the interaction is needed, an 'intuitive grasp' or whole understanding.
>
> *(Gendron 1994)*

THEORY DERIVATION FROM PARTICULAR CONTEXTS OF PRACTICE

Further into your career as a nurse, you may become engaged in the process of deriving and developing a theory or model of nursing *from* your practice, rather than applying a theory developed elsewhere by another nurse *to* your practice. During such a project you will need to consider contextual variables from another, reverse perspective. You will need to distill from your multifaceted local context the *a*contextual variables that constitute the superordinate level of theory development. Or, to conclude by using the tapestry analogy, you will need to unthread the contextual weft and lay bare the acontextual warp before inviting your colleagues worldwide to apply your theory in the context of their local practice.

SUMMARY

In this chapter you have been encouraged, indeed urged, to consider *context* as a crucial moderator in terms of the relevance and applicability of any nursing theory or model to the process of your clinical practice. The concept of context has been defined and addressed in terms of place, time and people as individuals. Place has been discussed in relation to *setting* (local, national and international) and *circumstances* (including those of culture, ethnicity, society, 'politics' and the environment). Time has been considered in relation to the currency of circumstances, ideas and philosophies; and to your work time. The individual people who become patients have been presented in terms of their unique contexts in regard to gender, age, attributes, capacity and background. Looming over all, it has been asserted, is the spectre of all-pervasive change.

It has been suggested that theories should be developed (and studied initially) at a superordinate level, where acontextual variables are addressed as abstract, general and inclusive. The subordinate level of theory utilisation requires a detailed elaboration of the variables in the context of contemporary local settings, circumstances and individual people. Guidelines for undertaking a detailed application of any nursing theory or model in a systematic fashion to your own practice context have been offered.

GLOSSARY

Acontextual: not in, or having, any context.

Case mix: the mixture of different illnesses, injuries and so on exhibited by patients in a particular hospital or other health care agency.

Currency: the state of belonging to the time actually passing.

Demographic: of, or pertaining to, the science of vital and social statistics, as of births, deaths, diseases, marriages etc. of populations.

Mores: customs or conventions accepted without question and embodying the fundamental moral views of a group.

Phenomena: the plural form of 'phenomenon': an immediate object of awareness in experience; a thing as it appears to, and is constructed by, us.

Subordinate: placed in, or belonging to, a lower order or rank.

Subsume: to consider (an idea, term, proposition etc.) as part of a more comprehensive one; to include in a larger or higher class or a more inclusive classification.

Superordinate: placed in, or belonging to, a higher order, level or rank; or described in general rather than specific terms.

QUESTIONS

As a focus for discussion, undertake the exercises suggested in the sections on the national setting (p. 110) and the international setting (p. 111). They are reproduced below.

1 Consider the particular State or territory where you live and work as an intermediate context between your local setting and the national Australian setting. Identify issues pertaining to your State or territory that distinguish this setting as a context from both local and national contexts.

2 Identify circumstances within the Pacific or Asian region, which are distinctive to one or other of those regions as compared to the world at large, and which might impact on both the Australian and your local context.

LEARNING ACTIVITIES

Identify a 'local context' of clinical practice for yourself, preferably one that includes an area within the health care system where you have undertaken clinical experience during your undergraduate program (and/or worked). Within this local context, identify all the variables of place and time suggested in this chapter, before undertaking the following activities.

1   Choose one of the theories or models in this book that originated in Australia. Using the details of the context variables you have identified, describe how these would influence (i.e. modify) the way in which you could utilise (i.e. apply) the theory in clinical practice within your 'local context'.

2   Choose one of the theories or models in this book that originated overseas. First, review the theory/model against the suggestions in the chapter sections entitled 'Philosophical assumptions' and 'Political assumptions'. Then, use the details of the variables you identified in your 'local context' to describe how these would modify the way in which you could apply the theory in clinical practice in this context.

3   Chose the theory or model described in this book that you think you would be interested in applying to your beginning practice as a registered nurse. Imagine that you are going to begin practice in the local context you identified for the purpose of these Learning Activities. Imagine some of the current variables you have identified in that context changing over the first two or three years of your practice there. Are the superordinate variables in the theory you have chosen sufficiently abstract, general and inclusive to accommodate these changes readily? Explain why, or why not.

7

SELECTING A NURSING THEORY FOR CLINICAL PRACTICE
Analysis and Critique

KAREN WOTTON

LEARNING OBJECTIVES

After reading this chapter you should be able to:

1 Understand nursing theories when you read them.

2 Be aware of theories and their application to clinical practice.

3 Undertake a collaborative approach in the selection of practice theories.

4 Undertake an analysis of the components of practice.

5 Understand the criteria to use for analysis, critique and evaluation of theory.

Karen Wotton, RN, RM, IW, DipED (Ns ED), BN, MMgt, is a lecturer in nursing at the The Flinders University of South Australia. She has taught Nursing Knowledge to undergraduate students for five years and coordinated this topic for three of those years. Her interest in nursing theory lies in promoting the discourse of clinicians concerned with the application of theory to practice and the subsequent involvement of clinicians in the process of selecting, implementing and evaluating models for practice. Karen, an acute care clinician, is also a member of the Department of Nursing Practice and teaches and coordinates topics in the third year of the preregistration nursing program. Current interests in this area are related to the development and refinement of a clinical reasoning model which is applicable to both the university and clinical settings.

INTRODUCTION

The purpose of nursing, a practice-based discipline, is to provide high-quality health care to individuals, groups and communities to assist them to retain, obtain and maintain a state of health. As a profession, nursing has the responsibility to provide comprehensive care and to incorporate current knowledge into practice. To achieve their goals, nurses must possess a theoretical foundation grounded in research. The future of theory-based practice depends on the involvement of clinical nurses in selecting, implementing and evaluating the goodness of fit between a theory and their practice.

Autonomous nursing practice has been difficult to achieve in the past, because of the restraint imposed by the medical model. At the present time, when there are nursing models to guide practice, autonomy is still restricted, because of a trend for nursing administrators and academics to impose and prescribe the approach by which practitioners work. If nurses are not allowed the autonomy to select approaches to care, and are forced to practise with a potentially opposing philosophy, then practice will be restrictive with resulting dissatisfaction with nursing; this could be counterproductive to caring and threaten nursing's professional existence (Holden 1991; Nagle & Mitchell 1991).

Nurse academics possess an important role within the nursing team. They work with clinicians and administrators in uncovering data which assist in the formulation of research questions that pertain to every-day clinical practice. It is only through the collaboration and collective action of clinicians, administrators and academics that the gulf between theory and practice will be bridged and the body of nursing knowledge extended for the benefit of clients and the nursing profession (Riehl-Sisca 1989). It is imperative that clinicians analyse and critique theories they believe are relevant and useful to practice.

The introduction of a nursing conceptual framework may necessitate a transformation in nurses' value orientations as well as in their thinking and problem-solving processes (Fitch et al. 1991), it is essential, therefore, that the process of selection be given as much attention as the process of implementation. It is therefore not prudent to select a particular model on the basis of a hunch, or because a model is popular, developed locally or developed by nurses who are currently in the limelight (Aggleton & Chalmers 1987). A judgement on the relevance and applicability of a nursing model for practice is best achieved when carried out systematically, incorporating subjective and objective components.

In this chapter the process of selecting a theory for use in practice will be discussed in several stages. First, an overview of the relevance of nursing conceptual models in clinical practice will be provided. Second, a review of criteria used by other nurses in selecting models for practice will be undertaken, to demonstrate some of the current inadequacies in both the process and the criteria. Third, the discussion will concentrate on identifying elements useful in an analysis of clinical practice, an essential process prior to the selection of a practice model. Fourth, criteria for analysing and critiquing a nursing model will be presented, with the view that nurses preparing to use a model in practice can select criteria that are appropriate for their needs.

Throughout this chapter, the terms 'nursing models', 'nursing conceptual models' and 'nursing theories' will be used interchangeably. The reason for this is the recognition that throughout the nursing literature inconsistent and tentative use of these terms is widespread (George 1990; Stevens Barnum 1994). They are defined and described in different ways by different authors and at the present time there appears to be no common acceptable definition.

WHY USE NURSING CONCEPTUAL MODELS?

Conceptual models provide a firm foundation, a scientific base, for practice, far removed from trial and error, guesswork or intuition (Fawcett 1989). Models provide guidelines for improvements in patient care, promote the uniqueness of the domain of nursing and put forward frameworks for thinking about nursing and reasoning and communicating in nursing.

The primary purpose of using a nursing model in practice is the improvement of the service to the consumer and of the care they receive (Clarke 1982; Storch 1986). The improvement of both service and care has been stimulated by the view inherent in nursing models that health is more than merely the absence of disease. Nursing models put forward the conviction that for nurses to make a difference they must view health care as a partnership, with the client assuming an integral role. It is partly because of the influence of nursing models that nurses are more aware of the wholeness of the individual, the integral relationship of the environment to people's health, and patients' capacity and need to control their own destiny (Storch 1986). The use of a model by members of a nursing team contributes to the sharing and coherence of purpose, leading to increased continuity of care (Pearson & Vaughan 1986; Ingram 1991), and ensures consistency in the delivery of nursing care (Ellis 1968; Allison, McLaughlin & Walker 1991). The sharing of common goals and a common philosophy does not mean that there will be reduced individuality or innovation in the provision of nursing care, but that nurses, patients and other health professionals will know the focus and domain of nursing.

Nursing's conceptual models make explicit the distinction between the activities of nurses and those of other health professionals by highlighting nursing's unique identity (Clarke 1982; Fawcett & Carino 1987). Models achieve this by identifying the focus, purpose and domain of nursing, explaining relevant events in the practice discipline of nursing and providing an organising framework on which to structure and develop nursing practice. Through the provision of a common body of knowledge, models enhance nursing's power and professional autonomy by guiding and directing the actions of the profession in practice, education and research (Fawcett 1989; Draper 1990; Ingram 1991; Meleis 1991; Sorrentino 1991).

The use of nursing models in practice increases communication among nurses, and between nurses and other professionals. The provision of a common base of theoretical knowledge has the potential to promote a common language, which increases communication between practitioners, researchers and theorists (Chinn & Jacobs 1987; Draper 1990; Allison et al. 1991; Gardner et al. 1991; Ingram 1991). Through the use of models in practice, nurses are more clearly able to identify commonalities and differences among the many facets of their role. This identification assists in demonstrating how the focus and contribution of nurses differs from, and articulates with, the service of other health care professionals (Allison et al. 1991).

With respect to guiding and directing thinking, nursing models provide divergent ways of viewing nursing procedure, the role of the nurse in the health care team and the decision-making process associated with the provision of nursing care. To assist in directing and facilitating decision-making, most nursing models:

- define the characteristics of legitimate recipients of nursing care;

- outline the general nature of the clinical problems to be considered;

- discuss the nature of assessment and provide guidelines for this process;

- demonstrate how problems are related under specific circumstances and indicate when nursing intervention may be required;

- state the aims of the planning and goal setting process;

- indicate the focus of nursing therapeutics and technologies during the implementation of the care plan;

- indicate the nature of the process of evaluation;

- identify criteria for ascertaining the quality and effects of intervention outcomes.

(Aggleton & Chalmers 1987; Fawcett & Carino 1987)

WHY ARE ANALYSIS AND CRITIQUE IMPORTANT?

Although a model may at first glance appear to offer a potentially useful guide for nursing practice, it should be remembered that the majority of conceptual models were constructed for the context, environment and health care of a particular country and era. Past popularity of a model therefore should not be an important criterion in selecting a model for practice. It is important to remember that the construction of models was dependent on the knowledge available at a point in time. If they have not been adapted to meet the current state of knowledge development they may promote the knowledge and values of an era long past.

A further point to consider is that models of nursing adapt some of their concepts and processes from other disciplines and thus there is the risk that the focus may not be closely linked to nursing. It is reasonable, therefore, to expect that some models may not be suited to the current trends in nursing and health care practices in Australia today. Birx (1993) clearly highlights the reason why concurrent validity and reliability of information and knowledge is important, and presents one of the reasons why any model should be critically analysed and evaluated before it is introduced. Birx (1993, p. 23) indicates that nursing knowledge is not static but a 'dynamic, ongoing process of awareness, inquiry, investigation, integration, imagination and openness to realities and possibilities'.

Over the past few years my discussions with clinical staff, concerning the use of a theory in their practice, showed that many of them could name the theory they were using in practice. Further questioning revealed, however, that they were in fact using an assessment tool and nursing care plan extracted from the nursing theory, without an understanding of the philosophy and concepts embraced by that theory. Often, clinical staff commented that, even though they knew the name of the theory, they had not been involved in its selection and were only educated in the use of the assessment tool and nursing care plan. Jennings (1987) strongly recommends that, for theories to make sense, practitioners must see theory as a process and not just a product. One of the reasons for a theory–practice gap is the failure of nurses using them to be involved in the analysis, critique and selection process of a theory prior to implementation. It is imperative that the selection and implementation be controlled by staff within the clinical domain.

The application and implementation of nursing theory require time and effort and, therefore, money. Nurses need to possess a sound understanding of the theory and the potential differences it will make to nursing care in order to justify the expense involved, in both time and money, to the cost-conscious health care administration team (Sorrentino 1991). The implementation of a theory is not to be taken lightly, for there will need to be a variety of adaptations and changes to the process and tools used in the practice area. For example, the implementation of a theory may require the redevelopment of documentation, policies and procedures, standards of patient care, patient classification systems, and job descriptions; and the development of staff education programs (Allison et al. 1991).

Careful selection of a theory will help to maintain critical thinking skills, individuality and innovation in practice. However, throughout this selection process, nurses must be mindful that some theories have the propensity to limit nurses' initiative and individuality in the provision of care, and may also have an inhibiting effect on nurses' ability to identify new knowledge (Birx 1993).

In order to select theories that relate more specifically to a clinical environment, a rigorous, systematic analysis is essential. Nurses need theories which relate more specifically to what they actually do, are based around core concepts which describe their practice and which have the potential to facilitate the further development of nursing knowledge (Clarke 1982). Decisions about which model to implement for practice should be made by nurses in a deliberate, systematic, criteria-based, objective and conscious manner (Meleis 1991). Although these evaluations may contain a component of subjective and experiential decisions, to use hunch and intuition as the only criteria is too simplistic for such a major element of practice (Aggleton & Chalmers 1987). Both types of evaluation, subjective and objective, are essential and neither is sufficient by itself.

CRITERIA FOR SELECTING A THEORY FOR PRACTICE

There exist several guidelines outlining criteria which can be used for analysis and critique of nursing theories. Table 7.1 details the author, date and criteria suggested by the different writers for evaluating nursing theories.

It would be logical to assume that nurses intending to select a theory for practice could consult literature written by those who had previously completed this task. The difficulty of this lies in the fact that, although many of the criteria listed in Table 7.1 are used by nurses in selecting theories for practice, their use is implicitly rather than explicitly stated in subsequent published reports. For example, nurses inform their readers that they selected a theory which was consistent with the health care unit's philosophy and mission but do not detail how they arrived at this decision. Clearly, the selection of a model based on its congruence with organisational philosophy and mission should increase the consistency and continuity of the provision of care. However, there are many aspects that must be taken into account to consider this an appropriate criterion for selection. The philosophy must express the collective and aggregate beliefs of all staff (Riehl-Sisca 1989). Thus a philosophy must be developed by all staff and be consistent with the beliefs of nurses about health and patient care today; it must not be one imposed by administration.

Nurses, in selecting a theory for practice, use a combination of criteria with the most frequent being that of congruency with unit philosophy and organisational mission. The following are examples of published criteria used by nurses for selecting a theory for use in practice.

Reed (1986) uses Fawcett's (1980) criteria for evaluation of conceptual models for clinical teaching and practice. Reed states that the criteria used in this evaluation consisted of examining the model for clarity, appropriateness for nursing, social relevance and logical congruence. Although Reed indicated that these criteria were used in delineating the conceptual elements of the model, she does not describe how this was achieved; she provides little assistance, therefore, to other nurses seeking to analyse a theory for use in practice.

Aggleton and Chalmers (1987), in their comparison of different types of models, use criteria which are very familiar to clinical nurses. They focus on analysing what developmental, interaction and systems models imply about nursing assessment, the planning of care, nursing intervention and evaluation. Sohn (1991) devised a simple method similar to that of Aggleton and Chalmers (1987) for comparing models. Sohn examines how models suggest that assessment data are managed in respect to physical, psychosocial, developmental and spiritual life dimensions. In addition, Sohn evaluates how models organise and manage nursing diagnosis, and plan, implement and evaluate care. Although the criteria used by Aggleton and Chalmers and Sohn are extremely relevant, they are limited to only one aspect of a model, that of decision-making processes; these criteria, therefore, are of limited utility if not used in conjunction with other criteria.

TABLE 7.1 CRITERIA EVALUATING NURSING THEORIES

AUTHOR	CRITERIA
Ellis (1968)	Scope, complexity, testability, usefulness, identification of implicit values, generation of information and use of meaningful terminology
Duffey & Muhlenkamp (1974)	Generation of testable hypotheses, guide for practice, presents a body of knowledge, complete subject matter, values of theorist made explicit, explicit relationships among propositions, and possess parsimony
Hardy (1974)	Meaning, logical, operational, empirical and pragmatic adequacy. Generalisability, understanding and predictability
Johnson (1974)	Social congruence, utility and significance
Chinn & Jacobs (1987)	Semantic clarity, semantic consistency, structural clarity and structural consistency; simplicity, generality, empirical applicability and consequences
Fawcett (1988)	*Analysis:* historical evolution of model, approach to model development, content and source of concern. *Evaluation:* explicitness of assumptions, degree of comprehensiveness of content, logical congruence, ability to generate and test theory, knowledge development in nursing, and social considerations.
Marriner-Tomey (1989)	*Evaluation:* clarity, simplicity, generality, empirical precision, derivable consequences
Stevens Barnum (1990; 1994)	*Analysis:* descriptions of model, and commonplaces. *Internal evaluation:* clarity, consistency, adequacy, logical development, and level of theory development. *External criticism:* reality convergence, utility, significance, discrimination, scope of theory, and complexity
Meleis (1991)	*Description:* structural components (assumptions, concepts and propositions) and function components (focus, client, nursing, health, nurse–patient interactions, environment, nursing problem, nursing therapeutics) *Analysis:* concept (differentiation from others, semantic, logic and context) and theory (theorist, paradigmatic origins and internal dimensions) *Critique:* Relationship between structure and function (clarity, consistency, simplicity, tautology, teleology) *Diagram of theory:* (visual and graphic presentation, logical representation and clarity), circle of contagiousness, and usefulness in practice, research, education and administration *External critique:* congruence with personal values, congruence with other professional values, congruence with social values, and social significance. Theory testing

Lewis's (1988) discussion is relevant for readers exploring the process of analysis and critique, as it provides an overview of the decision-making processes involved in selecting a model for an acute surgical ward. First, Lewis recognises that the most critical factor in model choice is its meaningfulness and practical utility to both registered nurses and student nurses. Prior to the selection process, Lewis classified the models into two main groups—those making use of natural science and those based on humanistic theory. He finally selected a systems model (natural science model), not because of its merits but because he was influenced by the view of Kershaw that humanistic models had little relevance to nursing care. Although Lewis's natural inclination was to use Roper, Tierney and Logan, a British model, because of its accessibility, it was rejected because it failed to pay sufficient attention to disease conditions.

Lewis reported that Roy's (1984) theory was chosen because:

- it used a nursing process approach;

- it was considered holistic in nature, because it accounted for the physical, emotional and social aspects of the individual;

- it could be used in a variety of settings;

- it had the assessment potential for prioritising potentially life-threatening functions;

- it used a problem-solving approach to care; and

- it could be used in conjunction with nursing diagnoses.

Lewis clearly shows that he analysed the current practices and value orientation of nurses in the acute surgical ward, and used the elements of this practice in conjunction with the criteria of clarity, purpose and applicability to clinical practice to direct the selection of the model.

McWilliams, Murphy and Sobiski (1988) selected Orem's (1985) theory for prevention, home care and long-term care for the Vancouver Health Department because it was the most compatible with departmental philosophy and community health nursing practice. Mayberry (1991) likewise advises that the models to be studied for application to practice should be those that seem to fit the mission, goal and philosophy of the nursing agency. These authors, like many others, fail to describe how they arrived at their decisions or whether they used any other criteria to evaluate the goodness of fit between nursing models and their practice.

Sullivan (1989) used Fawcett's analysis and critique to evaluate the Salutogenic Model (whose central concern is explaining how people stay well despite omnipresent stressors) developed by Antonovsky (a medical sociologist) in 1972. In the analysis the following areas were addressed:

- historical evolution of model;

- approach to model development;

- explication of nursing's four metaparadigm concepts;

- statement of relationships among the four metaparadigm concepts;

- content; and

- source of concern.

Elements of evaluation used by Sullivan were:

* explicitness of assumptions;

* degree of comprehensiveness of content;

* logical congruence;

* ability to generate and test theory;

* potential to promote knowledge development in nursing; and

* social considerations.

The work of Sullivan provides a good example of how criteria can be used to analyse and evaluate a model of nursing.

Fernandez et al.'s (1990) focus for theory selection was on utility and applicability to practice. They selected a theory, or practice model, for three health units in New Jersey, which was congruent with the Health Department's philosophy, the institution's mission and management style, application potential for nursing practice and the evolution of nursing practice. In choosing a model they also showed the importance of identifying and acknowledging new trends in health care. The trends these authors highlight are:

* shortened hospital stays;

* increased patient acuity;

* ageing population with complex needs;

* increase in ambulatory services;

* increased use of technology in home care; and

* the consumers' desire to participate in care decisions.

Fernandez et al. clearly show that they involved clinical staff in identifying criteria to assess models for their application potential for practice. Nursing staff identified the need for a model that described the domain of nursing; facilitated the use of a common nursing language; reflected the philosophy of nursing staff; provided direction for nursing actions; and allocated resources based on patients' needs.

Reynolds and Cormack (1990) developed and used a series of questions to assess the relevance of Johnson's behavioural model to psychiatric nurses. Reynolds (1993) further developed these criteria which include:

* utility in practice;

* clear delineation of scope;

* identification and understanding of clients' commonly occurring responses to health problems and the consequences of these problems to them;

* interventions that will help clients move towards optimal health;

* cultural and geographical portability;

* extent of testing and acceptance of theoretical constructs;

    ▓   freedom to use the theory within the constructions and ethical responsibility of clinical autonomy; and

    ▓   reliability and validity.

The significance of Reynolds' brief article is his inclusion of the criteria of clinical autonomy and cultural and ethical considerations as required variables when selecting a model for practice.

It is important when selecting criteria for analysing and evaluating a nursing model for use in practice that consideration is paid to both the criteria developed by theorists and those highlighted by nurses who have tried to implement a model in practice. In selecting a model for practice, there are three phases to be examined prior to any attempt to measure the goodness of fit between a model and practice. These stages are as follows:

1   Analysis of the essential components of clinical practice.

2   Analysis of theory.

3   Critique of theory.

ANALYSIS OF CLINICAL PRACTICE

Choosing a nursing model demands a close scrutiny of ourselves, our patients, other nurses and other health care workers. New ideas arrive, new concepts are identified and patients' needs change; so, then, does the possible choice of model. To introduce a new perspective into the work situation is, in effect, to introduce change. Planned change is inevitably easier to manage than change that is imposed, haphazard or misunderstood.

The first priority in selecting a theory for practice is for the nursing team to undertake an analysis of the nursing practice environment and to reach agreement on the central tenets of their practice. Although a large portion of this analysis will consist of objective information, a good portion will also consist of data from the nurses' personal models of nursing. All nurses possess their own personal models of nursing, developed throughout their professional lives and practical experience, and influenced by their own personal values, the environment, the values of their clients, feedback from clients and staff, and from perpetual observation, reflection and analysis of practice. However, at the present time this personal knowledge is 'perhaps one of the least recognised but most important sources of knowledge in nursing practice' (Sims 1991, p. 60). Failure to discuss the range of values and beliefs held about nursing, environment, person and health by different team members could also be one of the main reasons for lack of continuity and consistency in the provision of care, the cause of conflict within a team, and the basis of role confusion.

Before considering the selection of a model for practice nursing, team members will, therefore, require opportunities to explore their personal models of nursing and then to examine and discuss these within the nursing team. As the ability to identify underlying values, assumptions and perspectives is essentially a critical thinking skill (Birx 1993), the nursing team will require a person well versed in group work to facilitate this analysis. Nursing team members need to consider:

- their assumptions about people, health, environment and nursing;

- their goals for their practice;

- the assumptions made when approaching nursing in a particular way;

- the knowledge they have and the knowledge they need to achieve nursing goals; and

- the approach they use or want to use in the clinical reasoning process.

A consensus must be reached with respect to common beliefs and values, the goals of nursing, and an outline of the knowledge, skills, attitudes and decision-making processes that the team sees as fundamental in achieving the goals of nursing. It is also important for the nursing team to identify effective nursing strategies that staff would like to maintain (Johnson & Baumann 1992).

A further aspect requiring discussion within the nursing team is their current level of autonomy and the level of autonomy they deem appropriate for the level of work for which they believe they have been educated. This analysis involves, first, exploring nurses' current freedom in decision-making and the control they possess over important aspects of their work and, second, delineating professional standards of practice. The significance of this analysis is related to the view that a theory which is congruent with, and clearly delineates, professional standards of practice has the propensity to increase professional autonomy (Gruending 1985). As professional autonomy is linked to licensure, accreditation, certification requirements, and institutional policies and procedures, the nursing team will need to have a good understanding of these prior to selecting a model for practice (Buchanan 1987).

As nurses do not practise in isolation from other health care professionals, the nursing team will need to discuss (among themselves) the aims of their working relationship with other professionals. They may then choose to set up multidisciplinary team meetings to explore the common beliefs and assumptions of these groups about nursing, and examine the way in which these professionals see their roles and decisions interfacing with nursing. This process of analysis is essential, for it will help to ensure that theory selection allows for collaboration with other disciplines (Birx 1993).

Johnson and Baumann (1992) indicate the importance of categorising the attributes of the client population being served. These attributes include:

- patient classification system;

- components of service (e.g. medical conditions, surgical conditions, intensive care, midwifery, rehabilitation);

- short-stay or long-stay patients;

- variations in the age of patients;

- variations in the cultural background of patients; and

- the relationship between hospital and community services.

It is important in patient categorisation that nursing diagnosis and not just medical diagnosis, is included, in order to capture the full complexity of patient needs. The nursing team should also determine the method or the proposed method for delivering nursing care to patients. For example, this may be primary nursing, functional nursing, team nursing or patient allocation.

In the analysis of practice, it is important to identify the people who will be directly and indirectly involved in using the model. The staffing mix should be clearly stated in relation to both the numbers and the ratio of different levels of staffing. For example, the number of enrolled nurses, registered nurses, managers, clinical nurse consultants, clinical nurses, educators and nurse administrators in the clinical unit should be identified. Job descriptions that include statements about responsibility for nursing care should be obtained, so that nurses' differential involvement in patient care can be made explicit.

An analysis of the health care environment in which care is delivered, and the changes that may affect model introduction, should also be established. Possible changes which may need to be taken into consideration include:

■   decentralisation of nursing units;

■   implementation of case mix;

■   implementation of cost-reduction measures and budgetary constraints;

■   staffing decreases and changes in staffing mix;

■   shortened hospital stays;

■   increased patient acuity;

■   ageing population with complex needs;

■   increase in ambulatory services;

■   increased use of technology in home care; and

■   the consumers' desire to participate in care decisions.

(Fernandez et al. 1990)

Nurses must be politically astute if they are to gain the support of power groups such as hospital administrators and physicians to facilitate change within the turbulent fiscal environment. It is pointless to approach these groups for support without undertaking a careful analysis of the perceived benefits and costs of introducing conceptually based practice, and also, developing timelines for its implementation and evaluation. Thus, there is the need to articulate anticipated outcomes in measurable terms. This articulation of benefits will be helpful in gaining support from power groups but will also assist nurses to calculate what can be realistically accomplished.

There are other considerations to be borne in mind when selecting a model for practice. Who will it affect? What changes will it require in such things as work organisation, staff mix, ratio of patients to nursing staff and education of staff? What resources will be needed for such items as new assessment, care-planning and evaluation documentation? Are these resources available? A proposed budget should be prepared to assist in determining what financial resources are needed and what resources are available to support the project. It is also important to identify potential barriers to the introduction of the change and to outline strategies to overcome these problems when, and if, they arise. The most significant factor in the successful introduction of a nursing model for clinical practice is for the nursing team to work together throughout the selection, planning, implementation and evaluation stages.

WHAT CRITERIA TO USE?

The question the nursing team may ask is: Why not use one author's criteria for analysing and critiquing a nursing model? Nurses must be mindful that many of the published criteria were for the purpose of objectively delineating whether a nursing conceptual framework could be technically labelled a theory. In addition, although authors use similar criteria, they possess varying levels of complexity. What is required are criteria that possess meaning for the nursing team, criteria that are well defined, allow for comparative analysis, and take into account both subjective and objective processes.

Subjective processes refer to judgements that are personal and individual, and express the thoughts and emotions of a person or group. Meleis (1991) suggests that subjectivity is in evidence when it is difficult for a person to articulate the processes used to arrive at a judgement. *Objective processes* refer to concrete decisions made with the intent of dealing with things external to emotions, thoughts and feelings. An objective decision is one where the arguments can be clearly delineated and can therefore be evaluated by others. Subjective decisions may be combined with objective analysis, because nurses need to be convinced and feel comfortable that the theorist's assumptions and experiential background are congruent with their own thoughts and beliefs. Thus model analysis can be objective, and the decision process subjective (Meleis 1991). Subjectivity is as important as objectivity; however, neither can stand alone as the only process to be used. It is important for practitioners selecting a theory for practice to heed the warning by Meleis that: 'A highly objective decision with low subjectivity could result in theory use that is not true to the theory premises and propositions; and perhaps vice versa' (Meleis 1991, p. 215).

The criteria selected for use in the analysis and critique of theory in this chapter include those common to many of the metatheorists, those extracted from nurses who have previously evaluated models for practice (and elaborated upon), and those deemed relevant to the world view of nursing and health care today. You must be aware that the selection of criteria and the standards used to enable you to make a judgement of the fit between a theory and your practice will ultimately be your choice. What is presented in this chapter is an assortment of criteria that you can extend or delimit; it is not a definitive list of criteria for proving that a theory or model meets a set of prerequisites that enable it to be called 'a theory'.

ANALYSIS OF THEORY

Although a theory is accepted as a whole, it is composed of components which ideally should possess a relationship to one another. It is difficult to determine the true meaning of the theory and the strength of the relationship between the parts unless the theory is systematically examined. Analysis is a technique for separating a whole into its constituent parts in order to identify the essential features and consider the interrelationship of these elements. To do this, a knowledge of what constitutes the parts is needed.

It is only when the process of analysis and description has been completed that a critique of theory can be attempted—that is, where the theory can be evaluated against a number of identified criteria (Meleis 1991; Sims 1991).

COMPONENTS FOR ANALYSIS

Table 7.2 identifies the components to be used in this chapter for analysis of a theory.

TABLE 7.2 COMPONENTS OF THEORY ANALYSIS

COMPONENT DESCRIPTION	
BACKGROUND OF THEORIST	Sociopolitical context of theory development
	Experiential and educational background of the theorist
	Publications
ASSUMPTIONS	Implicit
	Explicit
PURPOSE OF THEORY	Overall
	Specific: descriptive, explanatory, predictive, prescriptive
CONCEPTS	Clarity, conceptual definitions, observable properties, boundaries, abstract/concrete
DEFINITIONS	Implicit
	Explicit
PROPOSITIONS	Types, existence, relationship
METHOD OF THEORY DEVELOPMENT	Inductive
	Deductive
	Retroductive
TYPE OF THEORY	Micro, middle range, grand
CLASSIFICATION OF THEORY	Interactional
	Systems
	Developmental

Background of theorist

As a conceptual model is formulated from the author's personal view of, and assumptions about, the world and nursing, the reconstruction of the sociopolitical context that influenced the theory's development is extremely important. Different theories mirror different realities, reflecting the nursing interests of the time, the sociocultural-political context and the particular scientific paradigm of the day. The first step in this analysis is to undertake a historical journey to expose the happenings in the particular era in which the theory was developed. This may mean using general historical texts as well as historical works in nursing to examine significant events that influenced societal trends, health care and nursing during that particular period.

The second step includes an analysis of the theorist's educational and experiential background and the view of science that surrounded the evolution of the theory. Such an analysis involves examining the theorist's experiential background for clues to experiences that may have stimulated the assumptions and concepts reflected in the theory, and exploring the theorist's educational experiences, including professional and academic networks, to identify the philosophical ideas that contributed to the theorist's view of the world (Fawcett 1989; Chinn & Kramer 1991; Meleis 1991).

As the content of models alters and evolves with changes in society and nursing, it is not unreasonable to find that a model's concepts and propositions are redefined as the theorist accommodates new ideas about health care and nursing (Fawcett 1989). It is important, therefore, to analyse the sociopolitical context that influenced the author's thinking—not just from the model's initial conception but right through to the present conception of the model.

This analysis can be achieved through a review of the references used by the theorist, a review of all his or her available publications and presentations, and a review of all available publications and presentations by other authors who have written about the theorist and the theory (Fawcett 1989; Meleis 1991). What you are setting out to achieve, through the analysis of the theorist's experiential and academic background, is information that can assist in determining whether the world view and philosophical basis of the model in question are relevant to currently dominant world views and philosophies.

Assumptions

The first element in the process of developing a theory is the theorist's identification of her or his own values, beliefs and goals, regarding aspects of person, health, environment, nursing and where nursing occurs. Theorists identify assumptions through reflection on, and analysis of, their values, beliefs and philosophical underpinnings (Meleis 1991). Assumptions 'evolve from a philosophical standpoint, from ideological positions, from ethical considerations, from cultural heritage, from social structure, or from previously tested and supported hypotheses' (Meleis 1991, p. 218). Assumptions are fundamental to theoretical reasoning as they are accepted as given; they are not tested but assumed to represent reality. Theorists accept assumptions as true in order to provide a philosophical framework to guide theory development (Duldt & Giffin 1985; Keck 1989; Chinn & Kramer 1991).

Assumptions can reflect value positions in that they assert or imply what is right, what is good or what ought to be (Chinn & Kramer 1991). The expectation is that assumptions are made explicit by the author, although a theory often contains both explicit and implicit assumptions. *Explicit assumptions* are those clearly identified and labelled by the theorist; they are precise and distinct in expression, and thoroughly formulated and developed, leaving nothing to be implied. *Implicit assumptions* may be central to the development of theoretical propositions but they are inherent, embedded in the writing although not succinctly expressed.

Assumptions should include the author's views about the central and unique concerns of nursing. Uncovering implicit assumptions is extremely important, as they will help you to understand what the theorist regards as valuable, right, wrong or worthwhile. An analysis of assumptions will allow you to make a more objective decision about the consistency of the theorist's beliefs with your own and with those of the nursing profession today.

To uncover implicit assumptions, you need to identify value-laden terms and phrases in definitions and supporting narrative. Ask yourself: What is the author taking for granted as truth or as an accepted value? What are the values the theorist holds true about nursing, health, environment and person? (Chinn & Kramer 1991).

Purpose of theory

Understanding the purpose of a theory is important for clarifying its usefulness for a particular clinical area.

The purpose of a theory, or why the theory has been developed, can be ascertained in terms of the level of theory developed—that is, whether the theorist intended the theory to be *descriptive* (factor isolating), *explanatory* (factor relating), *predictive* (situation relating) or *prescriptive* (situation producing) (Dickoff, James & Wiedenbach 1968; Stevens Barnum 1994).

A theory for the purpose of *description* looks at and identifies the major elements in nursing; it assists therefore in delineating, articulating and labelling concepts in nursing. This level of theory does not attempt to explain why the elements are present, or why and how they relate to each other, but provides clear descriptions of nursing-related phenomena and accurately identifies essential details about each of the variables, in terms that are comprehensible to nurses (Leedy & Pepper 1989; Meleis 1991; Stevens Barnum 1994). *Explanatory* theory, like descriptive theory, describes the concepts, but in addition shows how the concepts relate to one another. Thus, an explanatory theory requires the identification of possible relationships among the concepts but does not show how the concepts can be manipulated (Leedy & Pepper 1989; Meleis 1991; Stevens Barnum 1994). *Predictive* theories deal with cause and effect—that is, they demonstrate that certain conditions lead to others, and detail how interactions among variables can be manipulated in order to bring about change (Stevens Barnum 1994). *Prescriptive* theory is considered by many to be the highest level of theory development and prescribes nursing actions that will bring about desired goals (Dickoff et al. 1968; Meleis 1991).

Knowledge of the level of theory development may not provide sufficient information to enable nurses to make a decision on the congruency of the purpose of the theory to the purpose of their practice. In understanding the purpose of the theory, nurses also need knowledge of the theory's aims and intent. This can be achieved by examining the context and situation in which the theory applies—that is, the theorist's explanation of circumstances in which nursing occurs—and by determining what the theory highlights as nursing concerns related to the individual, family and community (Chinn & Kramer 1991).

A further aspect that will provide information about the purpose of a theory is an analysis of its recommended processes for nursing decision making. This analysis will reveal the role of the nurse as distinct from the role of the patient. *Process* is the way in which the theory advises nurses to demonstrate judgement in systematically applying their body of knowledge to the delivery of nursing care (Buchanan 1987). In examining the process of a theory, look at the theorist's recommendations for the organisation of decision making and the uniform procedures and behaviours suggested for your use when implementing the model in practice—for example, the use of the nursing process, nursing diagnosis and clinical decision making. An understanding of the process of decision making will facilitate your comprehension of the role of the nurse (Buchanan 1987).

Concepts

Concepts are the basic elements, the dimensions, aspects or attributes of nursing reality, that are of interest to the theorist. They are developed from the author's perception of reality and are complex abstractions or mental images of an object, property or event (Hardy 1974; Marriner-Tomey 1989). Concepts could be considered as the bricks that form the foundations on which the theory is constructed. Concepts are therefore labels, categories, or selected properties of objects to be studied.

In the past, concepts have been characterised by a rigid set of conditions, and seen to possess clear and distinct boundaries and some inherent truth value; they were perceived not to change over time or context. The problem with this view is that it presents a static view of the world; in nursing, concepts need to be considered as an abstraction whose attributes appear as a cluster, are continually subject to change and can be evaluated in reference to their resemblance, rather than strict correspondence, to their definition (Rodgers 1989). A dilemma experienced in theories with a high level of theoretical abstraction is the difficulty of relating theoretical concepts to operational phenomena (Hardy 1974).

In any given theory, concepts may be defined both theoretically and operationally. *Theoretical definitions* provide meaning to the terms in context of the theory and allow you to assess the validity of that definition. An *operational definition* shows how the concept is linked to concrete situations, provides a bridge between the theory and the practice environment, and describes a set of physical properties in order to assign a value for practical use of the concept (Hardy 1974).

Further knowledge development may be impeded when theorists are unable to articulate the definition and attributes of their concepts, or describe situations for their appropriate application to the essential tasks of nursing (Rogers 1970).

Concepts must be examined carefully for quantity, character, emerging relationships, and structure (Chinn & Kramer 1991). Concepts can be elicited by searching out words, or groups of words, that represent objects, properties and events in the theory, and then listing key ideas and identifying how they seem to relate to one another (Chinn & Kramer 1991). Chinn and Kramer (1991) suggest that questions you need to answer include the following:

- How many concepts are there?

- How many are major concepts and how many are minor concepts?

- Do the concepts represent abstractions of objects, properties or events?

- Is it possible to identify what they represent?

- What is the relationship between concepts?

- Are the concepts fairly discrete in meaning, or do several have similar meanings?

Definitions

Theorists tend to coin new words and redefine terms when constructing theories. As some terms may be new or used differently from normal, you should expect each concept, new term or derived term to be clearly defined in a way that is comprehensible to you. Definition of words and concepts is an essential component of theory construction, because words and concepts mean different things to different individuals. The potential user of a theory must know the meaning *intended by the theorist* for both words and concepts, in order to understand how the theory relates to practice (Keck 1989).

Many theorists carefully identify their central definitions and present them in a list. However, you will also discover that many meanings are implicit, not labelled as definitions, and are presented as part of the theory; hence they need to be teased out by the reader (Chinn & Kramer 1991). Definitions may also be classified as either denotative or connotative. A *denotative definition* outlines concepts in terms of what the concept represents and points out all those objects to which the term refers (Keck 1989; Stevens Barnum 1994). On the other hand, a *connotative definition* suggests or implies conceptual associations one might make with the concept. Connotative definitions express the characteristics of the object in terms of the meaning and worth bestowed on the object (Keck 1989; Stevens Barnum 1994).

The potential user of nursing theory must be cognisant that there are many abstract concepts in nursing theories for which the formulation of specific definitions is difficult. Nursing theory should not be devalued because of the abstractness of some of the definitions. Chinn and Kramer (1991, p. 113) warn that premature definition of abstract concepts may be counterproductive, as 'an early definition that is broad and non-specific encourages the exploration of many possible meanings' and can contribute to continued nursing knowledge development.

Propositions

Assumptions and concepts form the basis of theory development; however, a theory does not exist until the specific relationships between concepts are expressed (Keck 1989). This relationship is usually expressed in a relationship statement called a *proposition*. Although the word 'proposition' is commonly used in nursing theories, terms like 'propositions', 'hypothesis', 'axioms' and 'laws' can be used with reference to statements which link together and show the relationships between two or more concepts. Although often used in the same way, these terms do have different meanings in their degree of generality and empirical support—that is, they have been found to be an accurate representation of reality. Propositions and hypotheses possess a lower level of generality because they have not been empirically tested. They are, however, invaluable in aiding our understanding of events. Laws and axioms, on the other hand, are on the highest level of generality, have strong empirical support and state a constant relationship between two or more variables (Hardy 1974). The differences between these terms in relation to level of generality and empirical support is depicted in Figure 7.1.

A proposition is a relationship statement possessing a low level of generality and empirical support which provides links among and between two or more concepts. The nature and character of these relationships provide clues to the theoretical purposes and assumptions on which the theory is based. Thus, it is necessary for the nurse to describe

FIGURE 7.1 DIFFERENCES IN TERMS DEFINING THEORETICAL RELATIONSHIPS

LOW ——— LEVEL OF EMPIRICAL SUPPORT ——— HIGH

Propositions ————————————————— Laws

Hypotheses ————————————————— Axioms

LOW ————— LEVEL OF GENERALITY ————HIGH

the type of relationships between the concepts—that is, whether the propositions have the powers of description, explanation or prediction (Meleis 1991).

As a potential user of a theory, you should, therefore, determine whether the relationships are basically descriptive, explanatory or predictive, and whether the relationships are made clear by the author. Chinn & Kramer (1991) advise that, when a relationship is unclear, you should try to infer the possible relationships and their character; your own ideas may provide clues for further development of the theory.

Method of theory development

There are three ways to develop a theory: induction, deduction and retroduction.

Induction is a form of reasoning that proceeds from the specific to the general. Using the inductive method in research involves observing particular events and analysing these as a basis for formulating general theoretical statements—for example, nurses observe similar happenings over a period of time. The next step is the collection and examination of commonalities between these observations (Sims 1991). This exploration will lead to the formulation of theoretical relationships (Marriner-Tomey 1989; Meleis 1991; Sims 1991).

Deduction is a form of logical reasoning that proceeds from general to specific. This process involves a sequence of theoretical statements derived from a few general statements. Two or more relational statements are used to draw conclusions. Abstract theoretical relationships are used to derive specific empirical hypotheses. Evidence is then systematically sought in order to validate or contradict the initial relationships. Such a theory is substantiated if contradictory instances cannot be found (Sims 1991).

Retroduction combines induction and deduction (Marriner-Tomey 1989). According to Fawcett (1984), retroduction included a series of observations thought to be related (induction), searching for regularities of observations, deriving theoretical statements (deduction), and verifying hypothesised relationships other than those in which they were induced.

Types of theory

Theories differ in complexity and scope along a continuum from grand theories to micro theories (Table 7.3) (Keck 1989).

Micro theories are the least complex theories, dealing with a small number of variables and referring to specific, narrowly defined phenomena. Consisting of theoretical statements, micro theories are narrow in scope because they attempt to explain a small aspect of reality (Keck 1989; Marriner-Tomey 1989).

TABLE 7.3 TYPES OF THEORY

GRAND THEORY	MIDDLE-RANGE THEORY	MICRO THEORY
Broad in scope and complexity	Narrower in focus than grand theory	Specific focus—a set of theoretical statements
Requires further clarification	Most concepts and relationships clearly defined	Usually existence of hypothesis—clear links shown between concepts
Theoretical framework at general level of abstraction	Easier to link to reality than grand theory	Deals with narrowly defined phenomena
Difficult to link to reality	Can be used to explain complex life situations	Easy to apply to small units of reality
Contains summative concepts	Broader than micro theory	Narrower than both grand and middle-range theories

Middle-range theories are more complex than micro theories and present more variables for consideration (Keck 1989; Hardy 1990). Middle-range theories are primarily composed of relational concepts and possess greater scope than micro theories; they are not as abstract as grand theories and can be used to explain complex life situations. Middle-range theories consider a limited number of variables, possess a substantive focus, are more susceptible to empirical testing than grand theories, and can be consolidated into more wide-ranging theories (Meleis 1991).

Grand theories are the most complicated of the three types. They are broad in scope and complexity and attempt to explain everything surrounding a broad set of phenomena within a discipline. Grand theories state their theoretical formulations at a most general level of abstraction, which is why it is often difficult to link their propositions to practice. Grand theories contain summative concepts that incorporate numerous micro theories; in most instances, therefore, grand theories require further specification of theoretical statements for them to be empirically tested and theoretically verified (Keck 1989; Marriner-Tomey 1989). Figure 7.2 depicts the continuum of theories with respect to the criterion of abstraction.

CRITIQUE

Once the theory has been analysed a judgement can be made concerning its logical development and its relationship to the world of nursing. A critique consists of setting criteria in order to facilitate a critical examination and a judgement about how well a theory meets set standards and its stated purpose. The aim of a critique is to determine how adequately a theory meets criteria requirements and by this examination to highlight its merits, shortcomings and limitations (Chinn & Jacobs 1987; Meleis 1991; Stevens Barnum 1994). Critique can be further subdivided into internal and external (see Table 7.4). *Internal critique* evaluates the extent to which the theory components fit with each other and thus allows a judgement to be made about the soundness of theoretical

FIGURE 7.2 CLASSIFICATION OF THEORY

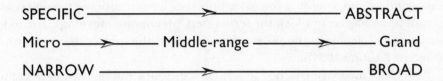

development (Chinn & Jacobs 1987). Internal critique will help you to understand the approaches used in theory development, and to determine whether those approaches are appropriate to the theory. This internal evaluation will also show strengths in theory development and will assist in delineating gaps in the theory. *External critique* evaluates the way that theory relates to the world to nursing's function in the world today (Stevens Barnum 1994). External critique could be said to contain a component of subjectivity in that some of the judgements can be derived from your own values about what the theory ought to achieve (Chinn & Jacobs 1987).

TABLE 7.4 GUIDELINES FOR CRITIQUE OF NURSING THEORY

INTERNAL CRITIQUE	EXTERNAL CRITIQUE
■ Clarity	■ Reality convergence
■ Generality	■ Cultural considerations
■ Simplicity	■ Utility
■ Consistency	■ Relationship to professional clinical practice, nursing education, research and administration
■ Adequacy	
■ Logical development	■ Ethical considerations
■ Level of theory development	■ Legal considerations
■ Empirical precision	■ Significance
	■ Capacity for discrimination
	■ Scope of theory
	■ Circle of contagiousness

INTERNAL CRITIQUE

Clarity

Clarity is the state or quality of being clear as perceived by the mind, and thus free of ambiguity or confusion (Kellerman 1973). In nursing theories clarity 'denotes precision of boundaries, a communication of a sense of orderliness, vividness of meaning, and a consistency throughout theory' (Meleis 1991, p. 231).

A nursing theory should possess both semantic (relating to the meaning of the language) and structural clarity. A theory should be presented in a way that you can easily understand, enabling you to identify the characteristics of the object and to point out all those objects to which the term refers (denotative meaning), and to identify the nuances of meaning and worth bestowed on the object (connotative meaning) (Stevens Barnum 1994).

Ask if the theory is 'couched in terminology which can be used meaningfully with, or applied to, phenomena observed in nursing?' (Ellis 1968, p. 221). This is an important question; frequently, theorists use terms borrowed from other disciplines and, although these may be 'expressive, descriptive and serve as a useful label for the phenomena, they may have lost their terminological meaning' (Ellis 1968, p. 221)—that is, the meaning initially intended for the term. Borrowed words should be carefully and cautiously defined, because words have multiple and competing meanings across disciplines and it is easy for clarity to be obscured. Theorists also coin words that are unique to their theory, and you need to assess whether these words enhance or impede the clarity of meaning (Chinn & Jacobs 1991). If new words and borrowed words are not clearly defined, you may be left to construct your own meanings, which may compete with those intended by the theorist (Chinn & Jacobs 1991).

In examining structural clarity, the aim is to ascertain whether the major concepts, subconcepts, assumptions, propositions, purpose and context of the theory are clearly expressed (Meleis 1991).

A model, or schema, may be used by the theorist as a visual description of the relationship between concepts. A *schema* allows the writer to express, by a combination of diagrams and words, the precise relationship between the main components. The diagrams used should be self-explanatory, enabling you to grasp the key points and see the relationship between them clearly. If schema, diagrams, tables and/or charts are used, you must evaluate whether they reflect the writing, whether they are clear and, ultimately, whether they enhance or impede your understanding of the theory.

The criterion of clarity varies within a range from high clarity to low clarity. To be able to make a final judgement, you should answer the following questions:

- Are sentences clear and meaningful?

- Are the basic terms clearly described?

- Can you identify the characteristics of the central concepts (denotative meaning)?

- Can you identify the nuances of meaning and worth bestowed on central concepts (connotative meaning)?

- If schema, diagrams, tables and/or charts are used, are they clearly presented and do they reflect the writing?

- Does the theory possess structural clarity?

- Is the context of the theory clearly identifiable?

- Is the theory presented in such a way that it is easily understood?

Generality

Generality is the state of being common to many situations and contexts, although not universal; it is not specialised and not limited to a precise application; it is applied to main elements or features rather than details or exceptions (Kellerman 1973). Hardy (1974) indicates that the more general a theory is, the more useful it will be in practice.

To determine generality, examine the scope of concepts and goals within the theory. A theory possesses generality when the concepts and goals are broad and non-specific and when empirical facts and situations to which the theory applies are not limited (Chinn & Jacobs 1987). Generality is often reflected in the scope of the theory, and assessed by inspecting the scope of the concepts and the propositions within a theory. In determining whether the theory is specific or general, you need to ascertain the groups to which the theory is directed. Does the theory apply to all health care professionals or just to nurses? Does it apply to nurses specialising in specific areas, or to all nurses independent of specialisation? Is it designed for specific classifications of patients, or for all patients? (Chinn & Jacobs 1987).

Simplicity

The criterion of simplicity refers to a theory which is not composed of many parts, and is not complex; it describes a theory that concentrates on fewer concepts. Debate exists as to whether simplicity is desirable for a nursing theory. Chinn & Jacobs (1987) state that practitioners need simple theory to guide practice, whereas Meleis (1991) suggests that, although simplicity may enhance utility, there must exist a balance between simplicity and complexity as nursing is a complex discipline. To achieve this balance, nursing theory should be comprehensive and concrete; without a degree of complexity, nursing theory would not possess significance (Ellis 1968; Argyris & Schön 1974; Meleis 1991).

Simplicity could be linked to the 'type of theory' in that Meleis (1991, p. 232) states that 'the more phenomena the theory considers the more potential relationships it can generate and the more complex the theory'. According to this statement, a micro theory should be considered to possess greater simplicity and a grand theory the greatest complexity. Simplicity can be ascertained by noting the number of concepts and the number of conceptual relationships. A large number of concepts and interrelated statements is indicative of complexity (Chinn & Jacobs 1987).

Complexity exists when a theory considers multiple variables or relationships, or the complexity of a single variable (Ellis 1968). The criterion of complexity may be seen as opposing simplicity and parsimony. Although parsimony is sometimes used synonymously with simplicity, if refers to a theory which seems to possess simplicity but which is generalisable in that it accounts for a broad range of phenomena (Chinn & Jacobs 1987). The argument for complexity in a theory is that it allows for explanation and interrelationship of more variables and enables a theory to account for the richness of its subject matter (Stevens Barnum 1994).

Consistency

The criterion of consistency refers to the coherence, congruity and agreement between the different components of the theory. In judging the consistency of the theory, you should examine the descriptions of each component of the theory and ask if there are any inconsistencies within, as well as between, these components (Chinn & Jacobs 1987).

Internal consistency examines whether components and concepts are defined and used consistently throughout the theory (Meleis 1991).

To satisfy the criterion of consistency, you should expect that terms will always be used in the same way and possess the same meaning throughout the theory. You are advised to search for simple shifts in the meaning of a term to determine any inconsistency (Stevens Barnum 1994). To maintain consistency, basic assumptions should be consistent with the goals of the theory and with other components, such as structure or relationships. Where the author makes use of diagrams, charts or examples of how to apply the theory to practice, you should examine the consistency between these and the theoretical narrative (Chinn & Jacobs 1987).

Adequacy

Adequacy indicates whether a theory is sufficient for a particular purpose. The purpose of nursing theory is to assist nurses to implement processes that ensure that desired outcomes are achieved. The usefulness of a theory (pragmatic adequacy) in achieving these outcomes is of major importance. The narrative of the theory will inform you of the anticipated outcomes and types of clients and processes. The adequacy of a theory is not related to the type of theory, for a theory is adequate if it carefully accounts for the subject matter claimed by the theorist, however broad or limited the subject matter may be (Stevens Barnum 1994). Thus a theory possesses adequacy if it is extensive enough to deal with the scope and subject matter claimed by the author.

Logical development

A theory should be logically developed and its structure based on well-researched premises. Stevens Barnum (1994, p. 90) states that the criterion of logical development requires that a 'theory develops naturally from its premises, that its propositions follow from application of the rules of logic, and that any assertion or conclusion flows reasonably from the groundwork laid for the assertion'. Logical development is judged on whether a conclusion is based on the reasoning that has preceded it, and not on whether the given premises or conclusions are themselves true (Stevens Barnum 1994). Thus, the logical development of a theory refers to the validity of its arguments. Further, if a theory is logically developed, you should not have to furnish missing links in the argument in order to arrive at the same conclusion as the theorist (Stevens Barnum 1994).

Level of theory development

The ultimate aim of any theory is to reach the stage of development in which it allows for purposeful nursing interventions leading to highly predictive patient outcomes (Hardy 1974; Chinn & Jacobs 1987; Meleis 1991; Stevens Barnum 1994). Stevens Barnum (1994) reminds us that, at its conception, every theory commences with the descriptive naming of its elements. She therefore suggests that it is important not to discard a theory just because it is at a descriptive phase of development, for it may possess more potential for future evolution of knowledge than another theory already in a prescriptive or a predictive phase of development.

Empirical precision

The criterion of empirical precision refers to the extent that the defined concepts are grounded in observable reality; this criterion thus examines the degree of agreement between a particular theory and objective empirical data. Empirical precision is related to the testability of a theory; if research, theory and practice are to be meaningfully related, then theory in nursing should lend itself to research testing, and knowledge developed through this testing should guide practice (Chinn & Jacobs 1987; Marriner-Tomey 1989).

EXTERNAL CRITIQUE

Reality convergence

The criterion of reality convergence examines how well a particular theory reflects the real world of nursing and health care. It can be considered from three perspectives—in terms of interpretation, principle and method.

With respect to interpretation, Meleis (1991) puts forward two questions to ascertain whether the beliefs, values and expectations of the model converge with the beliefs, values and expectations of the different societies and cultures within the world in which nurses practise. Is the role of nurses as portrayed by the model congruent with the role of nurses as perceived by society? Are the actions and outcomes suggested by the model congruent with societal expectations of nursing today?

You might assume that the answers to these questions must be positive; remember, however, that models might lead to nursing activities that are not congruent with society's expectations and, thus, society's expectations may need to change. An example of a theory requiring societal change was Orem's Theory of Self-care which was introduced at a time when consumers and nurses expected the patient to be dependent on nurses and the health care system.

You should also examine how the theory may be interpreted by nurses and other health professionals. Try to determine whether the values and beliefs encompassed by the theory are compatible with the values of nurses and other health professionals. This component of evaluation is important as awareness of competing or complementary value systems enhances the potential for collaborative work relationships and quality of patient care (Meleis 1991).

The reality convergence of a theory, in relation to principles, pertains to your acceptance or rejection of the basic premises of the theory and the method used in theory development (Stevens Barnum 1994). In the past, for example, scholars might reject a theory if its method did not readily lend itself to scientific research (Stevens Barnum 1994).

An examination of the criterion of reality convergence will help you to identify the *degree* of reality convergence in the theory, and also whether any societal education or societal change is required. It will allow nurses to judge whether such changes would be appropriate and warranted with respect to the health care needs of the world today.

Cultural considerations

Conceptual frameworks that recognise and incorporate cultural diversity are required for practice. The work of Leininger (1991) stresses the importance of nurses recognising the influence of culture on people's lives and their health status. Although Australia is a nation of cultural and linguistic diversity, at the present time nursing is dominated by a monocultural, Anglo-Australian approach. What is required is a nursing model to uphold a transcultural world view of nursing. A nursing model is needed which will facilitate the empowerment of individuals in the health care system by the promotion of a culturally sensitive approach to nursing care. It is only through the use of a model which provides a transcultural world view of nursing that individual health care needs can be identified. In response to these needs, nurses promote health, prevent illness and secure recovery from illness for their clients (Kanitsaki 1988).

You must evaluate a theory to determine whether it has the potential for developing in nurses a sensitivity to the cultural factors integral to their clients' care (Stevens Barnum 1994).

Utility

The criterion of utility requires that a nursing theory possess the potential for utility in clinical practice, education, research and administration (Meleis 1991; Stevens Barnum 1994). In order to be usable, or potentially usable, the theory's selected concepts must be pragmatic and the theory must include explicit rules and direction for research, clinical practice, education and administration (Ellis 1968). Utility is a prime characteristic in determining the significance of theories for nursing practice; even if theories possess significance by other criteria, they are not significant for nursing practice if they fail in their usefulness for developing or guiding practice (Ellis 1968).

To be able to be operationalised in clinical practice, the theory should:

- be generalisable, cost-effective and pragmatic;

- possess a framework which clearly shows how nurses are to view persons, health, nursing and the environment;

- clearly show the relationship within and between the above components;

- provide guidelines for clinical decision making with respect to assessment planning, implementation and evaluation;

- assist nurses to recognise that a nursing problem exists, and provide guidelines for prescribing and executing a course of action that achieves specified outcomes;

- provide guidelines for structuring nurses' work;

- show the relationship between nurses' work and that of other health care professionals.

(Meleis 1991; Stevens Barnum 1994)

To be useful in nursing education, a nursing model should provide a framework that helps to construct a curriculum appropriate to the health care needs of people and the philosophy of the nursing profession today. Although Stevens Barnum (1994) suggests that to be useful in nursing education a theory must suggest appropriate teaching methods, Meleis (1991) argues that this goal may not be feasible. Theories about teaching and learning, about the learner and about the educational environment will be required to complement nursing models.

Meleis (1991) suggests that for theories to be of utility in nursing administration they should be able to guide the organisation and delivery of nursing service. In addition, the use of theory in nursing administration should assist in clearly articulating nursing's role and contribution to the organisation's mission and goals (Allison et al. 1991). You must be aware, however, that organisational and managerial theories will be required to complement existing nursing models.

One of the aims of theory is to stimulate and guide research and, thereby, increase the knowledge of the profession. As Meleis (1991) suggests, this implies that theoretical evaluation should include testability which, in turn, implies the existence of observable or testable data. In determining the theory's potential to stimulate research, you should examine the literature to find whether or not research has been conducted using the theory, by the theorist or others. Examine, too, the research designs used to assess the degree to which they are congruent with research methods prevalent in nursing today.

Ethical considerations

Fawcett (1989) believes that nursing practice that is not theoretically sound could be ethically questionable.

Ethics puts forward the moral basis of theory and is concerned with values and value conflicts arising out of nursing practice and research (Yeo 1989). Nursing theories make assumptions about value issues in nursing and about nursing decisions, although often these are not explicitly identified as ethical issues (Yeo 1989). In determining whether a theory meets the needs of nursing in respect of ethical considerations, it is important to examine the way in which the theory promotes the concepts of patient autonomy, nursing autonomy, advocacy and paternalism (Yeo 1989).

Although there are relatively few theories that permit the professional to control phenomena, the future development of prescriptive theories is likely to increase. The ethics of using an essentially paternalistic approach which recommends control of personal behaviour should be examined in some detail (Hardy 1974). One of the ethical problems to be considered in using a prescriptive model in practice is that nurses may be uncomfortable with diagnosing and trying to control human beings and their experiences (Nagle & Mitchell 1991). You should also question whether control and manipulation are ethically sound in a profession that promotes collaborative decision making with clients. With the increased pressure for nurses to construct prescriptive theory, nurses may 'find themselves in situations where they are forced to practice according to values and beliefs that are incongruent with their personal and ethical standards' (Nagle & Mitchell 1991, p. 21). This could result in moral conflict for nurses who believe that every human being is a unique, dynamic entity rather than a sum of passive parts to be manipulated and controlled (Nagle & Mitchell 1991).

Legal considerations

A model is appropriate for use in practice if the roles of the nurse and the required nursing actions specified by the model are in harmony with licensure, accreditation, and institutional policies and procedures (Gruending 1985). Nursing theory purports to help delineate professional standards of practice, and professional autonomy is intrinsically linked to standards of practice (Gruending 1985). Nursing theory provides a focus to assist in the development of standards of practice; these standards are linked to Nursing Acts concerned with licensure, accreditation, certification requirements, and institutional policies and procedures; it could, therefore, be assumed that models have the potential to increase professional autonomy—that is, the freedom to make decisions and to control important aspects of nurses' work (Buchanan 1987). A model that is regarded as meeting legal considerations should allow for the application of those elements of law that provide direction for responsible nursing conduct during assessment, decision making, and intervention. A model which meets these elements ultimately translates into safe, effective nursing practice (Buchanan 1987).

Significance

To be judged as meeting the criterion of significance a theory should lead to nursing actions that make important differences and have significant positive impact on a person's well-being. According to Stevens Barnum, a theory meets the criterion of significance if it:

- addresses essential, not peripheral issues in nursing; and
- contributes to the development of nursing knowledge.

(1994, p. 95)

A theory is significant if it is capable of generating many hypotheses or researchable questions which could contribute to an understanding of the essential phenomena in nursing and further the development of nursing knowledge (Ellis 1968). Meleis (1991) also reminds nursing, as a profession, not to neglect the significance of its practice to humanity and society and, in relation to significance, to evaluate the benefit of the theory with respect to its impact on clients and other health care professionals.

Capacity for discrimination

A nursing theory should differentiate nursing from other health professions on the one hand and from other care-tending acts on the other (Stevens Barnum 1994). The important points in assessing capacity for discrimination are that the theory:

- explains role differences;
- highlights the essential decision-making role of the nurse;
- presents precise and clear boundaries between the roles of professional groups; and
- discriminates nursing practice through the development of concepts unique to nursing.

(Stevens Barnum 1994)

To make sense of the criterion of capacity for discrimination it must be remembered that nursing is a dynamic discipline in constant interaction with other disciplines; relationships or boundaries between disciplines may therefore not be clear or there may be an overlap between these boundaries.

Nurses throughout history have taken on the roles of other professionals as demand has dictated, or as roles were delegated by other professionals. Nurses, for example, may assume roles or functions traditionally carried out by medical staff when they are absent; thus the boundaries between nursing and medicine may be a source of conflict and confusion. To be able to discuss professional boundaries it is important not to confuse the task or function with the role of decision making. The boundary of a role is delineated by the decisions that can be made within the role, and not by the tasks and functions associated with the role. For nurses to be able to examine the decisions considered by them to be legitimately encompassed by their role, there must also be an examination of the decisions made by other health care professionals with whom they interact.

Scope of theory

The scope of a theory refers to the extent of application, operation or effectiveness and the breadth or range of phenomena in nursing to which the theory applies. A theory possesses scope when it:

- relates to a number and variety of concepts;

- encompasses both biological and behavioural observations;

- explains the relationships among and between concepts in terms of the generalisations pertinent to the patient's state of health; and

- provides a potential framework for ordering observations about a range of phenomena.

(Ellis 1968)

There are diverse points of view concerning the appropriate scope of theories in nursing. Jacob states that there is no pressing need to develop a grand theory; rather, theory-building efforts should focus on developing middle-range theories (Ellis 1968). In contrast, Chinn and Kramer (1991) believe that nurses should aim for theories that are broad in scope and achieve this by combining narrower theories or by initially formulating broad theory. The most appropriate answer to the question of scope is for you to recognise that theories of both broad and limited scope are needed. Theories with wider and broader scope tend to be more general and last longer, but nurses should be aware that the level of abstraction of these theories will make them more difficult to apply to practice. The broader the scope, in terms of the number of related concepts, the greater the significance of the theory (Ellis 1968).

Circle of contagiousness

Contagiousness is defined as the transmission of influence to the mind of others, communicated by contact (Kellerman 1973). Meleis coined the phrase and uses the criterion *circle of contagiousness* to help in the assessment of the theory's more general influence. Meleis uses geographical location and type of institution as units of analysis. In her explanation of the criterion, she suggests that it is usual, and often expected, that theories of nursing will be utilised within the geographical area in which they emerged. However, when the theory begins to influence theory and practice in more distant locations it is considered to be (relatively) contagious. This is a descriptive variable in a critique and will certainly help you to understand more about who is using the theory for practice and research. Be aware, however, that this criterion could be relabelled 'popularity', and the fact that something is popular does not necessarily mean it is the best model for every situation.

Evaluation

The last component of any analysis and critique is to arrange findings in an order that enables judgements to be made. Judgements can only be made after the criteria to be used are further defined with respect to findings from the analysis of practice. The intent of this is to provide standards for each criterion which are congruent with the model requirements of the clinical area in question. In this way, the criteria discussed in this chapter can be individualised to the particular needs of the clinical unit. Judgements can then be made as to the applicability of the model for practice, by providing an overview of the positive and negative aspects of the critique.

SUMMARY

This chapter has put forward suggestions for combining criteria and processes to be used in selecting a theory for clinical practice. The processes discussed as essential to the selection of a theory for practice are the involvement of clinicians in the selection process, an analysis of practice, and an analysis and critique of the theory or theories in question.

The involvement of clinical, academic and administrative nursing staff in selecting a practice model is strongly recommended. This collaborative partnership will ensure that nurses will be in a better position to articulate their practice needs, evaluate suitable models and justify the implementation of models into practice.

GLOSSARY

Metaparadigm: represents and serves as a global perspective, a total world view which is held by the majority of members of a discipline; provides a model for reality and a total view of the discipline.

Metaparadigm concepts: concepts which are central to the discipline of nursing. Currently outlined as the *person* receiving nursing, the *environment* within which the person exists, the *health* state of the person and *nursing*.

Metatheorist: distinguished authors who discuss, analyse and critique theory development—for example Meleis, Stevens Barnum, Chinn and Jacobs, Fawcett.

QUESTIONS

1   At the beginning of this chapter, the discussion concentrated mainly on the benefits of using models in practice. On the other hand, Birx (1993) suggests that some models could limit nurses' initiative in the provision of care and decrease the potential for further knowledge development. Undertake a literature review in order to discuss what you believe to be some of the problems associated with the introduction of nursing models into practice.

2   Write down your beliefs about nursing, people, environment and health. Think about what changes would be necessary if all staff were to use your beliefs as part of their philosophy. If this philosophy were used by all nursing staff, do you think there would be any improvements in the provision of nursing care? Describe the potential improvements.

LEARNING ACTIVITIES

1 Develop your own model of how you could portray the relationship between the territories of nursing and other professionals.

2 Choose an article which discusses the implementation of a model of nursing into clinical practice. First, identify the criteria the authors used in model selection. Second, identify the processes they used in model selection. Third, examine the appropriateness of the criteria and processes used. Give reasons for your findings, and suggest alternative criteria and processes they could have used.

FURTHER READING

Allison S.E., McLaughlin K. & Walker, D. 1991, 'Nursing theory: A tool to put nursing back into administration', *Nursing Administration Quarterly*, 15(3), pp. 72–8. An excellent article which examines the link between nursing administration and the use of nursing theory in a health care organisation. It uses the example of Orem's theory to show how administrators can structure nursing practice and make explicit nursing's role and contribution to the mission and goals of an organisation.

Field, P.A. 1987, 'The impact of nursing theory on the clinical decision making process', *Journal of Advanced Nursing*, 12, pp. 563–71. A very important article in light of the current focus on the development of clinical reasoning skills in nursing. Field explicates the role of nursing models in fostering nurses' decision making and discusses how nurses can be helped to translate clinical decisions into practice through the use of nursing theory.

Kanitsaki, O. 1988, 'Transcultural nursing: Challenge to change', *The Australian Journal of Advanced Nursing*, 5(3), pp. 4–11. An article that is extremely relevant for nurses looking at selecting a theory for practice as it analyses cross-cultural differences and the potential for value conflict in health care contexts. It provides ways in which nurses could be better prepared to adopt transcultural approaches to nursing practice.

Meleis, A.I. 1991, *Theoretical Nursing: Development and Progress*, 2nd edn, J.B. Lippincott Co., Philadelphia. This text assists in demystifying nursing theory. It contains a synthesis of the historical development of nursing theory and of the analysis and critique of theory. This is one of the most substantiative texts for students studying, analysing or developing nursing theory.

Rodgers, B.L. 1989, 'Concepts, analysis and development of nursing knowledge: The evolutionary cycle', *Journal of Advanced Nursing*, 14, pp. 330–35. This article provides interesting and relevant reading for students at both undergraduate and postgraduate levels. Rodgers provides a discursive definition of the relationship of concepts in nursing, discusses the relevance of concept development to the future of nursing knowledge and provides a framework to assist nurses in the explication, exploration and development of concepts relevant to nursing.

Stevens Barnum, B. 1994, *Nursing Theory: Analysis, Application and Evaluation*, 4th edn, J.B. Lippincott Co., Philadelphia. Written by a renowned metatheorist, Stevens Barnum's book is a must for nurses at both undergraduate and postgraduate level. This text provides a framework to assist students to learn the skills necessary to understand, analyse and evaluate nursing theory. The text also includes chapters on holistic and new age theories and captures new trends in nursing.

8

OREM'S SELF-CARE MODEL IN DIABETES HEALTH CARE

An Exemplar

MERILYN KING AND LYN GREEN

In memory of Madeleine who valued the dignity of self-care all the days of her life.

LEARNING OBJECTIVES

When you have read this chapter you should be able to:

1 Discuss the multidisciplinary nature of diabetes health care.

2 Identify the advantages and disadvantages of using nursing theory/models to guide practice.

3 Discuss how Orem's Self-care Model might be used in diabetes nursing practice.

Merilyn King, RGN, RM, MEdStds, is currently a Lecturer in Nursing at The Flinders University, Adelaide. Her background includes acute care nursing (in particular, orthopaedic and diabetes nursing), management, nurse education and midwifery. Merilyn presently teaches both undergraduate and postgraduate nursing courses in a range of clinical and theoretical nursing topics, for example, nursing practice, the development of knowledge and theory, and nursing research. As a contribution to clinical practice, Merilyn also coordinates the Diabetes Educators course, a continuing education program for health professionals employed in the area of diabetes health care.

Lyn Green, RGN, BN, DipAppSc, has worked as a clinical nurse in endocrinology and a clinical nurse consultant in hepatobiliary and pancreatic surgery. She is currently a clinical nurse consultant in diabetes education. Her principal areas of interest in nursing are the effect of psychosocial factors on diabetes management, wound healing and diabetes, team building and team work, and management of hypoglycaemia in the clinical setting.

INTRODUCTION

Self-care and **empowerment** are currently two important concepts being promoted in modern health care. Orem describes self-care as a deliberate action taken by mature and maturing people to maintain life, health and well-being. However, not all individuals are able to care for themselves—infants, children, the aged, the ill and the disabled. These individuals require complete care or assistance with self-care activities from responsible carers (Orem 1991, p. 117).

Client empowerment is facilitated through an educative process. The aim is to equip people with the relevant knowledge and skills to enable them to make informed decisions about their health and manage their own health care requirements.

Self-care and empowerment are also important concepts in contemporary diabetes nursing, and one of the ways that both concepts can be promoted by the diabetes nurse educator (DNE) is by using an appropriate nursing model to guide nursing practice. It is the purpose of this chapter to discuss how self-care and empowerment can be facilitated by using Orem's self-care deficit theory to guide diabetes nursing practice. This will entail some introductory material on diabetes mellitus and its effect on lifestyle, some notes on diabetes nursing, and a brief discussion of nursing models in general, and self-care models in particular. It will also entail a description of a South Australian diabetes care facility and the various responsibilities of the health practitioners employed in it. Lastly, it will entail an examination of the utility of Orem's theory to diabetic nursing practice in this care facility.

DIABETES MELLITUS

Diabetes mellitus is a complex metabolic disease that occurs in the body through an insufficient or total lack of insulin production by the pancreas. There are two types of diabetes mellitus—Type 1 (Insulin Dependent Diabetes Mellitus, known as IDDM) and Type 2 (Non Insulin Dependent Diabetes Mellitus, known as NIDDM) (Tattersall & Gale 1990; Haire-Joshu 1992).

Diabetes is regarded as a major health problem and 3 per cent of the Australian population are affected by the condition (Stepanas 1991). The disease is characterised by the disruption of normal carbohydrate, fat and protein metabolism and the development over time of microvascular and macrovascular complications and neuropathies (Cassmeyer 1987).

EFFECT OF DIABETES ON LIFESTYLE

Diabetic experts agree that there is overwhelming evidence that hyperglycaemia is the main factor in the genesis and progression of microvascular and macrovascular disease. The main tissues that are affected are the eyes, nerves, kidneys, heart and blood vessels (Tattersall & Gale 1990; Haire-Joshu 1992; Hillson 1992, 1994). Common complications that may occur are cataracts and diabetic retinopathy, loss of sensation or numbness in the hands or feet, impaired renal function, urinary tract and vaginal infection and, claudication, angina and hypertension.

Clearly, these pathological changes will impact on the lifestyle of the individual with diabetes. However, recent research indicates that complications associated with diabetes are significantly reduced in people with Type 1 diabetes (IDDM) who consistently follow the recommended medical regime for diabetes management (Diabetes Control and Complications Trial Research Group 1993). To achieve this positive outcome, people with diabetes need to be educated about the management of their condition, taught how to care for themselves and encouraged to take responsibility for their own health care.

THE DIABETES NURSE EDUCATOR

The diabetes nurse educator (DNE) plays a significant role in the health education of clients (the term used to designate people with diabetes and their significant others). It is the responsibility of this health professional to teach clients how to care for themselves on a daily basis (i.e. to self-care), how to solve health problems associated with diabetes and how to make decisions related to their health. The main aim behind diabetes nursing practice is to empower clients to make informed decisions about the management of their condition and, in so doing, assume responsibility for their own health care (Australian Diabetes Educators Association 1989). Thus, self-care and empowerment are two important concepts in contemporary diabetes nursing; these concepts will be discussed later in this the chapter.

Understandably, as a member of the diabetes health team, the DNE is always seeking ways to improve the standard of nursing services in some tangible way. One means of achieving this is through the use of a contemporary nursing model that provides guidelines to inform practice.

NURSING MODELS

Marriner-Tomey (1989, p. 21) defines a model as 'a schematic representation of some aspects of reality'; a more simple explanation of a nursing model, however, is suggested by Pearson and Vaughan (1986, p. 23). In their book entitled *Nursing Models for Practice*, the authors present a pictorial example of a nurse using a biophysical model of nursing that focuses on a hierarchy of nursing tasks. In an ascending order of importance is the 'emotional care' given by the nurse to the patient, 'the cleaning of sluices', 'baths and bedmaking', 'drugs and dressings' and, finally, the most important task, 'to carry out the orders of the doctor'.

Pearson and Vaughan's example represents their perspective on nursing reality—that is, the most important function of the nurse, according to the biophysical model, is to carry out the orders of a physician, and the least important is to address the emotional needs of patients (Pearson & Vaughan 1986).

Pearson and Vaughan believe that a nursing model has three basic components:

1 The beliefs and values on which the model is based.

2 The goals of practice or what the practitioner aims to achieve.

3 The knowledge and skills the practitioner needs to develop in order to gain these goals.

(Pearson & Vaughan 1986, p. 11).

They further state that these three components need to be considered before selecting a nursing model for use in practice (Pearson & Vaughan 1986, pp. 155–65).

Support for the use of nursing models to guide practice is well documented in the nursing literature. Examples of their use are King's model in gerontological nursing practice (Jonas 1987), Orem's Self-care Theory in preventative, home and long-term care (McWilliams, Murphy & Sobiski 1988), and Roy's adaptation model in oncology nursing (Samarell & Fawcett 1992) and chronic illness (Pollock 1993).

Of particular interest to the DNE is the fact that several nurse researchers have found Orem's Self-care Model to be credible and useful in diabetes nursing practice (Frey & Denyes 1989; Mulkeen 1989; Keohane & Lacey 1991; Smits & Kee 1992; Estes & Hart 1993). In a study on adolescent clients with Type 1 diabetes, Frey and Denyes (1989) confirmed the credibility of Orem's theory—that is, they found that self-care actions are necessary to meet requirements related to health (universal self-care) and illness (health-deviation self-care). In addition, Smits and Kee (1992) found that there was a relationship between **self-concept** and self-care among independent elderly individuals with diabetes who resided in the community.

Mulkeen (1989) and Keohane and Lacey (1991) reported that Orem's Self-care Model could be used effectively to teach nursing students and clients about diabetes health care. Mulkeen (1989) used Orem's Self-care Model to teach a student district nurse and a newly diagnosed diabetic patient about self-care. The model enabled the teacher to assess the learning needs of both individuals and then to plan and evaluate the aims and objectives of the teaching session.

Keohane and Lacey (1991) reported the successful use of a Structured Teaching Plan (STP) that was based on a framework devised by Fitzgerald (1980) but adapted from Orem's Self-care Model. The STP promoted the use of Orem's 'supportive-educative system' and it was used to teach staff nurses how to educate women with gestational diabetes (Keohane & Lacey 1991, p. 189).

Lastly, Estes and Hart adapted Orem's Self-care Model to form a framework that would predict the health promotion needs of adolescents. This innovation was found to be particularly useful by the authors because it enabled the Clinical Nurse Specialist not only to predict, but also to recognise and meet adolescent health care needs (Estes & Hart 1993).

Pearson and Vaughan (1986) also advocate the use of nursing models to guide practice because they believe that models:

1 lead to consistency in the sort of care received by patients and thus to a continuity of care patterns and treatments;

2 give rise to less conflict within the team of nurses as a whole;

3 make sense of the nursing given by the team; the other health care workers involved, such as doctors, physiotherapists and ancillary staff, will understand better the logic behind the care;

4 give direction to nursing care within the area, since the goals of nursing work will be understood by the whole team;

5 act as a major guide in decision- and policy-making because the components of the model chosen can act as a guide against which to check decisions;

6 act as a guide for the criteria on which new team members are selected.
(Pearson & Vaughan 1986, p. 5)

To illustrate the significance of the points raised by Pearson and Vaughan (1986), it is useful to give an example from diabetes nursing practice. For instance, if the DNE decided to adopt Orem's Self-care Model to guide practice in the Diabetes Centre, then the nursing goal would be to assist clients to self-care, whenever possible. Using Orem's model, the DNE would concentrate on helping clients to do things for themselves, rather than just doing everything for them. This would be clearly understood by all the other members of the multidisciplinary team. Thus, even when a client was not able to be independent, the multidisciplinary team would understand that the DNE or another carer would perform the required self-care until such time as the client was able to assume responsibility for his or her own self-care.

Similarly, when using this model to guide practice, each DNE in the same team, or working from the same diabetes centre, would value knowledge and skills related to promoting self-care, and they would all work towards their clients achieving this important health outcome. As a result, there would be minimal conflict between the nurses over the type of care the client should receive because the goal of nursing is to promote in clients self-care and independence, not dependence. Other advantages of using Orem's Self-care Model within diabetes care are that the outcomes of diabetes care reflected in Orem's model are consistent with the goals of the multidisciplinary team (i.e. self-care and empowerment) and that the DNE can clearly demonstrate to all interested parties that the model does guide and inform nursing practice.

Not all nurses, however, are convinced that nursing models can enhance and guide practice and their arguments should be examined carefully. Key points made by 'unbelievers' are as follows:

- Models present only the subjective view or views of those who construct the model and these views do not necessarily reflect the views of those who use the model (Hardy 1986).

- Models reflect the view that everyone's world view is the same and that all people may be assessed in the same way (Hardy 1986).

- Models that are adopted rigidly restrict questioning and change (Hardy 1986).

- Models may uncover multiple problems in clients that cannot always be dealt with by nurses (Hardy 1986).

- Models use language that is not always clear and, as a result, nurses are confused about its meaning (Chalmers 1990).

- Many models have not been validated by research and, therefore, there is no rational explanation for their use (Chalmers 1990).

- Nursing models promote a theory-practice gap because models taught in an academic setting are not practised in the practical setting (Speedy 1989).

These reservations indicate clearly that nursing models should be critically assessed before introducing them into the clinical setting. The clinical setting that provides the context for the discussion of diabetes nursing practice in this chapter is the Adelaide Diabetes Centre.

THE ADELAIDE DIABETES CENTRE

In 1986, a metropolitan teaching hospital in Adelaide established the Diabetes Centre to teach clients how to manage their disease. The Centre is located in a pleasant building, a short distance from the main hospital buildings, and it services clients who come from diverse ethnic backgrounds. The age range of clients varies from mid adolescence to old age. Referral to the Centre is through the various departments of the hospital or from the general practitioners and medical specialists in the community.

A multidisciplinary approach to health care is in operation in the Centre because it enables clients to benefit from the expertise of a range of health care professionals. The multidisciplinary team is comprised of the client, three diabetes nurse educators (DNEs), several endocrinologists, a specialist dietitian, a podiatrist, a social worker and general practitioners/medical specialists from the community. Both general practitioner (GP) and medical specialist are acknowledged as significant members of the health team and their contribution to the care of the client is readily sought by the health team. First, the

GP and the medical specialist may have access to information that should be known by the other members of the team, since such information may affect the treatment given to the client. Second, when the client is discharged from the Centre, it will be the responsibility of the GP or the medical specialist to provide the ongoing care of the client in the community. To facilitate continuity of care, the medical personnel need to be kept informed about the care given to the client by the multidisciplinary team at the Diabetes Centre.

The aims of the multidisciplinary team are to:

- educate clients about the management of their condition;

- encourage self-care and independence in clients; and

- empower clients so that they can make informed decisions about the management of their condition.

Because of the complex nature of diabetes and its effect on the lifestyle of the client, each member of the diabetes health team has an important role to play in the management of this condition. It is the responsibility of the endocrinologist/physician to diagnose and prescribe the client's treatment. The dietitian advises on dietary management, the podiatrist assesses and treats foot problems and educates the client about foot care, and the social worker focuses on the social welfare of clients living with diabetes. The DNE teaches the client the skills and knowledge required to manage the condition and, in doing so, reinforces the important advice given by other health professionals in the multidisciplinary team.

To summarise: because of the complex nature of diabetes and its critical effect on lifestyle, it is important to recognise that the person with diabetes requires the contribution and commitment of a multidisciplinary health team to maintain health.

Members of the multidisciplinary team work together as a cohesive unit to teach clients how to manage diabetes. Their intention is to promote the belief that people with diabetes who live within the constraints of their disease can cope with the limitations imposed on their lifestyle. To do this, clients need to be educated about diabetes, and taught the skills of problem solving and decision making, so that they can make informed decisions about their health care and how to care for themselves. In short, team members wish to empower clients to undertake their own self-care.

EMPOWERMENT

The notion of client empowerment has been progressively and generally promoted in contemporary health care and not just in diabetes health care. Connelly and associates (1993) report that client empowerment has been promoted successfully in the following areas: the disabled elderly (Cohen 1990), the hospice patient/family (Bailey 1990), women with diabetes (Anderson 1991) and in mental health (Connelly et al. 1993).

The word 'empower' means 'to give power or authority or to authorise' (*The Macquarie Dictionary* 1991, p. 302). In a general context, Rappaport (1987) defines empowerment 'as a process by which people gain mastery over their affairs'. Funnell and associates (1991) state that empowerment is not just a sudden increase of power that is used to dominate or change the lives of people; rather, it is a process that seeks to improve the quality of life for people by enabling them to take charge of their health through informed choices and personal goals.

In addition, Funnell and associates believe that the aim of empowerment is preferable to the more traditional, medical view of the aim of patient education and even to the aims of patient education reflected in consumerism. The traditional medical view of patient education is one that seeks to promote client compliance with medical treatment. However, this approach often leaves clients feeling helpless, awed or resigned and, as a result, they tend to withdraw from involvement in their care (Funnell et al. 1991, p. 38).

The consumer view arose as a reaction to the traditional medical view of client education. It seeks to involve clients as active participants in their own care; however, it can leave clients dissatisfied because they feel a burden of responsibility for their health care (Funnell et al. 1991, p. 38). Client empowerment is now considered by many health care professionals as the preferred aim of patient education.

Funnell et al. (1991) believe that an empowerment approach to patient education views the person with diabetes as an equal and active partner in the treatment program. Individuals are seen as experts on their own lives and the professional is seen as the expert on diabetes care. Funnell et al. (1991) also believe that the role of the diabetes educator is to help patients to acquire the skills to manage their disease and to overcome barriers to such disease management through education, self-exploration and emotional support.

Key concepts of empowerment are:

- an emphasis on the whole person;

- emphasis on personal strengths, rather than deficits;

- patient selection of learning needs;

- patient setting of learning needs;

- setting of shared or negotiated goals;

- transfer of leadership and decision making to the client;

- self-generation of problems and solutions;

- analysis of failures as problems to be solved rather than as personal deficits;

- discovery and enhancement of internal reinforcement for behaviour change;

- promotion of escalating participation;

- emphasis on support networks and resources;

- promotion of patients, networks and resources;

- promotion of patients' inherent drive toward health and wellness.

(Funnell et al. 1991, pp. 38–9)

In a study undertaken on chronically mentally ill clients from a drop-in centre, Connelly and associates found four distinct levels of empowerment. The four levels were identified as participating, choosing, supporting and negotiating. From the clients' perspective, these differing levels of empowerment meant they participated more in the community, their choices were increased, they provided support for each other and they negotiated on a more equal basis with health care personnel (Connelly et al. 1993, p. 297).

Connelly and associates also found that each level presupposed the achievement of previous levels and, therefore, if clients were at the supporting level they would also be participating in the community and exercising choice (Connelly et al. 1993, p. 300).

To illustrate: clients at the first level of empowerment participated either by calling in at the drop-in centre for casual advice on current health problems or by taking part in organised educational sessions. At the second level, clients had the freedom to choose options and to make decisions about their care. At the third level, clients received support in the form of caring, relating, accepting, coaching and sharing behaviours. At this level, support may be given by other clients, significant others and health professionals. Examples of this level could be coaching a client to handle a situation that was problematic, listening and giving suggestions to a client to assist with decision making and the sharing of resources. The fourth level is one of negotiating, which is characterised by mutual respect between client and the health professional. An example of this level of empowerment would be clients who stand firm on issues they think are important and, thereby, influence their health care management (Connelly 1993, pp. 300–1).

A similar view of empowerment is reflected in the Nursing Philosophy (and, therefore, the nursing practice) of the Adelaide Diabetes Centre.

NURSING PHILOSOPHY OF THE DIABETES CENTRE

The diabetes nurse educators working in the Diabetes Centre believe the following:

1   Clients have the right to access health care and to be accepted without bias or prejudice.

2   Clients have the right to make informed decisions about their care.

3   The DNE is responsible for:

(a) providing a safe, calm and harmonious environment that will enable clients to acquire the skills and knowledge required to manage their health care;

(b) involving clients in the planning of their own health care needs;

(c) providing clients with accurate information about diabetes health care so that they can make informed decisions about their health;

(d) tailoring individual educational programs that will meet the health care needs of clients and their families;

(e) teaching clients the essential psychomotor skills required to manage their activities of living and their medical condition (i.e. to self-care);

(f) teaching clients decision-making and problem-solving skills so that they can make informed decisions about their own health care (i.e. empowerment);

(g) assisting people to take responsibility for their lives;

(h) providing ongoing educational programs for clients about diabetes health care; and

(i) evaluating educational programs on a regular basis to ensure that programs are maintained at a high standard and client needs are met.

(Diabetes Centre Philosophy of Nursing 1994 and the ADEA 1989, pp. 1–4)

Client empowerment is primarily facilitated by the DNE through an educative process. To be effective in this process it is essential that the DNE has an educational background that includes specialist training in diabetes management, human development theory, medical/surgical nursing, teaching and learning methodologies and curriculum development. The DNE also needs to possess the appropriate communication and 'people skills'.

There are several reasons why the educational preparation of the DNE is important and they are related to client empowerment.

- The DNE requires specialised training in contemporary diabetes management and education in order to teach clients about their complex health care requirements.

- As clients come from a range of ethnic backgrounds, it is important that the DNE has the appropriate training in 'people skills' to effect meaningful communication.

- The age of clients ranges from adolescence to the elderly, so the DNE must be familiar with the problems and needs of each development stage, in order to tailor the teaching to their specific needs. This means that the DNE requires a knowledge of developmental psychology.

- The DNE is expected to deliver holistic nursing care, and clients often present with medical conditions other than diabetes; this means that the DNE needs an adequate knowledge of medical/surgical nursing.

- The main responsibility of the DNE is to teach clients across the life span about diabetes health care.

To do all this effectively, the DNE also needs to know how to develop, implement and evaluate educational programs that meet the learning needs of all ages, and then how to effectively teach those people about diabetes management.

SELF-CARE AND DOROTHEA OREM

Pearson and Vaughan (1986) believe the notion of self-care originated in the 1960s through the reaction of the consumer movement to 'professionalism' and 'intellectualism'. As discussed above, the consumer movement believes that people and families should have the right to take the initiative and responsibility for their own health care. People should be able to identify their own self-care needs, establish their own health care goals and evaluate their self-care behaviour (Pearson & Vaughan 1986, p. 69).

Contemporary diabetes health care seeks to promote client empowerment and self-care. As a result, any nursing model that seeks to guide diabetes nursing practice must accommodate the two concepts. One model that does this is the Self-care Deficit Theory, constructed by Dorothea Orem.

Dorothea Orem was born in Baltimore in the United States. She was the first nurse to think about using self-care in nursing practice and she began developing her theory between 1956 and 1960 while employed as a curriculum consultant by the US Department of Health, Education and Welfare. In 1971, Orem published her Self-care Deficit Theory of Nursing in a book entitled *Nursing Concepts of Practice*; since then she has published a further three editions, in 1980, 1985 and 1991 (Eben et al. in Marriner-Tomey 1994).

With the exception of Eugenia K. Spaulding, who was a great friend and teacher, Orem believes that no particular nursing leader had a direct influence on her work. Instead, Orem believes that her association with many nurses over the years provided her with learning experiences that contributed to her greater understanding of nursing in general. She also acknowledges the influence of work with graduate students and collaborative work with colleagues (Eben et al. in Marriner-Tomey 1994). Similarly, she acknowledges the contribution made by the members of the Nursing Development Conference Group (Orem 1991).

However, we believe that other likely influences on Orem's theorising were Maslow's hierarchy of human needs, and the consumer movement, which focused on the rights of individuals to be involved in decisions about their health care. Eben and associates suggest that other influences include the work of Virginia Henderson, which lists 14 patient needs, and that of Abdellah, which lists 21 nursing problems (Eben et al. in Marriner-Tomey 1994).

We also believe that Orem's Self-care Deficit Theory is a middle-range theory (i.e. the theory covers a broad range of nursing situations) and that Orem utilised deductive reasoning (from the general to the specific) to create her theory. Meleis (1991, p. 399) classifies Orem as a 'needs theorist'—that is, nursing care is based on the needs of the patient.

AN OVERVIEW OF OREM'S SELF-CARE DEFICIT THEORY

Nurse authors Foster and Janssens (George 1990) and Eben et al. (Marriner-Tomey 1994) describe Orem's Self-care Deficit Theory as a general theory of nursing that comprises three related theories: self-care deficit, self-care and nursing systems. The theories are outlined below.

1   *The Self-care Deficit Theory* postulates that people benefit from nursing in that they have health-related limitations in providing self-care (Chinn & Kramer 1991). In other words, the client is unable to meet some aspect of care, such as personal hygiene, and needs the services of a nurse.

   A typical example of a self-care deficit in diabetes nursing are clients with Type 1 diabetes (IDDM) who are unable to care for themselves by administering the insulin required by the body to metabolise glucose. As a result, the services of the DNE are required to teach the clients how to administer insulin, so that they can continue to self-care.

2   *The Self-care Theory.* Orem (1991, p. 3) defines self-care as 'the personal care that individuals require each day to regulate their own functioning and development'. This theory postulates that self-care and care of dependents are learned behaviours that purposely regulate human structural integrity, functioning and development (Chinn & Kramer 1991).

   An example of self-care in diabetes nursing is the young male client with Type 1 diabetes (IDDM) who wants to learn everything he needs to know to manage his own health care, so that he can care for himself.

3   *The Nursing System Theory* postulates that nursing systems form when nurses prescribe, design and provide nursing that regulates the individual's self-care capabilities and meets therapeutic self-care requirements (Chinn & Kramer 1991).

Orem contends that 'on the principle that nurses and/or patients can act to meet patients' self-care requisites, three basic variations in nursing systems are recognized:

- the wholly compensatory nursing system;

- the partial compensatory nursing system; and

- the supportive–educative (developmental) system'.

(Orem 1991, p. 287)

These systems are discussed later in the chapter.

CONCEPTS OF OREM'S SELF-CARE DEFICIT THEORY

The main concepts of Orem's theory are self-care, human beings, health, environment, nursing and nursing systems.

SELF-CARE

Orem's (1991) theorising commences with this concept because she believes that self-care is basic to the understanding of the theory of self-care deficit and the theory of nursing systems. She defines self-care as 'the practice of activities that individuals initiate and perform on their own behalf in maintaining life, health and well-being' (Orem 1991, p. 117).

Moreover, Orem (1991) believes that self-care is normal behaviour for adults and that self-care is performed on a continuous basis. She states that adults achieve self-care through the provision of self-care requisites. Conversely, infants, children, the aged, the ill and the disabled require complete care or assistance with self-care requisites from a responsible individual.

Orem also believes that self-care is a deliberate, learned, goal-oriented activity that is undertaken by individuals to promote and maintain health. She states that self-care is conduct that is influenced by various factors—the self-concept and maturity of the individual, culturally derived goals and practices, position in the family, membership of social groups and lack of access to scientifically derived knowledge about self-care (Orem 1991).

She further believes that self-care has an important role to play in health and disease. To begin with, self-care is necessary for a 'person's integrity as a psychophysiologic organism with a rational life' (Orem 1991, p. 120). If individuals are to remain healthy, they must either perform, or have performed for them, a minimum of activities each day. In the advent of disease, individuals require both a scientifically derived fund of knowledge about self-care goals and practices, and related skills and habits. In addition, Orem states:

disease, injury and mental or physical malfunctioning may limit what a person can do for himself, since such states may limit his ability to reason, to make decisions, and to engage in activity to accomplish self-care goals.

Disease, injury and malfunctioning may involve structural changes as well as functional changes, which may necessitate the use of specialized self-care measures, some of which may be medically prescribed.

(Orem 1991, p. 120)

Orem (1991) believes that self-care measures are influenced by:

- a general knowledge of self-care goals and practices. To access this information, an individual may need the expertise of health care professionals;

- access to medical care prescribed by the physician;

- access to resources that will promote a healthy environment.

To self-care, an individual requires the provision of self-care requisites. Orem (1991) states that there are three categories of self-care requisites or requirements—universal, developmental and health-deviation self-care requisites.

Universal self-care requisites

Universal self-care requisites are those associated with the life processes that are common to all human beings during each stage of their life cycle. Orem maintains that all human beings require eight universal self-care requisites in order to self-care. They are as follows

1 The maintenance of a sufficient intake of air.

2 The maintenance of a sufficient water intake.

3 The maintenance of a sufficient intake of food.

4 The provision of care associated with elimination processes and excrements.

5 The maintenance of a balance between activity and rest.

6 The maintenance of a balance between solitude and social interaction.

7 The prevention of hazards to human life, human functioning and human well-being.

8 The promotion of human functioning and development within social groups in accord with human potential, known human limitations and the human desire to be normal.

(Orem 1991, p. 127)

Orem states that when the eight universal self-care requisites are provided for, the individual experiences positive health and well-being (Orem 1991, p. 127). Conversely, if any of the universal self-care requisites are absent, there is a self-care deficit that may need nursing services.

The framework of the universal requisites provides the DNE with a useful tool for directing the assessment, planning, implementation and evaluation of client care (see example on next page).

Example

The DNE knows that it is important for the newly diagnosed Type 2 (NIDDM) client to eat the correct diet to maintain health but realises that the client does not know the appropriate dietary requirements for Type 2 diabetes. Identifying this self-care deficit, the DNE is able to plan the care required to meet this deficit—that is, to provide advice on appropriate diet.

Developmental self-care requisites

Orem (1991) states that there are also two types of developmental self-care requisites that an individual requires for self-care.

1 Those requisites that bring about and maintain 'conditions that support life processes and promote the processes of development, that is, human progress toward higher levels of the organisation of human structures and toward maturation during the intrauterine stages of life . . . or adulthood' (Orem 1991, p. 131).

Here is an example of this type of developmental self-care deficit.

Example

A young pregnant woman has just been diagnosed as having gestational diabetes. The 28-week developing foetus requires the universal self-care requisites provided by the maternal placenta in order to develop normally to term. After assessing the mother's knowledge about gestational diabetes and its effect on the developing foetus, the DNE realises that the young woman does not know how to care for herself or her developing foetus. If this knowledge deficit is not addressed by the DNE and the endocrinologist as a matter of urgency, foetal development may be seriously compromised. To meet this developmental self-care deficit, the DNE teaches the young woman how to manage her diabetes by eating the correct diet and administering the correct insulin dose, and shows her how to monitor her blood glucose level. This action by the DNE facilitates an environment that will promote the healthy development of the foetus to term.

2 Those requisites that can adversely affect human development if they are lacking. Orem identifies two subtypes:

(a) those that prevent the occurrence of deleterious effects;

(b) those that mitigate or overcome existent deleterious effects.

Examples of self-care deficits could include:

- educational deprivation;

- problems of social adaptation;

- failures of healthy individuation;

- loss of relatives, friends, associates;

- loss of possessions;

- loss of occupational security;

- abrupt change of residence to an unfamiliar environment;

- status-associated problems;

- poor health or disability;

- oppressive living conditions;

- terminal illness and impending death.

(Orem 1991)

Orem herself provides an example of a developmental self-care requisite. She refers to a 66-year-old diabetic who had never been to school. The man can think only concretely; he cannot read; he can distinguish colours but not name them. He has fairly good motor ability. Recently he was asked by the nurse to begin testing his urine at home and the nurse began to teach him. The content had to be broken into small units and presented slowly. After two sessions, the man could test his urine accurately and he was very pleased with his progress. The man regarded this as an important self-development (Orem 1991).

Health-deviation self-care requisites

Orem states that 'self-care requisites exist for persons who are ill or injured, have specific forms of pathology including defects and disabilities, and who are under medical diagnosis and treatment' (Orem (1991, p. 132).

The theorist believes that significant changes to human function (e.g. oedematous extremities, presence of tumours, difficulty in breathing) cause people to begin focusing attention on themselves. As a result, they begin to ask questions: What is wrong? Why is this happening to me? What should I do? Family members and friends may also ask similar questions. These questions and observable changes to the health state of individuals result in some dependence on others to sustain life or well-being; this, in turn, leads society to express a demand for medical diagnosis and treatment.

Thus, Orem states that 'seeking and participating in medical care for health deviations are self-care actions' (Orem 1991, p. 132).

Orem identifies six categories of health deviation self-care requisites:

1 Seeking and securing appropriate medical assistance . . . ;

2 Being aware of and attending to the effects and results of pathological conditions and states . . . ;

3 Effectively carrying out medically prescribed . . . measures . . . ;

4 Being aware of attending to or regulating the discomforting or deleterious effects of prescribed medical care measures . . . ;

5 Modifying the self-concept (and self-image) in accepting oneself as being in a particular state of health and in need of specific forms of health care;

6 Learning to live with the effects of pathological conditions and states and the effects of medical diagnostic and treatment measures in a life-style that promotes continued personal development.

(Orem 1991, p. 134)

Example

A client with a health deviation self-care requisite in diabetes nursing could be a 68-year-old woman with Type 2 diabetes (NIDDM) who has just developed a small ulcer on her big toe. She has been warned previously about the consequences of diabetes and peripheral vascular disease and, consequently, seeks an urgent appointment with the DNE and the endocrinologist for advice concerning the treatment of her foot ulcer.

HUMAN BEINGS

Orem states that 'human beings are distinguished from other living things by their capacity to (1) reflect upon themselves and their environment, (2) symbolise what they experience, (3) use symbolic creations (ideas, words) in thinking, in communicating and in guiding efforts to do and to make things that are beneficial for themselves or others' (Orem 1991, p. 180). Furthermore, human beings take deliberate action to 'maintain a state of health for themselves and their dependents by undertaking self-care' (Orem 1991, p. 180).

Orem prefers to use the word 'patient' instead of client. She states that 'patient means someone who is under the care of a health care professional' or 'a receiver of care'. On the other hand, the term 'client' implies a recognition of a contractual agreement between a professional and an individual with a view to employing or retaining the services of an attorney or counsel for advice and assistance. The word 'client' also means a customer who regularly buys from another or receives services from another (Orem 1991, p. 30).

HEALTH

Orem conceptualises 'health' and 'healthy' as 'terms used to describe living things—plants, animals, human beings—when they are structurally and functionally whole or sound'(Orem 1991, p. 179). She accepts the World Health Organisation's definition that 'health is a state of physical, mental and social well-being and not merely the absence of disease or infirmity' (Orem 1991, p. 181).

ENVIRONMENT

Orem conceptualises the environment as the factors that make up the context in which people live. Moreover, she states that human beings are never isolated from their environment. 'They exist in them' (Orem 1991, p. 38). She believes that human environments should be analysed and understood in terms of the physical, chemical, biological and social factors that affect them.

The *physiochemical factors* comprise the atmosphere of the earth, the gaseous composition of the air, pollutants, smoke, weather conditions and the geologic stability of the earth's crust (Orem 1991, p. 39).

Biological features include pets, animals in the wild, infectious agents (e.g. viruses), people or animals that under natural conditions act as reservoirs for infectious agents, and people or animals that harbour infectious agents with manifest disease or 'unapparent' infection (Orem 1991, p. 39).

Socioeconomic–cultural features include all aspects of the family, the community, the availability of resources for daily living and health services (Orem 1991, pp. 39–41).

To summarise, the environmental factors that make up the individual's environment must be considered because that is where the person lives. If nursing care is to be meaningful, relevant and holistic in diabetes nursing, then the DNE must also consider the factors that comprise the client's environment.

NURSING

Orem states that:

> nursing, a specialized health service, is distinguished from other human services by its focus on persons with inabilities for continuous provision of the amount and quality of time-specific care that is regulatory of their own functioning and development, whenever inabilities that limit care are associated with their states of health or the complex, specialized nature of required regulatory care measures.
>
> *(Orem 1991, p. 4)*

Orem identifies five behaviours that nurses use to help their clients meet self-care deficits. They are called helping behaviours and are as follows.

1 Acting for or doing for another;

2 Guiding and directing;

3 Providing physical or psychological support;

4 Providing and maintaining an environment that supports personal development; and

5 Teaching.

(Orem 1991, p. 9)

Orem believes that helping behaviours are met by all health professionals, according to their particular expertise. She asserts that 'nurses help others because of action limitations that are within the domain of nursing' (Orem 1991, p. 13).

Acting, or doing, behaviour

Orem (1991, p. 9) states that 'acting for another is a helping method that requires the helper to use developed abilities toward achieving specific results for persons in need of help'. An acting behaviour in diabetes nursing practice might be a DNE who acts on behalf of an obese client interested in participating in an appropriate exercise program. The DNE makes the necessary enquiries for the client and, having found out the facts, assists the client to make decisions about the suitability of the program. Similarly, a doing behaviour is illustrated in the action of a DNE who performs glucose monitoring for a mentally or physically incapacitated client.

Guiding another

Orem suggests that guiding another person is considered as a method of helping in situations where a person must choose one course of action in preference to others, or decide whether to pursue any course of action (Orem 1991, p. 10). Guiding behaviour is expressed in the advice given by the DNE in consultation with the endocrinologist, concerning the expected behaviour of clients when unwell. To illustrate: in good health the client is advised to eat a well-balanced diet as recommended by the Australian Dietary Guidelines, and to administer a prescribed dose of insulin. However, when unwell, and to cope with the effects of illness, the client may need to make informed choices about the amount and type of food eaten and to vary the dose of insulin prescribed by the endocrinologist. These choices are made possible for clients because the DNE and endocrinologist guide and supervise them.

Supporting behaviour

Orem (1991, p. 10) states 'to support another person means to "sustain in an effort" and thereby prevent the person from failing or from avoiding an unpleasant situation or decision'.

Supporting behaviour in diabetes nursing is apparent in the action of a DNE who actively assists a woman with gestational diabetes throughout her pregnancy to the healthy delivery of her infant. Supportive behaviour from the DNE may variously take the form of physical assistance, encouragement and wise advice (Orem 1991, pp. 10–11).

Providing a developmental environment

Orem suggests that 'this method of assistance requires the helper to provide or help to provide environmental conditions that motivate the person being helped to establish appropriate goals and adjust behaviour or achieve results specified by the goals' (Orem 1991, p. 11).

She also believes that all the developmental needs of the client should be considered when providing a total environment. Included would be issues that are important to the client—for example, psychosocial and physical factors, attitudes and values, and the opportunity to interact and communicate with significant people about relevant issues. In other words, all the factors that are important to the client should be completely addressed by the DNE when creating a developmental environment for the client (Orem 1991).

Example

A developmental environment may be facilitated by the DNE who considers the needs of a young male client who has Type I diabetes (IDDM) and is about to be married. The client is worried about potential impotence and how that possible complication might be addressed by the couple. To create an environment that is meaningful for the client, it would be appropriate to include the fiancée in discussions and also the endocrinologist. This action would assist the client and his fiancée to set relevant health goals related to potential impotence and to plan how those goals might be met.

Teaching another

Orem states that 'teaching is another valid method of helping a person who needs instruction to develop knowledge or particular skills' (Orem 1991, p. 12). Successful teaching depends on several factors, the most important of which are the teacher's knowledge and ability to teach a specific topic, and the learner's ability and readiness to learn (Orem 1991).

As mentioned above, education is an important part of the role of the DNE (ADEA 1989). An example of a teaching behaviour could be seen in the DNE who teaches the pre-adolescent child about the relationship of insulin to diet. Clearly, the DNE needs to know all about juvenile diabetes and be able to recognise the readiness of the child to learn. The DNE also needs to have the skills to teach the child.

NURSING SYSTEMS

Orem defines a nursing system as:

> something constructed through actions of nurses and nurses' patients. It is a product that should be beneficial to persons with patient status in nursing practice situations when the time frame for production fits the time of occurrence of requirements for nursing.
>
> *(Orem 1991, p. 63)*

Orem (1991) describes three nursing systems or actions.

1 The *wholly compensatory nursing system* is required when clients are unable to meet their self-care requisites for any of the following three reasons:

(a) the client is in a coma;

(b) the client is fully aware of the necessary self-care requirements but is unable to perform them for some reason;

(c) the client is unable to make rational decisions about his or her self-care requisites or to perform those activities.

For example, an unconscious female client with Type 1 diabetes (IDDM) is admitted to hospital with a diagnosis of diabetic ketoacidosis (DKA). It is obvious that the client is not able to self-care and that the nurse will need to meet all her self-care requisites.

2   The *partial compensatory nursing system* is required in 'situations where both nurse and patient perform care measures or other actions involving manipulative tasks or ambulation' (Orem 1991). In this instance, the amount of care provided by the nurse will depend on the abilities and limitations of the patient to undertake care. Either nurse or patient will have the major role in the performance of care measures (Orem 1991, p. 291).

For example, an arthritic and elderly woman with Type 2 diabetes (NIDDM) is able to perform most of her self-care requisites, but is unable to carry out glucose monitoring because of a lack of coordination and dexterity. The woman needs the assistance of the DNE to perform this task.

3   The *supportive–educative system* is 'for situations where the patient is able to perform or can and should learn to perform required measures of externally or internally oriented therapeutic self-care but cannot do so without assistance' (Orem 1991, p. 291). Support, guidance, the provision of a developmental environment, and teaching are components of this system. Orem states that this system is the only one where the patient's requirements for help are confined to decision making, behaviour control, and acquiring knowledge and skills (Orem 1991).

With reference to the role of the DNE, the supportive–educative system is the most commonly used nursing system in diabetes nursing practice.

For example, a male adolescent client with Type 1 diabetes (IDDM) has a behaviour problem, especially when partying with his friends. In an effort to be seen as normal by his peers, the youth refuses to adhere to a healthy diet, preferring to eat 'junk' food. He also refuses to take his insulin when prescribed. Clearly, the youth is able to comply with the recommended diabetes regime but, because of peer pressure, he needs the wise assistance of the DNE to help him make decisions about the type of food he can/will eat when he parties, the relationship of insulin therapy to 'junk' food and how he might modify his behaviour to comply with his treatment.

All nursing systems utilise the nursing process to assess, plan, implement and evaluate patient care (Orem 1991).

To summarise the main points of Orem's Self-care Deficit Theory: all people require self-care requisites in order to self-care; when they are unable to meet the self-care requirements for healthy living, a self-care deficit arises and there is a need for a nursing system; nursing actions are provided according to client need or self-care deficit—that is, care may be complete, partial or merely supportive through an educative process.

ASSUMPTIONS OF OREM'S SELF-CARE THEORY

Orem (1991) disagrees with some nurse scholars, such as Fitzpatrick and Whall (1989) and Marriner-Tomey (1994), who state that she bases her theory on a set of assumptions. Orem prefers to use the word 'premise' rather than assumption, because premises were and are advanced as true and not merely assumed. Orem offers five premises for her theory.

1 Human beings require continuous deliberate inputs to themselves and their environments in order to remain alive and function in accord with natural human endowments.

2 Human agency, the power to act deliberately is exercised in the form of care of self and others, in identifying needs for [inputs] and in making needed inputs.

3 Mature human beings experience privations in the form of limitations for action in care of self and others, involving the making of life-sustaining and function-regulating inputs.

4 Human agency is exercised in discovering, developing, and transmitting to others ways and means to identify needs for and make inputs to self and others.

5 Groups of human beings with structured relationships cluster tasks and allocate responsibilities for providing care to group members who experience privations for making required deliberate input to self and others.

(Orem 1991, p. 67)

Nurses should resist the temptation to incorporate nursing models uncritically into practice and education (Greenwood 1988) because, quite simply, they may not fit. Models should be examined for the appropriateness of their possible introduction into practice and education against relevant criteria.

CRITIQUE OF OREM'S SELF-CARE DEFICIT THEORY

Meleis (1991) and Eben et al. (Marriner-Tomey 1994) offer criteria that could be used in model critique:

■ *Credibility* of the theory.

■ *Internal components.* The theory/model should have clarity, consistency, simplicity/complexity, a circle of contagiousness, and be useful in practice, research and education.

■ *External components.* The theory/model should address the congruence of the personal, professional and social values of the theorist and the professionals who plan to implement the theory (Meleis 1991, pp. 237–8).

We have examined the utility of Orem's theory against these criteria.

CREDIBILITY OF OREM'S THEORY

Both Meleis (1991) and Eben et al. (Marriner-Tomey 1994) testify to the credibility of Orem's theory. They cite reports from various nurse researchers who have devised instruments or undertaken research that has enabled them to successfully utilise or validate Orem's theory. Meleis cites reports that have included measuring self-care agency and the patient's perception of self-care (Meleis 1991). Other authors have focused on self-care practices, identified categories of self-care consequences, self-care activities and self-care needs, established the relationships between propositions, nursing systems and self-care behaviour, and the effect of self-help and groups (Meleis 1991).

We also believe that Orem's Self-care Deficit Theory is a credible theory to guide diabetes nursing practice.

INTERNAL COMPONENTS

We believe that Orem has clearly identified and defined the major concepts and assumptions of her theory. There is also a consistent relationship between the concepts and assumptions in her theory. Orem's theory is logical, credible and not difficult to follow—the main themes and ideas in it are simple and easy to understand.

There is ample evidence that Orem's theory has been examined and adopted by nurses in the United States, the United Kingdom and Australia. Eben and associates, for example, report that Orem's theory has been translated into several languages and has been used worldwide (Eben et al. 1994). Orem's theory, therefore, can claim both a circle of contagiousness and usefulness.

The theory has been used as a basis for clinical practice in a wide range of health care settings. Eben and associates (Marriner-Tomey 1994) refer to its successful use in outpatient care, cardiac clinics and diabetic clinics, the acute care setting, clinics dealing with adolescent alcohol abusers, in women and children's health, maternity care, paediatrics and hospice care.

Orem' Self-care Deficit Theory has also been used successfully in the development of nursing curricula in the United States (Eben et al. in Marriner-Tomey 1994). However, Meleis (1991) cautions against the use of just one theory in any nursing curriculum.

In the light of all this evidence, we believe that the use of Orem's Self-care Theory in diabetes care is justified.

EXTERNAL COMPONENTS

Meleis states that any theory/model should be congruent with the personal, professional and social values of the people who are expected to implement it (Meleis 1991). We believe (and, indeed, we hope we have demonstrated) that Orem's Self-care Theory reflects the values of the multidisciplinary team employed in the Adelaide Diabetes Centre and that it could guide and improve nursing practice. In our view, it facilitates client empowerment and self-care across the life span.

SUMMARY

There are advantages in using Orem's Self-care Model to guide nursing practice in the Adelaide Diabetes Centre.

- The model provides a clear framework from which the DNE may assess, plan, implement and evaluate the client's care.
- The model promotes the mutual planning, implementing and evaluation of health goals by the DNE and the client.

- The model provides an educational structure that may be used by the DNE in education.

- The model promotes self-care and client empowerment, which are the health goals of primary importance to the diabetes health care team.

- The model enables the DNE to articulate clearly what it is that nurses do within contemporary diabetes health care.

GLOSSARY

Empowerment: 'a process by which people gain mastery of their affairs' (Rappaport 1987).

Self-care: 'the practice of activities that individuals initiate and perform on their behalf in maintaining life, health and well being' (Orem 1991, p. 117).

Self-concept: (self-regard) 'the overall perception of self that includes self-satisfaction, self-acceptance, self-esteem and congruence or discrepancy between self and ideal self' (Mercer in Marriner-Tomey 1994, p. 393).

QUESTIONS

1 What factors would you need to consider before you implemented Orem's theory in your health care setting ?

2 How would you use Orem's Self-care Deficit Theory to guide practice in your health care setting ?

3 What might be some of the advantages of using Orem's theory to guide practice in your health care setting ?

LEARNING ACTIVITY

Select one patient from among those you are currently nursing. Using Orem's model, assess the patient's care needs and plan his or her care for one shift.

FURTHER READING

Frey, M.A. & Denyes, M.J., 1989, 'Health and illness self-care in adolescents with IDDM: A test of Orem's theory', *Advances in Nursing Science*, October, 12(1), pp. 67–75.

McWilliams, B., Murphy, F. & Sobiski, A. 1988, 'Why self-care theory works for us', *Canadian Nurse*, October, pp. 38–40.

Mulkeen, H. 1989, 'Diabetes: teaching the teaching of self-care', *Nursing Times*, 18–25 January, 85(3), pp. 63–5.

Orem, D.E. 1991, *Nursing Concepts of Practice*, 4th edn, Mosby-Year Book Inc., St. Louis.

Smits, M.W. & Kee, C.C. 1992, 'Correlates of self-care among the independent elderly: Self-concept effects well-being', *Journal of Gerontological Nursing*, 18 September, (9), pp. 13–18.

9

PARSE'S HUMAN BECOMING THEORY OF NURSING

JOHN DALY AND JENNIFER WATSON

The authors of this chapter convey their appreciation and gratitude to Professors Rosemarie R. Parse and Jennifer Greenwood who provided helpful critiques of earlier versions of the work.

Excerpts from R.R. Parse (1981) Man-living Health: A Theory of Nursing *are reprinted with permission of the copyright holder, Rosemarie Rizzo Parse.*

LEARNING OBJECTIVES

When you have read this chapter you should be able to:

1 Define the key concepts used in Parse's human becoming theory.

2 Describe the evolution of the theory of human becoming.

3 Explain the principles of human becoming and relate these to nursing practice.

4 Appreciate how the human becoming theory may be applied in nursing practice.

John Daly, RN, BA, BHSc, MEd (Hons), PhD is Associate Professor of Nursing at the University of Western Sydney, Macarthur. He is an experienced critical care nurse, nurse educator, researcher and administrator. John has had work published in the areas of critical care nursing, nursing research and nursing theory. He is currently President of the Australian Parse Interest Group and a member of the International Consortium of Parse Scholars. John utilised Parse's theory and research methodology in his doctoral thesis which investigated the lived experience of suffering.

Jennifer Watson, RN, BA, MEd (Admin), is Senior Lecturer and Dean of the School of Nursing at The Flinders University of South Australia. She has practised nursing for 30 years. For the last decade Jennifer has been teaching and supervising research students in the areas of nursing theory, nursing knowledge, ethics and research. She is currently completing a PhD in Nursing. Jennifer's interest in Parse's theory has evolved from her research into knowledges and domains of nursing.

INTRODUCTION

As many of the ideas considered in this chapter will be new to many readers, we have included a brief definition of key terms in the glossary at the end of the chapter. You are encouraged to become familiar with these terms before reading the chapter. It may be of interest to note that the theorist Parse (1981, 1987, 1992, 1995) intended her work to be used by graduate students in nursing, that is, students who are studying at the masters or doctoral level. The theory of human becoming is complex, its roots are in abstract scientific and philosophical theories. Also, the language of this theory is unique and, for some, difficult to comprehend initially. The theory is presented in this chapter with an undergraduate audience in mind. We encourage you to approach exploration of the chapter's contents with an open mind and a sense of adventure. We believe that Parse's work has much to offer the discipline of nursing, in enhancing and enriching relationships between nurses and those they care for, and enhancing quality of life.

The nurse theorist Rosemarie Rizzo Parse is currently Professor and Niehoff Chair in Nursing Research in the Marcella Niehoff School of Nursing, Loyola University, Chicago, Illinois, in the United States. She assumed this appointment in 1993. Prior to this she was Professor and Coordinator of the Centre for Nursing Research at Hunter College, The City University of New York, in New York. Parse held this position for 10 years. During her

30-year career in nursing, Parse has held positions in clinical nursing, nursing management, educational administration and education. She served as Dean of Nursing at Duquesne University, Pittsburgh, United States, in the late 1970s. In addition, Parse has been a visiting professor at numerous universities in the United States, Finland, Sweden, Germany and Canada. In 1991 she was a visiting Fellow in Nursing at the University of Western Sydney, Hawkesbury, in Australia. She was also an Honorary Fellow of the Faculty of Health Sciences at the former University of New England (Northern Rivers), Australia, which is now Southern Cross University. Parse has been active in contributing to the literature in nursing for a considerable time. Her publications include *Nursing Fundamentals* (1974), *Man-Living-Health: A Theory of Nursing* (1981), *Nursing Research: Qualitative Methods* (1985) (co-authored with Coyne & Smith), *Nursing Science: Major Paradigms, Theories and Critiques* (1987), and the recently published *Illuminations: The Human Becoming Theory in Practice and Research* (1995). She is founder and editor of *Nursing Science Quarterly*. Parse is also active in nursing research, with a focus on universal lived experiences of health and development of her **human becoming** research methodology.

A group called the International Consortium of Parse Scholars was established some years ago in North America. This group has a membership representing nursing in the United States, Canada, Japan, Korea, Sweden, Finland, Australia and the United Kingdom. The purpose and goals of the consortium are to:

- contribute to human health and quality of life through practice and research guided by Parse's human becoming theory;

- provide a forum for nurses committed to practice and research with the human becoming theory;

- provide venues for learning and discussing the integration of Parse's theory in nursing practice, research, education and administration; and

- advance nursing science from a human becoming perspective, through the presentation and publication of work related to nursing philosophy, practice, research, education and administration.

The international group also operates an active e-mail network, publishes a quarterly newsletter, 'Illuminations', and holds an annual human becoming theory conference.

In the development of her theory, Parse was exposed to the ideas of the psychologist and phenomenologist Amadei Giorgi (1970, 1985). He is credited with contributing a human science perspective to the discipline of psychology in the United States. Other influences on Parse's theorising include her practice as a nurse, the nurse theorist Martha Rogers (1970, 1987, 1990) and several philosophers including, in the main, Heidegger (1962), Dilthey (1988), Sartre (1966) and Merleau-Ponty (1963, 1974). A reading of Parse's theory will show that she drew on an extensive range of additional sources, which also exerted influence on the construction of her human becoming theory—for example Tillich (1952) and Buber (1965, 1970). As is the case with many theories, it is difficult to judge precisely the degree of influence each minor source has had on the overall development of Parse's theory. The human becoming theory has been used as a guide for nursing practice and research (Parse 1995), with recent research activity focusing on the use of the human becoming research methodology. This method investigates lived experiences of health; it is qualitative and phenomenological (see Parse 1987, 1992).

Parse's theory was first published in 1981 as Man-Living-Health (Parse 1981) and in 1992 it was renamed Parse's Human Becoming Theory of Nursing (Parse 1992). This name change reflected a general alteration in the use of the term 'man' to include only the male gender. 'Human' reflects Parse's intent to include all human beings. When Parse named her theory in 1981, she structured and linked the words Man-Living-Health by the use of hyphens to establish a conceptual bond between the words, and thus created a unity representing a construct unto itself (Parse 1981). Parse (1992) states that 'the name, human becoming, reflects the unity of the construct Man-Living-Health which is still the focus of the theory' (p. 37). 'Human becoming' as a construct is the name of the theory in the simultaneity paradigm, the focus of which is the 'human-universe-health process' (Parse 1992, p. 41). The concept of human becoming flows from the existential notion that the human being never sees self as complete (Barnum 1990).

For Parse (1981, 1987, 1992, 1995) nursing is a basic, human science with a unique knowledge base. The philosophical basis of this 'human science' can be located in the work of the philosopher Dilthey (1988). According to Dilthey, human science seeks an 'understanding of the connectedness of life itself which can never become wholly accessible to the understanding' (Dilthey, cited in Parse 1992, p. 37). Seeking 'understanding of life itself' calls for a focus on experience as it is humanly lived. The human science perspective that is embraced by Parse (1981, 1985, 1987, 1992) sees the human being as unitary, which means that people cannot be separated from something termed 'objective reality'. From this perspective, 'the focus of scientific activities is the humanly lived experience of the world, in which subjectivity is primal' (Mitchell & Cody 1992, p. 58).

PARSE'S VIEW OF PARADIGMS IN NURSING

Parse has identified two competing **paradigms** in the discipline of nursing—the totality paradigm and the simultaneity paradigm (Parse 1987). The term 'paradigm' is synonymous with the term 'world view'; this includes the general beliefs and values that constitute or underpin such a perspective (Nagle & Mitchell 1991). Essentially, world views represent philosophic claims which incorporate ideas about the nature of being (**ontology**). This has implications for the way in which nursing, and its related concerns, can be constructed in theory and 'actioned' in practice. In nursing, for instance, these assumptions are quite different when we compare one paradigm with another. For example, the relationship between the person and the environment is described or conceptualised in a number of ways, and ideas like health are viewed in different ways. Each paradigm incorporates a number of theories which are said to be 'holistic'. This can also mean different things, a point which is clarified in our discussion of paradigms below. The underpinning values and beliefs of each paradigm have important implications for practice and research in nursing. Each paradigm in nursing knowledge provides a focus for nursing practice that encompasses a view of health.

THE TOTALITY PARADIGM

The totality paradigm is based on a number of assumptions about human beings, the environment and health, and their interrelationship. In this perspective, human beings are seen as made up of biological-psychological-social-spiritual parts. Parse (1992) refers to this as a central triad of body, mind and spirit. From this perspective, the person is seen as 'the sum of the parts', and an entity that can be separated from the environment. This **particulate** view of the human being is one way of conceptualising 'holism'—that is, the whole is the sum of the parts. The beliefs that human beings interact with the environment by coping, and respond to stimuli in the external environment, are fundamental to the totality paradigm, as is the idea of cause–effect relationships. Health status in this paradigm is judged in relation to norms for well-being, including physical, mental, social and spiritual aspects of the person.

Dynamic equilibrium is also an important concept in this paradigm. For example, it is accepted that successful positive coping in the face of challenging environmental stimuli will maintain health. In both practice and research, the totality paradigm directs nurses towards discovering interventions or variables that will generate consistent outcomes according to predefined definitions of health or quality of life. This is seen as possible because of the belief that people are shaped, in effect, by cause–effect relationships with the environment. This is a closed system view in which people are seen as predictable and confined by their situation (Jonas et al. 1992). Ideas regarding space–time are fixed in this perspective and consistent with the notion of **linear causality**.

In the totality paradigm, the nurse is placed in the position of expert authority and decision maker in relation to the health needs of the person (Parse 1987, 1992). Essentially, the nurse is in control of the situation and has the decision-making prerogatives. There is an imbalance of power here in the nurse's favour. The goal of nursing from this perspective is to shift the person to a position of health relative to accepted 'norms'. Here the nurse is required to identify the patient's problems and devise ways of correcting them to restore the person, as far as possible, to a state of health. This is reflected in the use of nursing diagnosis and the nursing process (Parse 1992). In the totality paradigm, health is regarded as a static state, is linked to well-being, or harmony, self-care and adaptation.

Critics of this paradigm take issue with its mechanistic, reductionistic and normative view of the person and health and prescriptive nursing practice methods. Here the person is regarded as similar to a machine with parts that can be fixed. A further major issue is the way in which totality-paradigm approaches to nursing often see the patients' values subordinated to a set of 'norms' defined by the nurse (Parse 1995). Many nursing theories can be classified as totality-paradigm theories—for example, Orem (1991) and Roy (Roy & Andrews 1991).

THE SIMULTANEITY PARADIGM

Pioneering work in this paradigm was undertaken by Rogers, who published her account of the science of the **unitary human being** in 1970. Parse has further explicated and developed this paradigm (Parse 1981, 1987, 1992) with a different focus from Rogers. Values and beliefs supporting this paradigm differ radically from those underpinning the totality paradigm. Parse and Rogers look to a 'non-particulate human being who cannot be known by a study of the biopsychosocial parts' (Nagle & Mitchell 1991, p. 19). In this paradigm, 'the person is more than and different from the sum of the parts, changing mutually and simultaneously with the environment' (Rogers 1970). Here there is a belief that people have a relationship with the environment based on mutual process.

For the human becoming theory in this perspective, the human is held to be 'free to choose in mutual rhythmical interchange with the environment' (Parse 1987, p. 136) and, further, the human 'gives meaning to situations and is responsible for choices in moving beyond what is' (Parse 1987, p. 136). The human and environment may be distinguished, one from the other, according to their respective **patterns** (Parse 1981, 1987, 1992; Rogers 1987). Space–time becomes a relative dimension of life from the simultaneity perspective—the human 'lives in a relative Now experiencing the what was, is and will be all-at-once' (Parse 1987, p. 136).

Differences exist, however, within the nursing perspectives of the simultaneity paradigm (Parse 1992). These differences relate to specific perspectives of the human being, health, the central phenomenon of nursing, the goal of nursing and practice, and research methodologies related to each of the theories of the paradigm. These differences are summarised in Table 9.1.

For Parse, nursing focuses on quality of life from the perspective of the individual (Parse 1981, 1987), not the perspectives of the nurse, physician or society. Further, the existence of disease states as defined by 'societal norms' is not held to be a 'significant factor' (Parse 1987) in determining a person's health from the simultaneity perspective. In this paradigm, health is construed as a value (Rogers 1987) or a process of becoming (Parse 1987, 1992), not an entity which is adjudged relative to societal norms. Parse states:

Health is the human being's unfolding. It is experienced by the individual and can only be described by that individual. There is no optimal health; health is simply how one is experiencing personal living.

(Parse 1987, p. 136)

She sees health as:

a process of becoming uniquely lived by each individual. It is [the human beings'] lived experience, a non-linear entity that cannot be qualified as good or bad, more or less. It is not the opposite of disease or a state [the human] has, but rather a continuously changing process [the human] cocreates.

(Parse 1981, p. 39)

From this perspective there are no standards of normality by which to assess the person. The person is the expert and ultimate authority on his or her own health (Daly, Cody & Romanini 1994). The role of the nurse from Parse's perspective is similar to that of 'nurturing gardener as opposed to that of technician or mechanic' (Parse 1990, p. 139). For Rogers (1970, 1987), health is an expression of life process. She asserts that health and illness are not dichotomous but continuous (Rogers 1980). Moreover, Rogers claims that terms such as 'health' and 'illness' are poorly defined, embody varying definitions across cultures, and are value-laden (Rogers 1970). She regards health as a value, sees the central concern of nursing as unitary human beings and the goal of nursing as well-being and optimal health (Parse 1992). In contrast to totality paradigm practice methodologies, within the simultaneity paradigm Parse's theory guides approaches to nursing practice in which the recipient of nursing is regarded as the 'authority figure and prime decision maker in regard to nursing' (Parse 1987, p. 137).

TABLE 9.1 PARADIGMATIC PERSPECTIVES IN NURSING THEORY (ADAPTED FROM PARSE 1992)

	TOTALITY PERSPECTIVE	SIMULTANEITY PERSPECTIVE	
		ROGER'S LIFE PROCESS THEORY	PARSE'S HUMAN BECOMING THEORY
Human being	biopsychosocial-spiritual organism interacting with the environment	energy field in mutual process with the environmental field	open being cocreating becoming with the universe
	recognised by physiological, psychological, sociological and spiritual attributes	recognised by field pattern	recognised by patterns of relating
	interacts by coping with or managing the environment	participates knowingly relative to power index	freely chooses in situation
Health	physical, mental, social and spiritual well-being as defined by norms	a value	process of becoming as experienced and described by the person
Central phenomenon of nursing	self-care, adaptation, goal attainment, or caring	unitary human beings	human becoming
Goal of nursing	prevention of disease and promotion of health	well-being and optimal health	quality of life from the person's perspective
Primary mode of practice	nursing process with nursing diagnoses	pattern manifestation appraisal; deliberate mutual patterning	true presence in all-at-once: *illuminating meaning* through explication; *synchronising rhythms* through dwelling with; *mobilising transcendence* through moving beyond

In summary, within the simultaneity paradigm, the human being is regarded as an open being (inextricably one with the environment for Rogers, and one with the universe for Parse) who is recognised through patterns. Patterns are manifestations of the mutual human-environment or human-universe process. The simultaneity view of wholeness is quite different from the view embraced within the totality paradigm (Parse 1992). The simultaneity paradigm does not accommodate the principle of linear causality. This principle is rejected together with other closed-system concepts such as homeostasis, adaptation and dynamic equilibrium. Change from a totality paradigm view is causal, while change from a simultaneity paradigm view is mutual and unpredictable. In opposition to the totality paradigm, individual perceptions and differences are valued from the simultaneity perspective (Nagle & Mitchell 1991). Finally, there are no 'norms' within the simultaneity paradigm. This allows for acceptance of diversity and change in the patterns manifested by individual human beings in living, including respect for individuals' values, hopes and dreams.

UNDERPINNINGS OF THE THEORY OF HUMAN BECOMING

A survey of the underpinnings of the human becoming theory calls for examination of the work of the nurse theorist Martha Rogers (1970, 1980, 1987, 1990) and several philosophers. Rogers created the science of unitary human beings. Her perspective is very abstract and has its roots in microphysics and a vast array of other sources (Meleis 1991). A comprehensive examination of Rogers' work is beyond the scope of this chapter. Her theory is comprised of three principles, known collectively as the principles of homeodynamics. 'Homeodynamic' implies a process of evolving towards greater diversity and complexity. Change is a constant aspect of this process. Rogers sees human beings as irreducible wholes and open energy fields in mutual process with the environment, which is also held to be an energy field. For Rogers, both the human being and the environment exist in a universe of open systems, and change is continuous for the human and environmental energy fields, and unpredictable. The continuous interchange between the human and environmental energy fields is expressed in a rhythmical pattern that evolves always towards greater diversity. Rogers believes that the human being and the environment manifest unique patterns, which allows for differentiation between the human field and the environmental field. Shared adherence to the fundamental tenets of the simultaneity paradigm provides common ground for Rogers and Parse.

A number of significant existentialists and phenomenologists also had a major influence on Parse's theorising. Noteworthy are Kierkegaard (1958, 1959), Husserl (1976), Merleau-Ponty (1962, 1963), Heidegger (1962) and Sartre (1966). **Existentialism** holds human existence as its fundamental focus (Sarter 1988). It is a philosophical perspective that focuses on individual existence. Major beliefs in this perspective are that the individual is free and responsible for personal choices in determining how to live our lives. A number of major thinkers in philosophy contributed to the development of this theory including Nietzsche, Kierkegaard, Sartre, Merleau-Ponty, Heidegger, Tillich and Camus (Sarter 1988).

Phenomenology may be defined as 'the study of phenomena as they unfold' (Parse 1981, p. 178). Husserl, a German philosopher, was a non-existentialist phenomenologist. He is credited with creating phenomenology (Parse 1981). His focus was 'on the nature of human consciousness, which he characterized as exhibiting intentionality, or objective reference, in other words the mind is always actively encountering the world' (Sarter 1988, p. 57). Husserl was echoing the thesis of his teacher, Brentano, when he described 'intentionality', a state where the mind exhibits directedness-to-objects (Urmson & Ree 1991). The most profound insight of phenomenology is that consciousness is always consciousness-of-something. Husserl was interested in how objects are constituted in pure consciousness.

The German philosopher Heidegger (1962) is credited with merging phenomenology and existentialism to create **existential-phenomenology**. Existential-phenomenology is concerned with phenomena encountered in living and the meaning of human existence, including interpretation of experiences in life. This requires exploration of subjective, individual experiences in life. In this view, it is accepted that knowledge can be developed through advances in understanding of lived experiences (human experiences such as suffering, grief or hope). Of the philosophers who influenced Parse, Heidegger (1962), perhaps more than others, is reflected in her theoretical perspective. Heidegger was preoccupied with the question of being. He contributed a landmark work to philosophy, *Being and Time* (1962). This important work is concerned with ontology and human 'being', which Heidegger called *Dasein* (this translates from the German as being-there or existence). Heidegger posited concernful being-in-the-world as the unitary structure of human existence. Also he questioned the notion of time as linear, and the notion of linear causality (Parker 1991). Parker notes succinctly Heidegger's perspective on time:

> What Heidegger has helped us to understand is that [the] linear notion of time is itself historical. That is to say, it is a construct of our particular epoch. Humans have constructed this notion of time as linear and have used this construct to explain human events in a causal way. Heidegger recognised that time is directional and relational. The now is taken as the point of departure. The past exists as it comes into being for us now. The future also exists only now in terms of possibilities.
>
> *(Parker 1991, p. 292)*

Heidegger also believed that human beings are perpetually defining and redefining themselves through interpretation. From his perspective, life for humans is a relentless interpretive process through which we develop knowledge. Heidegger also saw humans as being future-oriented, free to choose in situations and pushing towards future possibilities—that is, towards the not-yet (Heidegger 1962). Also he theorised that anxiety was an inescapable part of human living as the human being in living is 'being-toward-death'.

These tenets and concepts from existential-phenomenology, which Parse synthesised with Rogers' science of unitary human beings in creating the theory of human becoming, are examined next.

INTENTIONALITY

This tenet suggests that human consciousness is intentional (Husserl 1976)—that is to say, consciousness is never reduced to the status of subject without consideration of object (Kockelmans 1978). Subject and object are always linked. Husserl's position is that intentionality gives meaning to the world (Husserl 1976). Consciousness-of-something is consciousness of meaning and therefore the world as apprehended by consciousness is a meaningful world. Parse (1981) defines intentionality as the human being's 'nature of knowing and being present to the world' (p. 177). This tenet 'posits that [the human] is by nature an intentional being' (Parse 1981, p. 18). The human being is intentional and 'involved with the world through a fundamental nature of knowing, being present and open' (Parse 1981, p. 18). The concepts of coexistence and situated freedom emerge from the tenet of intentionality (Parse 1981).

HUMAN SUBJECTIVITY

Parse (1981) defines subjectivity as a 'wholistic phenomenon referring to man' (p. 178). By this she means that it is a unitary phenomenon. It incorporates the human's personal view of a situation, but this emerges from, and with, the views of others. This process is dialectical. **Human subjectivity** is therefore intersubjective in a sense. Parse (1981) believes that the human being 'grows through this relationship giving meaning to the projects that emerge in the process of becoming, ... coparticipates in the emergence of projects by choosing to live certain values ... and participates with the world in the cocreation of self' (p. 19). The concept of coconstitution flows from this tenet (Parse 1981).

Parse abstracted three assumptions from the tenets of intentionality and human subjectivity which relate to human beings; 'one coconstitutes situations with the world, ... experiences existence as coexistence, and ... has freedom in situation' (Parse 1981, p. 20). The concepts of coconstitution, coexistence and situated freedom are explained below.

COCONSTITUTION

The notion of **coconstitution** relates to emergent meaning in context as 'related to particular constituents of that situation' (Parse 1981, p. 20). Parse (1981) states that the human being 'interrelates with the various views of the world and others and indeed cocreates these views by a personal presence. [The human being] by nature is present to the world and all-at-once, open to possibilities and, as such, participates in the creation of the world' (p. 20). This means that individual meaning is unique in some respects, but also includes shared meaning. And that humans collectively build the situations they share in life.

COEXISTENCE

The notion of **coexistence** relates to the human always becoming with the world and others. Parse states the human is:

> an emerging being, is in the world with others, indeed even the act of coming into the world is through others. [The human being] knows self in the comprehension of dispersed concrete achievements and through the perception of others. Without others one would not know that one is. To exist, then, is to coexist as the possibility of transcending self to be more than one is at a given point in space–time.
>
> *(Parse 1981, p. 20)*

This means that, in Parse's view, we are never alone, we coexist with others, but know how self is different from others. This comes from interrelating with others.

SITUATED FREEDOM

Parse (1981) asserts that 'freedom in situation means that reflectively and prereflectively one participates in choosing the situations in which one finds oneself as well as one's attitude towards the situations' (pp. 20–1). Humans choose within situation and choosings cocreate these situations. We can only choose from options that unfold in situation. The term 'situated freedom' means that options are limited by the situation one is in. Choices always reflect personal values. This idea means that human beings live with **situated freedom** as opposed to radical freedom; options or choices in context are always limited.

THE HUMAN BECOMING THEORY OF NURSING

Any accepted theory in nursing is based on key assumptions or 'givens'. Theoretical principles can be developed from these assumptions by creating concepts and linking them in a meaningful way. The assumptions underpinning the human becoming theory are written at what Parse terms the 'philosophical level of discourse' (Parse 1987). She describes a hierarchy in language which takes as its pinnacle highly abstract terms, while its base is language which is concrete. *Abstract concepts* are notions that are not directly experienced through the senses, and *concrete concepts* are those that are more readily experienced in reality, like height. Parse's assumptions are very abstract; her theoretical principles are also abstract but less abstract than her assumptions. She states that her principles are written at the theoretical level of discourse. Theoretical principles can be shifted down the hierarchy and linked with concrete experience. An example of how this can be done is provided later in this chapter.

When Parse published her theory in 1981, it was based on nine assumptions. Over time these were condensed into three assumptions. In 1992, Parse's three assumptions were stated as follows, reflecting the changes in the theory as discussed above:

1 Human becoming is freely choosing personal meaning in situations in the intersubjective process of relating value priorities.

2 Human becoming is cocreating rhythmical patterns of relating in open interchange with the universe.

3 Human becoming is cotranscending multidimensionally with the unfolding possibles.

(Parse 1992, p. 37)

These assumptions represent the philosophical tenets of the theory of human becoming.

The beliefs advanced in the three assumptions listed above are supported by ideas which can be located in the work of Heidegger (1962), Husserl (1976), Merleau-Ponty (1962), Sartre (1966) and Rogers (1970, 1980, 1987). In Parse's first assumption the unitary nature of being is reflected in the construct 'human becoming'. This view is consistent with Rogers' (1970) science of unitary human beings, where human and environment are seen as being in mutual process. The existential–phenomenological tenets of intentionality and human subjectivity are also reflected in the first assumption. Intentionality relates to the unity of the human and the universe and the all-at-once perpetual bestowal of meaning in context. The idea of human subjectivity also provides a view of the human being existing in mutual relationship with others and the universe. Heidegger's (1962) perspective is congruent with the view Parse expresses in her first assumption. According to Heidegger, the human is 'a performer of intentional acts which are bound together by the unity of meaning' (1962, p. 73). Parse asserts that freely choosing personal meaning is an aspect of human becoming. This view is consistent with Sartre's (1966) perspective on being and freedom. Sartre (1966) states 'to be free is to choose one self' (p. 568). The essence of this position may be extrapolated to encompass personal choice related to meaning and 'being-in-the-world'. Relating value priorities is also reflective of personal choice. The concepts of coconstitution, coexistence and situated freedom are also reflected in the first assumption.

Parse's second assumption also presents a unitary view of the human-universe-health process. This view is consistent with the view expressed in her first assumption and as such is supported by many of the sources discussed previously. In addition, there is concurrence between Parse's second assumption and Rogers' (1970, 1987, 1990) science. This is related to the view of the mutual human-environment process in part and the notion of **rhythmicity** related to pattern. The concept of becoming 'in open interchange with the universe' reflects a belief which is grounded in Rogers' conceptual system. The concept of cocreation is included in the second assumption. This concept evolved from existential-phenomenological thought (Parse 1981) and relates to how humans cocreate rhythmical patterns of relating in a unitary way.

Parse's third assumption suggests that the human is cotranscending—that is, transcending in a unitary way with others and the universe all-at-once. **Cotranscendence** relates to moving beyond with others (Parse 1981). That the human is held to cotranscend 'multidimensionally' means that the human lives at many realms of the universe simultaneously (Parse 1981), unbound by temporal or spatial limits. The view espoused in the third assumption is consistent with Rogers' (1970) belief that humans live in a relationship with the environment which is not confined by temporal or spatial attributes. The concept of cotranscending with the unfolding possibles reflects beliefs which are congruent with Heidegger's notion that humans are oriented towards future possibles—that is, towards the 'not -yet' (Heidegger 1962).

Three major themes emerge from Parse's philosophical assumptions: meaning, rhythmicity and cotranscendence (Parse 1981, 1987, 1992). Each theme leads to a principle of her theory and each principle is specified by three related concepts (Smith & Hudepohl 1988). Each principle posits a complex process assumed to be pivotal in the overall process of human becoming (Parse 1981). Parse wrote the theoretical concepts of the theory using present participles—words ending in 'ing'—to emphasise the process orientation of her theory. The three principles, which are presented in the following discussion, are written at the 'theoretical level of discourse'. That is, the language is less abstract than that used at the 'philosophical level of discourse'.

> *Principle 1:* Structuring meaning multidimensionally is cocreating reality
> through the languaging of valuing and imaging.
>
> *(Parse 1981, p. 69)*

This principle describes the process of constructing meaning. Meaning can be thought of in two ways—ultimate meaning, and meaning in the moment. Ultimate meaning has to do with our view of the purpose of life, while meaning in the moment is the day-to-day meaning of living. Meaning changes constantly in living through new experiences. What is suggested in this principle is that human beings structure **meaning** from many levels of the universe, the tacit and explicit simultaneously. Parse believes that living many levels of the universe means living in the now moment, with the past and future simultaneously. This relates to the concept of **multidimensionality**. The individual creates personal meaning and a view of reality together with others. Meaning is conveyed through languaging, valuing and imaging. *Languaging* is the process of self-expression, involving speech, silence and movement. *Valuing* is living life showing our precious beliefs and desires. *Imaging* is the process of picturing reality, including events and ideas. Through imaging, the human being constructs a view of reality, including precious beliefs which are made known through languaging.

> *Principle 2:* Cocreating rhythmical patterns of relating is living the paradoxical unity of revealing–concealing and enabling–limiting while connecting–separating.
>
> *(Parse 1981, p. 69)*

Parse's second principle describes the way in which the human being, with others, creates and lives rhythmic patterns in interrelating. 'Rhythmicity involves human beings living recognisable, rhythmic patterns in relationship with the universe' (Jonas et al. 1992, p. 33). This principle suggests that these rhythmic patterns of relating are paradoxical, that is, they possess what appear to be contradictory aspects. Parse has identified three rhythmical patterns of relating: revealing–concealing, enabling–limiting and connecting–separating. *Revealing–concealing* is the process of showing some aspects of self while hiding others in interrelating with others and self. Human beings cannot tell all that is known about self. There is always more to the other than is seen in being with a person. *Connecting–separating* is another 'paradoxical unity'. 'This rhythm is moving in one direction and away from others, yet always towards greater diversity' (Jonas et al. 1992, p. 34). *Enabling–limiting* is a process of choosing; with each choice the human being makes, there are possibilities and limitations available simultaneously.

> *Principle 3:* Cotranscending with the possibles is powering unique ways of originating in the process of transforming.
>
> *(Parse 1981, p. 69)*

Parse's third principle suggests that human beings, with others and the universe, are constantly moving forward in life towards new possibilities. This involves a struggle which possesses contradictory aspects. Parse believes that day-to-day life involves a rhythm of pushing–resisting, a tension experienced in striving with new goals and values. *Powering* is the term Parse uses to describe this process. *Originating* is a process of finding ways of expressing unique aspects of self. This involves choosing ways of living that are unique. *Transforming*, the third concept in this principle, is the process of struggling to move forward in life towards new possibilities and greater diversity by looking at what is familiar in life in a new way. Cotranscendence involves the processes of powering, originating and transforming.

Parse (1981) has developed a number of theoretical structures to guide nursing practice or research. She has done this by linking theoretical concepts. For each structure one concept is taken from each of the theoretical principles of the theory of human becoming. These structures are 'non-directional propositions. They are non-causal in nature and are consistent with the assumptions and principles of the theory' (Parse 1992, p. 39). The structures are stated below.

1 Powering is a way of revealing–concealing imaging.

2 Originating is a manifestation of enabling–limiting valuing.

3 Transforming unfolds in the languaging of connecting–separating.

(Parse 1987, p. 166)

These propositions are written at the theoretical level of discourse. Written at a less abstract level of discourse, these propositions may be restated for guiding research and practice as follows.

1 Struggling towards dreams discloses and hides the significance of the situation.

2 Creating anew uncovers cherished beliefs that lead in a particular direction.

3 A different view of the familiar emerges through speaking and moving, while being close to and away from others.

(Parse 1987, 1992).

NURSING PRACTICE GUIDED BY THE THEORY OF HUMAN BECOMING

For Parse the goals of nursing practice are (1) to enhance the quality of life from the person's perspective and (2) to preserve the dignity of the person (Parse 1989, 1992). A central assumption here is that nursing practice mandates valuing the person and the family (Parse 1981). In this practice methodology, 'the person is never viewed as an object to be manipulated or controlled on any level, but is viewed uncompromisingly as *an experiencing, choosing, subjective unity to be revered* [emphasis added]' (Daly, Cody & Romanini 1994, p. 147). Here, the nurse is with the person/family in considering decisions and activities regarding the person's health which come from their perspective. The focus in this coparticipation is the hopes, dreams and beliefs of the person/family receiving nursing. Central to this are the personal meanings, cherished beliefs and patterns of relating of the person and family. The human becoming practice methodology takes as its primary mode 'true presence in all-at-once illuminating meaning through explication, synchronizing rhythms through dwelling with [and] mobilizing transcendence through moving beyond' (Parse 1992, p. 36).

For Parse, nursing practice happens in true presence—'It is a subject-to-subject interrelationship, a loving true presence with the other to enhance the quality of life' (Parse 1987, p. 169). The Parse nurse focuses on the person's hopes, dreams, beliefs and views in true presence with the recipient of nursing care (Parse 1981). True presence is defined as 'a nonroutinized, nonmechanical way of "being-with" in which the nurse is authentic and attentive to moment-to-moment changes in meaning for the person or group. These changes in meaning lead to changes in commitment and may occur through the creative imaging, affirming self, and glimpsing the paradoxical as the nurse is present to the person' (Parse 1990a, p. 139).

There are many examples of the use of Parse's theory in practice in the literature. The examples provided in this chapter have been taken from Daly, Cody and Romanini (1994), who demonstrate how Parse's theory of human becoming can be used to guide nursing practice in the acute or critical care setting. The dimensions and processes of Parse's practice method are sequenced in concept only. Parse believes that they happen all at once.

Illuminating meaning

The first dimension of Parse's practice method is *illuminating meaning*. Here, the nurse is with the patient as the patient explores the personal meaning of their situation. New insights and meanings emerge through this process. The patient's understanding of the situation grows as the familiar is seen in new ways. The related process is *explicating*, which is 'making clear what is appearing now through languaging' (Parse 1987, p. 167). The nurse participates with the person/family in this process, seeking to clarify such questions as: What is the person's/family's life situation like now? How do they live from day to day? What is most important to the person/family?

Example

Peter J., a 68-year-old retired railway engineer with a long history of congestive heart failure and emphysema, is admitted to a coronary care unit (CCU) with respiratory insufficiency and fluid overload. He has been in and out of hospital for years but recently has been able to live at home, using portable oxygen, cardiac medications and diuretics, with the help of a community health nurse. He tells the nurse in the CCU that he enjoys visiting his children and grandchildren, but that he misses his wife, who died a year ago. He says he keeps going by 'just taking things as they come' but that he 'doesn't know how much more he can take'. He says that he knows the end of his life is near and that he 'hated' the two previous times he was intubated. After intensive medical treatment he continues to experience hypoxia and hypercapnia, and the physician advises intubation and mechanical ventilatory assistance.

The nurse, centring on the concerns of Peter and his family as these are expressed in the nurse–person/family relationship, is with them as they clarify the meaning of the present situation and identify the value priorities that underpin their decision making.

Synchronising rhythms

The second dimension of the practice method is *synchronising rhythms*. Here, the nurse goes with the ups and downs of the patient's story as they are in true presence with the other (Jonas et al. 1992). The related process is *dwelling with*, which is 'giving self over to the flow of the struggle in connecting–separating' (Parse 1987, p. 167). The nurse goes with the patient and does not try to influence what the individual wishes to discuss or reveal or experience. The nurse participates with the person and family in this process by centring self on their unique meanings and concerns, and by seeking with them to clarify such questions as: Who does the person/family feel most comfortable with? Who can help to cocreate comfort with the person/family? Who is most important to the person/family now?

Example

Jenny B., a 45-year-old factory worker, is admitted to the neurosurgical ICU, having suffered the 'worst headache of her life' and collapsed at work. She has received the medical diagnosis of a ruptured cerebral aneurism.

Since her admission to the ICU, cerebral vasospasm unresponsive to treatment has resulted in paralysis of her right side. Jenny is divorced and has two sons, aged 14 and 16, who see their father only occasionally. Jenny has been working overtime every week to save for her sons' university education. In the time away from her job, she has been busy running her house, relaxing by visiting a few close neighbours or playing with her pet cat, Ginger.

She undergoes a craniotomy to clip the aneurism, but afterwards her right side remains paralysed. She says that she is worried about the boys, and expresses doubt that they are taking good care of Ginger or keeping up with the housework, although on their visits they assure her that they are 'managing all right' at home. She also worries about her sons' future now that she cannot do her usual job in the factory. Jenny wonders how she will ever be able to keep her house or support her family again but she is determined 'to get back to her own home' and to 'see the boys get through university'.

The nurse in this situation listens to the concerns voiced by Jenny, and participates with her in exploring the changing patterns of relationships in her life as the new situation is integrated with existing patterns. As Jenny discusses the boys, their father, the neighbours and Ginger in light of her own value priorities, the nurse moves with her as the possibilities for rearranging activities and responsibilities become apparent.

Mobilising transcendence

The third dimension of the practice method is *mobilising transcendence,* and the related process is *moving beyond,* which is 'propelling towards the possibles in transforming' (Parse, 1987, p. 167). Here the patient is guided to consider hopes and dreams for the future. Through this process, ideas regarding change are considered, to enhance quality of life from the patient's perspective. The nurse participates with the person and family in this process, attending to such questions as: What are the person's/family's hopes and dreams relating to this situation? What are their plans? How does the person/family intend to make these plans a reality?

Parse has developed three standards for nursing practice guided by the human becoming theory. They can be used in evaluating quality of nursing practice and are as follows:

1   A *personal health description*—this is recorded by the nurse as given by the person or the family. It includes meanings the person ascribes to relationships, choices, and the person's/family's hopes and dreams.

Example

Alice T., a 25-year-old physical education teacher, is admitted to a general intensive care unit after a motor vehicle accident in which she sustained multiple fractures, cerebral contusions and internal haemorrhaging. After weeks of intensive treatment, including several surgical operations for orthopaedic and abdominal injuries, prolonged intubation and extensive antibiotic therapy, she is beginning to talk about her situation and her concerns. The orthopaedic surgeon has advised that her left leg will require traction for six weeks, followed by another operation.

Alice says that she has no contact with her immediate family and does not wish to see them. She lives with her partner, Brenda, and their two dogs, in a country house, where they have enjoyed a lifestyle focusing on sports and the outdoors. Brenda comes to be with her every day and has taped photographs where Alice can easily see them of the two of them together, of their dogs, and of Alice's soccer team. Alice talks with the nurse about her enjoyment of coaching the girls' soccer team and her love for the life she and Brenda lead in the country. She says she feels that she 'let the girls down' by getting injured. She also worries about Brenda taking the time to travel from the country every day to be with her.

The nurse participates with Alice and Brenda as ways of living with the new situation are explored, and their hopes for the future are interrelated with the possibilities as they appear now. Planning for the future emerges from the perspective of Alice and her partner, and activities directed towards the achievement of personal goals are decided on, based on their beliefs and values.

---

2   *Emerging patterns of health-becoming*—these are identified through nurse-person dialogue. Documentation here reflects the paradoxical nature of the rhythms of interrelationships in that both aspects of the rhythm are considered (e.g. both opportunities and limitations). The nurse-person-family activities in which these patterns unfold are decided on by the person and the family.

3   *The directional movement of specific plans* formulated by the person/family in dialogue with the nurse are documented from the person's perspective. Documentation here reflects striving with intentions as progress in a chosen direction is described by the person or family.

(Parse 1981, pp. 72–3)

Parse's theory has been used to guide nursing practice in a number of settings in North America (see Parse 1995). Evaluation studies of human becoming in practice have been undertaken by Santopinto and Smith (1995), who investigated use of the theory in nursing practice with adults and children, Jonas (1995), who evaluated theory-guided practice in family practice, and Mitchell (1995), whose focus was theory-guided practice in acute care. All these reports suggest that the human becoming theory enhances nursing practice both for recipients of nursing and nurses. For example, Santopinto and Smith report that the major changes they noted in practice were 'greater inclusion of client's perspectives of feelings, wishes and hopes; less use of ritualized phrases in charting; and more focused accounts of how patients describe their life situations' (Santopinto & Smith 1995, pp. 328–9). Mitchell reports the following patterns in her data:

> [C]hanged nurses' perspectives of the patient from problem to patient as human being, changed morale in nurses, less judging and labelling of patients, more talking and listening to patients, respecting the patient's right to choose [and] enhancing the quality of [the] nurse–person relationship.
>
> *(Mitchell 1995, p. 388)*

Introducing Parse's theory in traditional nursing practice settings may not be smooth sailing. It requires intensive education and mentoring of nurses who are new to the theory by a nurse who has appropriate expertise. The major challenge for those who are new to the theory is shifting values and beliefs in order to change views of nursing and patients and ways of being in practice. This process can be painful and rewarding all-at-once. Some nurses will not be able to live the theory in their practice because their values and beliefs are inconsistent with the theory.

The literature also discusses the massive organisational change that may accompany introduction of this theory in practice, which may involve casualties among the nursing staff (Santopinto & Smith 1995). Infrastructure issues are involved here too—economic and human resource factors, among others—which would require the commitment and support of the senior members of the health care institution involved in using the theory in practice.

Perhaps another issue that could be problematic are the attitudes and values of medical practitioners who practise with the nurses who wish to use the human becoming theory as a guide to practice. Successful implementation of the theory would require, at the very least, education of medical colleagues to ensure that they do not seek to undermine its use in practice. (We are all aware of the existence of the 'conservative medico' who does not believe that patients should be allowed decision-making prerogatives.)

CRITICAL PERSPECTIVES ON THE HUMAN BECOMING THEORY: A SYNOPSIS

A number of critiques of Parse's work have been published in book chapters or scholarly journals. Some scholars have taken issue with the language of Parse's theory (Holmes 1990; Limrandi 1982; Winkler 1983), not realising that theory should be written in unique language at a theoretical level. The issue here is the use of what is regarded by some as esoteric, abstract language. It has been suggested that articulating a theory of nursing in this way limits access to what it may have to offer practice (Holmes 1990). Of those who have been critical of the language of the theory of human becoming in print, a number have nonetheless appreciated its value to nursing knowledge (Levine 1988; Limrandi 1982). The theory, it has been noted, has fascinating potential (Limrandi 1982) and, further, it 'uses the language of passion and compassion' and 'recreates the reality of the human experience . . . the exaltation and anguish of a lived life' (Levine, cited in Cody & Mitchell 1992, p. 61) On the other hand, a number of scholars who have critiqued Parse's theory have not found her language problematic (Phillips 1987; Pugliese 1989; Smith & Hudepohl 1988). There is no consensus on this issue.

Another polemical issue raised in the literature is that the theory of human becoming lacks operational propositions amenable to testing (Limrandi 1982). Such a comment reflects the critic's lack of understanding of the philosophical base of Parse's theory. Cody and Mitchell (1992) assert that early critiques of Parse's theory reflect ignorance of the unitary view of reality, and minimal understanding of human science and its related practice and research methods. The notion of testing propositions is antithetical to the theory of human becoming. Research with Parse's theory is designed to expand the theory (Cody & Mitchell 1992, p. 62).

A further issue in the literature was raised by Winkler (1983)—that Parse's theory fails to consider biological dimensions of the person. This claim has been contested by Phillips (1987), who contends that Parse's theory considers all aspects of the person because of its focus on wholeness and lived experience. Other aspects of the theory have been discussed in the literature: its process orientation (Cowling 1989); its potential for viewing nursing in a new way (Cowling 1989); its repudiation of linear causality and vigorous approach to science (Phillips 1987); its potential for developing appreciation of the science and art of nursing (Pugliese 1989); and its inclusion of the humanity of the person (Smith & Hudepohl 1988).

THE AUTHORS' VIEWS

We acknowledge that, initially, Parse's language can be challenging for some. However, in our view, this can be rewarding as your familiarity with the work grows. Words used by Parse all have a source—the addition of 'ing' to some words may concern some of you, as for example, in power-ing. Its purpose, though, is to emphasise the process orientation of the theory.

Parse's language has its roots in human science philosophy. If you wish to build your knowledge and understanding of Parse's theory, but are unfamiliar with this knowledge base, you will need to go to appropriate sources in order to do so (these could include Parse, Dilthey and the existential-phenomenologists). Cody and Mitchell (1992) have suggested that the nurse who wishes to learn to use the theory of human becoming in practice or research not only has to become familiar with Parse's distinctive language, but develop a new way of thinking about nursing. Remember, Parse believes that nursing is an autonomous science and performing art. Any science has a unique body of knowledge and a language of its own, which is usually abstract.

We also wonder whether it is reasonable to expect to feel comfortable with theoretical information which is picked up and readily understood at the first, second or even third reading. If this were the case, would interest, creativity and opportunities for learning be stifled? We also acknowledge openly that not all nurses will want to develop expertise with, or even consider using, the human becoming theory in nursing practice or research. This is often because of an inability to live the values and beliefs of Parse's theory. Many nurses will be more open to, and comfortable with using, a totality paradigm theory.

In our experience the number of Australian nurses who are interested in Parse's work appears to be growing. We can only speculate as to why this is so. However, the theory often appeals because of its emphasis on valuing people for who they are, and a willingness to reconsider traditional nursing practice because of perceived shortcomings in the area of patients' rights. Often the theory appeals to nurses because they see it as a vehicle for enhancing quality of care for patients or clients. The relationship between nurse and patient/client is balanced when the theory is used in practice. Where questions of quality of life are concerned, the patient is the expert. This can be liberating for the patient/client and the nurse.

Parse's theory also attracts interest and commitment because of its emphasis on the meaning of lived experiences of health. Exploration of these experiences can enhance the nurse's understanding of nursing phenomena, thus enriching appreciation of the humanity of patients/clients and nursing practice. Another consideration is the ethical stance of many nurses who believe in autonomy as a patient right. The nurse using the theory of human becoming in practice believes in respect for the individual values, hopes and dreams of patients; in a person's right to choose in relation to their health and in their responsibility for those choices; in the value of exploring the personal meaning of the patient/client situation; and in the value of true presence in practice with patients/clients as they find their own way of becoming.

Another fascinating aspect of the theory is its recognition of paradox in lived experience. This helps nurses to understand that life is complex, and that situations in which patients find themselves are rarely black and white (Jonas et al. 1992). Nurses can appreciate the complexity of being human, lived experiences of health and the mystery of life, using Parse's theory as a 'lens on life'. Understanding this, and having the courage to be with patients as they confront life's experiences, can be enriching for the nurse and the patient or client. We recognise also that the theory of human becoming can assist the discipline of nursing in humanising nursing practice.

Parse has developed a unique theoretical perspective which is a human science in terms of its philosophical orientation. This theory is unlike other nursing perspectives in that it focuses on subjectivity, the meaning of personal reality and the experience of 'being-in-the-world' (Smith & Hudepohl 1988). Transcendence, or 'moving beyond what-is by pursuing valued hopes and dreams' (Smith & Hudepohl 1988, p. 48), is another unique area of concern for Parse. Further, the theory of human becoming is

> concerned with health as a subjective experience of the quality of living, illuminated through personal description; patterns in the person-environment relationship that reflect health; health as transcendence and transformation; personal choice and commitment as health; and the paradoxical nature of the lived experience of health.
>
> *(Smith & Hudepohl, 1988, p. 48)*

Its focus on moving forward in life in pursuit of hopes and dreams is also unique. Many would argue that the ultimate test of a theory in nursing is its usefulness in practice. Despite the criticisms of Parse's theory, the major difficulty being its inaccessibility, there is much evidence to show that the human becoming theory is making a significant impact on nursing practice in numerous settings (Cody & Mitchell 1992; Fawcett 1993; Parse 1995). The nurse using Parse's theory in practice accepts patients for who they are, exercises compassion and a commitment to being with patients as they struggle to enhance their quality of life. Central to this is not judging patients, being open and accepting of their individual values, hopes and dreams, and focusing totally, when in true presence in practice, as a patient tells her or his story.

That patients are open to the nurse in this way is a practice privilege that is valued from Parse's perspective. A fundamental belief held by the Parse nurse is that as patients speak about the meaning of their situation, this meaning changes. These insights can see patients making progress in their understanding of their situation. Often this allows or facilitates transcendence, with the patient moving forward in life (Mitchell 1991). Change is a central aspect of this process, and this is chosen by the patient.

Though she does not use the term, Parse appears to have developed what could be considered 'nursology'. Her theory provides a knowledge base for the discipline that may be used in guiding practice and research.

SUMMARY

This chapter presents Parse's human becoming theory of nursing. Its relationship to paradigms in nursing knowledge, and its theoretical and philosophical underpinnings have been examined. We have also presented examples of how Parse's theory can be applied in clinical nursing practice. A number of perspectives or views of the human becoming theory, documented by nurse scholars, have also been considered.

Several issues related to the theory have been acknowledged and addressed. We believe that the theory makes a significant contribution to nursing knowledge, practice and research. We emphasise that the nurse who wishes to use the human becoming theory in practice must make a commitment to its values and beliefs, undertake the study necessary to build knowledge and understanding of the theory, and develop requisite skills in order to live it in practice.

GLOSSARY

Coconstitution: relates to meaning in context, which is unique in some respects but also includes shared aspects. Meaning is constituted, or comprised, of multiple shared aspects.

Coexistence: a state where one is seen to exist with others and the universe at all times. This relates to Parse's notion of the human being as always becoming with the world and others.

Cotranscendence: a process identified by Parse (1981, 1987) which involves powering, originating and transforming. This relates to the way in which the human being, against resistance, pushes forward and onward in life with others, expressing unique aspects of self. This movement with others and the universe is towards new possibilities and greater diversity.

Existential-phenomenology: a combination of ideas from existentialism and phenomenology. Existential-phenomenology is concerned with phenomena encountered in living and the meaning of human existence including interpretation of experiences in life. This requires exploration of subjective, individual experiences in life. In this view, it is accepted that valid knowledge can be developed through advances in understanding of lived human experiences, such as suffering, grief or hope.

Existentialism: a school of thought or theory in philosophy. Existentialism takes human existence as its basic focus, including personal experience (Sarter 1988). It is a philosophical perspective or theory that focuses on individual existence. Major beliefs from this perspective are that human beings are subjects, not objects, that the individual is free up to a point, chooses meaning in life and is responsible for choices. Existentialism also places emphasis on open examination of the experiences that individuals have in life, including what may be regarded as tragic. This requires consideration of personal meaning in living through human experiences, like suffering, grief, loss and hope. A number of major thinkers in philosophy contributed to the development of this theory, including Nietzsche, Kierkegaard, Sartre, Merleau-Ponty, Heidegger, Tillich and Camus (Sarter 1988).

Human becoming: a construct (highly abstract concept) which is the central focus of Parse's (1981, 1992, 1995) theory of nursing. Like Rogers, Parse has a unitary view of reality. For Parse, human becoming is living health with the universe (rather than environment) in a unitary way. Health in this view is simply how one is experiencing living. Human becoming is constant, something which is ongoing.

Human subjectivity: a term from existential-phenomenology. It refers to our personal world view, something that is largely private. However, the meaning of life for us, or the meaning of a situation, has unique and shared aspects. This is because we can only form such views by considering the views of others. Meaning is cocreated—that is, it is created by self in concert with others and the universe. Parse believes that the human being exists in a dialectical relationship with the world. She defines subjectivity as a 'wholistic phenomenon referring to the human being' (Parse 1981, p. 178), by which she means that subjectivity is a unitary phenomenon. Here, subjectivity and objectivity are not separate categories but are linked or merged.

Linear causality: the empirical notion of cause and effect, commonly believed to occur in a logical, rational way, closely related in time and space. It is a principle which is fundamental to positivism. In that world view, 'human beings are shaped by cause–effect relationships with the environment . . . [they] are like machines, that can be broken into parts for analysis and fixing; like machines they are predictable. They are confined by their situation' (Jonas et al. 1992, p. 21).

Meaning: Parse (1992) defines meaning as the 'whatness' of a situation. Meaning occurs on two levels: the ultimate meaning of life, and meaning in moments of living—which constantly changes.

Multidimensionality: Parse (1981) believes that human beings live multidimensionally—that is, at a number of realms of the universe all-at-once (simultaneously). This means that human beings live in the now moment, with the past and the future simultaneously. Living in the now is relative; it includes what has gone before and what is ahead in living. Living in the future is explained by the assertion that human beings are future-oriented, always considering their intentions for the future.

Ontology: a term from metaphysics, which is a branch of philosophy. Ontology 'deals with the nature of being' (Australian Concise Oxford Dictionary). Central to this is consideration of the relationship between the human being and the world. The term 'world view' is commonly used in nursing knowledge to capture how this relationship may be conceptualised. World views are concerned with 'philosophic claims about the nature of human beings and the human–environment relationship' (Fawcett 1993a, p. 56). A world view may be called an 'ontological perspective', because it is based on ontological assumptions, which are beliefs about the nature of human beings and the human–environment relationship.

Paradigm: this term is synonymous with the term 'world view'. A paradigm is a construction which is comprised of values and beliefs (that is, philosophical claims). Paradigms in nursing theory capture supposed aspects of the discipline which are shared by its community (Meleis 1991). This includes assumptions regarding human beings, health, the environment and their interrelationship.

Particulate: comprised of, or in the form of, separate particles or minute portions of matter. The term may be used to capture the reductionistic view of human beings, as posited in the totality paradigm, where the person is seen as comprised of parts.

Pattern: an abstract concept, used in the simultaneity paradigm. When speaking of human beings, pattern refers to the distinguishing characteristics, or form, the individual takes in living. The environment/universe has distinguishing characteristics or form also. Health patterns are unique and show considerable diversity. Individuals' health patterns can be explored through patients/clients describing what health is in their life as they live day-to-day.

Phenomenology: may be defined as 'the study of phenomena as they unfold' (Parse 1981, p. 178). The term 'phenomena' may be defined as circumstances or events that capture our attention. Husserl, a German philosopher, is credited with creating phenomenology. His focus was 'on the nature of human consciousness, which he characterized as exhibiting intentionality, or objective reference, in other words the mind is always actively encountering the world' (Sarter 1988, p. 57). Intentionality is a state where the mind exhibits directedness-to-objects (Urmson & Ree 1991). Husserl was interested in the way in which objects are constituted in consciousness. The most profound insight of phenomenology is that consciousness is always consciousness-of-something. Thus, there is always a link between subject and object.

Rhythmicity: refers to the cocreation of rhythmical patterns of relating, a process involving human beings and the universe. Rhythms, according to Parse, are paradoxical and recognisable; for example, enabling–limiting.

Situated freedom: from the perspective of existential-phenomenology, we are free to choose from a range of options in any situation. These options are limited by our situation. Therefore, we live with situated, as opposed to radical, freedom.

Unitary human being: a concept from Rogers' (1970, 1987, 1990) science of unitary human beings. In Rogers' theoretical perspective *the human being is an energy field that is one with the environment* (also considered an energy field). This is the crux of what is meant by the notion of 'unitary human being'; the human and environment are indivisible. The human being therefore cannot be viewed as split in parts, or separate from the environment, as occurs in some theoretical perspectives in nursing. For Rogers, the human being is irreducible, more than the sum of the parts, and can only be known by consideration of pattern. Pattern is a manifestation of the whole.

QUESTIONS

1   Has Parse made a unique contribution to nursing practice? If so, what are the dimensions of this?

2   Introducing the human becoming theory as a guide to nursing practice in any clinical setting requires a rational and prudent plan. How should this plan be constructed?

3   Can the human becoming theory be used in all nursing practice settings?

LEARNING ACTIVITY

Collect and critique five journal articles which discuss the application of the human becoming theory in practice. Use the critique in a group discussion to stimulate critical analysis of Parse's theory in practice.

FURTHER READING

Parse, R.R. 1981, *Man-Living-Health: A Theory of Nursing*, John Wiley, New York (reprinted 1989, Delmar, New York). Contains Parse's theory of nursing in its original form. In addition to comprehensive presentation of the theory, this text also explores the theory's potential use in nursing practice, research and education.

Parse, R.R. 1987, 'Parse's man-living-health theory of nursing', in *Nursing Science: Major Paradigms, Theories and Critique*, ed. R.R. Parse, Saunders, Philadelphia, pp. 159–80. Presents Parse's theory and expands discussion of its use in practice and research. Parse's practice methodology is related to the man-living-health theory, incorporating discussion of its dimensions and processes. This chapter also presents the research method which was developed using Parse's theory.

Parse, R.R. (ed.) 1995, *Illuminations: The Human Becoming in Practice and Research*, Pub. No. 15–2670, National League for Nursing, New York. Presents updated information on Parse's theory. It includes theoretical conceptualisations of unitary phenomena from a human becoming perspective and examples of the theory in practice and nursing research. The work also contains a number of evaluation studies of Parse's theory in practice.

10

USING THE NEUMAN SYSTEMS MODEL AS A CURRICULUM ORGANISER

ALISON BALLANTYNE AND ANITA LANGE

LEARNING OBJECTIVES

When you have read this chapter you should be able to:

1 Describe the components of the Neuman Systems Model.

2 Apply the Neuman Systems Model to curriculum development, program design and organisation.

3 Recognise the value of using a nursing model as a framework for organising curriculum, planning teaching and learning, and the linking of theory to practice.

Alison Ballantyne, RN, GerNursCert, DipT(Nurs), BEd, MEdAdmin, is a Senior Lecturer in the Faculty of Nursing, University of South Australia. Alison has had extensive experience in curriculum development, subject development and coordination at both undergraduate and postgraduate levels, as well as writing distance learning for subjects in graduate courses. Her teaching experience extends over 20 years and has involved teaching in hospital programs and, since 1987, in the higher education sector. Her responsibilities have included teaching in both undergraduate and graduate courses for nurses as well as in multidisciplinary courses including gerontology. Alison's research experience has focused mainly on issues concerning nursing in aged and extended care. She is currently a doctoral student undertaking research about nursing work in nursing homes.

Anita Lange, RN, DipT(NursEd), BEd, GradDipEd(Comp), MPH, is currently Head of the School of Nursing (City and Whyalla campuses), Faculty of Nursing, University of South Australia. Anita has vast experience in program design and development, and has coordinated and taught in nursing programs at both the undergraduate and postgraduate level. She has taught extensively in multiprofessional education courses in collaboration with the Department of Community Medicine, University of Adelaide. Anita's research experience has centred on an examination of the smoking behaviours, risk perception and health practices of nursing students. Her current research for her doctoral studies is in the area of policy development related to planning the nursing workforce.

INTRODUCTION

This chapter describes the implementation of a curriculum using the Neuman Systems Model as a curriculum organiser for a Bachelor of Nursing program in Australia.

Nursing programs prepare professional nurses (registered nurses) who will practise and are responsible and accountable for nursing and health care in a dynamic and changing society. This program needs to challenge and develop creativity, and prepare graduates for their emerging roles and the evolving health needs of the community they serve.

Health care in Australia, as in many other countries, is the product of numerous social, cultural and political factors. It is essential that nursing students gain a comprehensive knowledge base of the multifaceted nature of the context in which they will practise nursing. Rapid advances in medical technology and the changes in the patterns of disease may pose a dilemma for nurse curriculum planners. It is inappropriate to teach nursing students everything about nursing and health care in a 'now' mentality. More importantly, nursing curricula should facilitate role induction into the profession, be adaptive to future trends, and facilitate lifelong learning based on sound problem-solving and reflective and critical thinking. Using models and conceptual frameworks facilitates this process. Sipple (1989) suggests that the Neuman Health Care Systems Model provides a systematic framework for assessing, planning, organising, managing and controlling curriculum change activities.

NURSING EDUCATION IN AUSTRALIA

In the late 1960s and 1970s, nurses and professional organisations were lobbying the Commonwealth Government for nursing education to be transferred to the tertiary education system. In the late 1970s, the first pilot nursing education program was established in a number of the States (Russell 1990).

In the early 1980s, nurses continued to lobby the government for the total transfer of undergraduate nursing education into the tertiary sector. At the same time the nursing profession was also involved in developing a career structure for nurses, which was progressively implemented in different States and territories from the mid 1980s.

Finally, in the 1980s, a decision was made by the Commonwealth Government in Australia to transfer nursing education from the hospital-based system to the tertiary arena, which meant educating nurses in Colleges of Advanced Education and Institutes of Technology, with the exception of one course taught within a university. At the time of the transfer of nursing education, Australia had a binary system for tertiary education with Colleges of Advanced Education and Institutes of Technology being one aspect of the system, and universities the other. Universities were funded at a higher level than Colleges of Advanced Education and Institutes of Technology.

In the 1990s, the binary system was dissolved, and Colleges of Advanced Education and Institutes of Technology became universities in their own right, or merged with established universities. Therefore, in the 1990s, all students studying to become registered nurses are studying at university.

Nursing education in Australia has experienced many changes and challenges during the last 25 years. In conjunction with the developments in nursing, science and technology as well as a knowledge explosion, nurses are requiring additional skills and knowledge in order to function effectively and deliver a high standard of nursing care and service to their clients. Nurses are also being encouraged to develop and use nursing theories and other theories in education, practice and research. It is recognised that theory can evolve from practice and theory can guide practice.

The concept of a curriculum has undergone marked changes over the past 20 years, without any agreement on what an appropriate definition should be. Essentially, curriculum can be viewed as any or all of the following:

- a means of organising knowledge;
- a vehicle for reflective thinking;
- a guided learning experience;
- an instructional plan;
- a technological system of production.

Perhaps the best way to view, or define, a curriculum is as a dynamic living structure, one that adapts, changes and reflects those for whom it is intended—that is, the student, those who teach within the nursing profession and the consumers of the service that the graduates will provide.

Before the transfer of nurse education, the nursing curriculum was very much determined by the setting in which the teaching of nurses took place. The training hospital settings all varied in size, acuity, geographic location and autonomy of school. The hospital service needs took precedence over the students' learning needs. Anecdotal evidence suggests that many nurses were taught survival techniques related to their first clinical exposure following the initial study block. A lot of this was information based on very little theory and possibly even less regard for the students' learning experiences. Much of what was taught within a hospital school really was reinforced by the setting. As a result, the focus was definitely an illness/medically dominated model that lacked appro-priate sequencing and was unable to facilitate an integrated approach to theory and practice.

This chapter describes how the Neuman Systems Model was used as a framework for curriculum development in a new nursing program at the University of South Australia, formerly the South Australian Institute of Technology, Adelaide.

WHY CHOOSE THE NEUMAN HEALTH CARE SYSTEMS MODEL?

In 1987 the School of Nursing was established in the South Australian Institute of Technology at the City Campus, and later at Whyalla, the rural outreach campus. The School of Nursing at City was planning an intake of 240 undergraduate students, while Whyalla campus would have an intake of 50 students each academic year. The School of Nursing is now part of the Faculty of Nursing, University of South Australia. The Faculty of Nursing came into being in July 1992 as a result of the formation of the University of South Australia in 1991.

The first nurse academics employed in the School of Nursing recognised the need to use a nursing model as the organising framework for the undergraduate program. A decision was made to use the Neuman Systems Model as a curriculum organiser for the Diploma in Nursing and later the Bachelor in Nursing. The Neuman model was chosen after several models had been examined. Each model was carefully examined in the context of the foundation academic staff's own professional experiences, and philosophical position. Models were eliminated if they were perceived as too esoteric or ephemeral, or if they applied to one particular nursing context only. Adoption of a particular model and/or theories as the basis of curriculum development was, in many instances, supported by broad consultation with nursing leaders and clinical colleagues and a careful review of the available literature (McCulloch 1995).

The Neuman Systems Model was selected as the conceptual framework on the basis of its congruence with the School of Nursing's philosophical statements on nursing and education, and the intended aims and graduate outcomes of the proposed program (see box on p. 206). The selection of a single model of nursing as the curriculum organiser was not without its critics. Concerns were raised about the exclusivity of using one model of nursing only, and these were addressed by the foundation lecturers. Subsequently, many models of nursing were used in teaching when they best demonstrated an aspect of nursing practice. The rich debate engendered by the process of model selection raised the educational process to a level that continues to stimulate thinking, exploring and testing by both staff and students. This debate assisted the curriculum planners in identifying how Neuman's model could be used to explore the learning process and the relationship between students, teachers and patients, and this became a useful illustration of open systems at work.

The philosophy of the School, the course aims and graduate outcome statements guided the choice of the model to be used as a curriculum organiser, as well as guiding academic staff in developing the teaching process and learning experiences. These three factors are detailed in the box on p. 206.

DESCRIPTION OF THE NEUMAN SYSTEMS MODEL

The Neuman Systems Model has a holistic approach to the viewing of potential and actual health problems. The model essentially represents an individual as an open system with input, process/throughput and output, which can be characterised in terms of two components—stress and reaction to it. (However, the system can be a family, community or organisation.) Health is viewed as the system being in harmony with the environment and the person's total needs being met. Illness is the state of disharmony that occurs when the person's needs are not met, which could result in death. It is important to note that by enabling the individual's total needs to be met, the model implies that Neuman views health as an outcome of a variety of events or processes that are not just biological in nature—rather, they are spiritual, developmental, psychological, social and cultural.

The Neuman Model brings together the physiological, psychological, sociocultural and developmental components of a person. The person is depicted graphically (see Figure 10.1) as being composed of a basic structure, or central core, common to all human beings, surrounded by a series of concentric circles. The basic structure consists of physiological, psychological, sociocultural, spiritual and developmental variables. Systems models focus on discrete parts and their interrelationship which make and describe the whole, that being the system. The Neuman model focuses on individuals and their reaction to stressors. Individuals are seen as composites of physiological, psychosocial, developmental and spiritual variables, who are open systems in a state of dynamic interaction with their environment. Stressors in the internal and external environment create a process of interaction and adjustment. Any stressor is capable of creating the potential for a disturbance in the individual, resulting in illness. Nursing interventions can begin at any point at which a stressor is suspected or identified. Nursing interventions are aimed at maintaining, attaining or regaining a state of wellness. The subsystems of the individual, stress and the nurse interact dynamically within the larger system of the Neuman Model (Lowry 1988).

Philosophy of the School of Nursing

On nursing

Health is a dynamic state of well-being and a fundamental human right. Nursing's goal is to assist individuals and groups in society in the promotion and maintenance of health, health restoration in illness and to provide support and comfort for those who are dying. Nursing is concerned with all the variables affecting an individual's response to the stresses of living. Nursing, therefore, requires the development of interpersonal, intellectual and technical skills in order to meet human needs.

The practice of nursing is an expressive art and an applied science based on concepts and theories derived from the biophysical, social, behavioural and nursing sciences. Nursing respects and supports the rights of individuals to participate in decisions affecting their health care.

Nursing is responsible for generating and sharing knowledge regarding nursing practice. Nursing recognises that society is continually changing and, through research, education and practice contributes to the development of planned change in health care and to nursing as a profession.

On education

Education is that process, directed towards the development of inner resources, which enables individuals to fulfil a social and vocational role; live and interact with other human beings; appreciate fully the richness of life and understand the meaning of their existence and experience.

Such educational processes facilitate the discovery of inner power and control and the maintenance of personal integrity in response to diverse environmental factors.

Learning is best facilitated when the individual is self-directed, goal-oriented and studies in an environment in which resources are compatible with the aims and objectives of the chosen course of study.

Course aims

To prepare nurse practitioners who are competent to work in a variety of settings at beginning level, and who will be eligible to register with the Nurses Board of South Australia on successful completion of the course.

To prepare nurse practitioners whose decision-making skills will demonstrate a sound knowledge of nursing, social and biophysical sciences.

Graduate outcomes

The course design anticipates the following graduate outcomes:

- Professional practice according to current and approved standards, and legal and ethical parameters of society relating to health care.
- Effective and objective decision-making, based on current knowledge and sound principles derived from the nursing and biophysical sciences and the humanities.
- Positive interaction through the use of effective communication and interpersonal skills.
- Demonstration of caring behaviours and appropriate action, evidenced as companionship, support, concern, nurturance and empathy.
- The ability to identify values and behaviours within the workplace and to use these in professionally astute and discriminating ways to enhance the practice of nursing.
- The taking of responsible action in relation to issues and trends which affect the practice of nursing.
- Demonstration of a commitment to the process of continuing education.

(University of South Australia, Bachelor of Nursing Curriculum 1991, City Campus)

The Neuman Model builds on a range of concepts familiar to those working in the health care field. In particular, it draws on theories which suggest that, in order to understand people and their behaviour in health and illness, we need to understand the relationship between them and their environments (Edelson 1970).

Figure 10.1 is a diagrammatic representation of the Neuman Systems Model.

Neuman describes her model as a set of concentric circles surrounding the basic structure. These circles are protective and they comprise the following.

Lines of resistance, or the organism's internal mechanism for defence against stress—for example, the inflammatory and immune responses, and previous life experiences.

Normal line of defence, or what the individual has become over time; an adaptational state which includes, for example, the individual's response, learned emotional response, coping mechanisms and problem-solving behaviours.

Flexible line of defence, which is the protective buffer around the normal line of defence and which can, after time, become the individual's normal line of defence; for example, the body's rest/activity levels, hormonal levels, lifestyle or role changes.

Stressors are either harmful or beneficial and are seen as being derived from three sources, as is the system's response or reaction to the stressors. The sources of the stressors and responses are viewed as:

intrapersonal—refers to those factors within the individual, elements of the basic structure;

interpersonal—refers to those factors between individuals and others, such as family groups; or

extrapersonal—refers to factors outside the individual, such as community and societal influences.

The goal of nursing is to assist individuals, families and groups to attain a maximum level of wellness by assessing all the variables that affect people's response to stress, and intervening appropriately to meet their needs. *Intervention* has been used to replace the term '*prevention*' and can occur on three levels.

1   *Primary intervention* focuses on identifying actual or potential stressors and is aimed at health promotion and maintenance; for example, immunisation programs, health education activities related to improving lifestyle, and other environmental factors.

2   *Secondary intervention* focuses on treatment of clients who are experiencing signs and symptoms of illness because stressors have penetrated the normal line of defence; for example, reducing symptoms and promoting comfort.

3   *Tertiary intervention* focuses on re-adaptation and re-education to prevent further occurrences of illness and to maintain stability by strengthening the lines of resistance; for example, rehabilitation programs.

While nursing intervention is organised on three levels, it is recognised that more than one level of care can be implemented at any one time.

FIGURE 10.1 THE NEUMAN SYSTEMS MODEL (REPRODUCED WITH PERMISSION FROM B. NEUMAN)

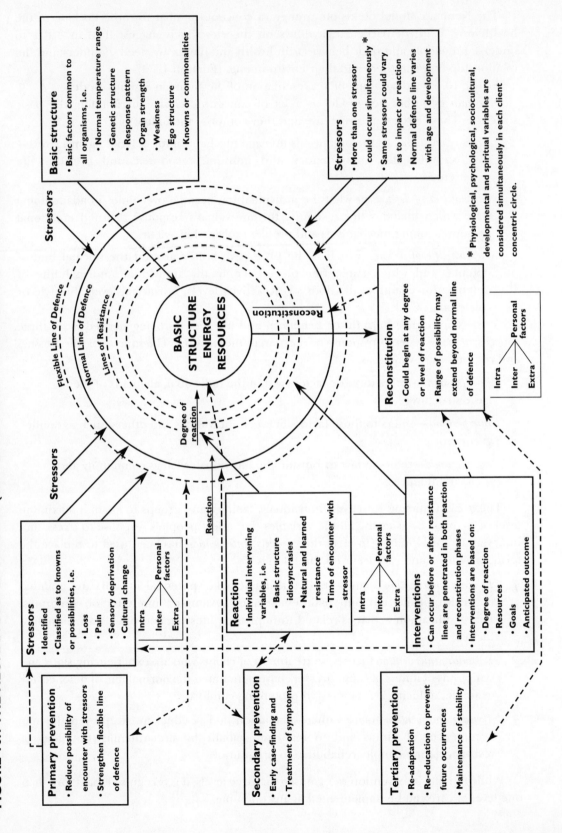

FRAMEWORK FOR CURRICULUM DEVELOPMENT AND DESIGN

The Neuman Systems Model provided a framework that was holistic and incorporated concepts that were familiar to nursing as well as to other disciplines. The model offered a focus on care, arising from the analysis of the primary, secondary and tertiary health needs of individuals, families and communities. A number of characteristics had to be considered in the delivery of the theoretical content when using this specific model. The chosen model had to:

* be holistic and have a focus on health;

* utilise concepts familiar to a wide variety of disciplines (i.e. not exclusive to nursing);

* be applicable across the spectrum of health care, ranging from wellness to ill-health, and able to be used in a variety of health care services;

* facilitate a life-span approach to nursing;

* promote a primary health care approach;

* provide a framework for understanding and interpreting the complexity of the health care system in which students of nursing and graduates of the program would work;

* provide a useful teaching tool;

* be practical (not too esoteric or ephemeral), with concepts that would be easy to understand and apply to the practice of nursing at all levels;

* facilitate problem solving;

* enable students to develop a well-connected knowledge network;

* foster a positive attitude to the use and development of nursing models and theory;

* facilitate nursing research.

The Neuman Systems Model addressed what were regarded as the essential building blocks for an undergraduate nursing curriculum, as well as being expressed in language that could be readily understood by students, nursing academics and other academics. As the model could appear complex, it was recognised that there was a need to articulate the model clearly to academic staff.

* The Neuman Model clearly met the requirements of the teaching program; in particular, it gives a holistic framework for providing care and determining clients' needs. Neuman considers the client as a being—that is, physiological, psychological, sociocultural, developmental and spiritual.

* These are considered to be the five variables that make each client a unique individual. It is recognised that these five variables interact with each other and cannot be viewed in isolation. The Neuman Model is a fine example of a model that has broadened the focus of traditional health care (which tended to emphasise a biomedical approach) to include the patient/client and his or her attributes as an individual. The biomedical approach to health care and definitions of health has

tended to dominate the health system. The biomedical model tends to focus on disease as the presence of physical symptoms and views health as the absence of the same. The Neuman Model defines the five-step nursing process well and guides nurses in clinical practice to consider the interactive nature of the client variables in relation to the clinical situation.

▪ The Neuman Model utilises concepts familiar to a wide variety of disciplines. It was believed that a systems model would provide a useful integration device.

▪ The model can be used across the spectrum of health care. Therefore, it facilitates a primary health care approach which is essentially multidisciplinary. The model has been used widely in a variety of countries and health care settings with different client groups, and there is considerable evidence to support its successful use (Neuman 1982; 1989; 1995).

▪ The model facilitates a life-span approach. This is evidenced in the holistic approach based on the five variables, which can be applied to any stage of human development.

▪ Lastly, the model provides a framework for understanding and interpreting the complexity of the health care system. Health care systems are becoming more and more complex, ambiguous and paradoxical. They are composed of interrelated parts that act together as a whole. By using systems theory it is possible to examine the multifaceted character of organisational life, describe the relationships between each subsystem and suprasystem, and solve some organisational problems (Sauber 1983). A systems theory is a most useful tool for any nurse practitioner.

APPLICATION OF THE MODEL TO CURRICULUM ORGANISATION

The curriculum was designed to cover three academic years of full-time study for the award of Diploma of Applied Science (Nursing) and subsequently the Bachelor of Nursing accreditation document. In designing the curriculum, the School of Nursing employed an adaptation of the Neuman Systems Model which had been validated through use in many areas of clinical practice (Neuman 1982; 1989; 1995). Even though this model reflected the philosophical viewpoint of the School and would be a useful pedagogical device, other models and theories of nursing were discussed and used throughout the program when they best illustrated an aspect of nursing practice.

The conceptual framework was sequenced to provide experiences that flowed from simple to complex, from self to others, and from wellness to illness. Students were encouraged to reflect on wellness and illness as progressive and dynamic states of function and dysfunction at cellular, individual and social levels. The curriculum was organised so that the first year of the course introduced concepts of humanity, health and nursing, focusing on five dimensions: the biological, psychological, sociological, spiritual and developmental. These studies within the first year helped students to understand the physiological, psychological, sociocultural, developmental and spiritual processes identified in the Neuman Model and represented accepted views of the human species. The nursing units introduced the concept of primary intervention, which focused on healthy individuals and identification of risk factors associated with stressors. Nursing actions were aimed towards promoting and maintaining the individual's health status, and thus strengthening the lines of defence (see Figure 10.1).

During the second year, the course built on previous experiences and focused on secondary and tertiary intervention with individuals and families who are experiencing illness. The role of the nurse as it relates to other therapies, including medical, surgical and pharmacological, was developed and enhanced through clinical placement. Students applied nursing care to reduce the effect of stressors, and to facilitate the rehabilitation process.

During the second and third years, the content was organised according to categories of stressors, resulting in specific human dysfunction. Clinical dysfunction focused on the concepts of trauma—obstructive, inflammatory, developmental and degenerative. Clinical experience was organised so that students gained experience in acute care settings, extended care and community agencies (see Table 10.1). A clinical rotation of students was designed so that they all experienced contact with children and adults in a variety of settings. Supporting studies extended students' understanding of the forces in society that impinge on health states and the professional role.

During the third year of the course, student experiences were designed to facilitate the synthesis of knowledge in the application of nursing interventions with clients at all levels of dependence and in a variety of settings. The focus was on individuals, families and community groups experiencing stressors which had resulted, or may result, in major complex health problems. An excellent example of using the model to illustrate the application of nursing interventions to community groups is discussed by Procter and Cheek (1995).

Throughout the course, opportunities existed for students to identify and debate political, ethical, legal, professional and occupational issues related to nursing, health care and health service provision in Australia.

When used as a framework, the Neuman Systems Model facilitated the provision and acquisition of new knowledge and skills that were seen as being in line with demands in the health service industries. Skills were developed which enabled the graduate to interact confidently at the computer interface and to address issues related to other technologies. The computer skills, initially introduced as simple word processing skills, were developed to include database management, spreadsheets and computer statistical packages. The skill development in this area was particularly evident, as one of our primary responsibilities was the teaching of computing. Many of the students who commenced the program in 1987 were female and mature age entry students and, as a consequence, had little experience of computers. The confidence of the students grew dramatically with the initial skill development and many of these early students graduated and were working in health agencies when patient management systems were being introduced. Employer feedback suggests that these graduates were well prepared for this challenge.

Throughout the course, a focus on the nurses themselves and the environment in which they worked was maintained through the teaching of the principles of ergonomics and occupational health and safety.

The curriculum design embodied an adult learning approach in which students' life experiences were utilised and self-directed learning was encouraged. Opportunities for critical analysis, values clarification, evaluation, and reflective practice were provided to encourage development of the professional role of the nurse. As suggested by McCulloch (1995), the Neuman Systems Model assisted students and staff in defining nursing itself.

TEACHING AND LEARNING USING THE NEUMAN SYSTEMS MODEL

The focus throughout the program is on wellness, restoration and maintenance of health. During the second year of the program, major pathophysiological concepts were introduced. Throughout the program students were encouraged to utilise a problem-solving approach to identify the specific stressors that can result in an alteration in health status, and specific levels of nursing interventions to strengthen lines of defence. Tutorials provided students with the opportunity to interact with the model and develop nursing assessments (see Appendix A at the end of this chapter) and care plans (see Appendix C) that focus on the holistic nature of nursing.

The practical sessions in the Nursing Skills Laboratory provided the opportunity to put into practice the assessment of the client and planned interventions. The practicals were enriched by the contribution of the Friends of the School of Nursing. The Friends of the School participated in simulation sessions, enabling students to experience first-hand the impact of their nursing interventions and to receive feedback in a non-threatening environment. The nursing assessment and care plans were used in these sessions based on the Neuman Systems Model (see Appendices A and C). The Friends of the School of Nursing is a group of people of all ages from diverse social and cultural backgrounds who wish to participate in activities that will facilitate nursing students' learning about health. Friends have the opportunity to choose the activities they wish to take part in. These may include interviews regarding health, role playing a patient/client in simulated exercises, or undertaking health assessment activities in practice sessions. This enables nursing students to interact with people of all ages in different settings, and in a variety of ways, thus enhancing their personal and professional development.

TEACHING STRATEGIES

The teaching strategies used included lectures (see Appendix B) in which the Neuman Systems Model was applied, and which focused on alterations in health status. Case studies were used for tutorial sessions and students were expected to use the Neuman Systems Model to assess, plan, implement and evaluate care (see Appendix A for an Assessment Tool and Appendix C for a Nursing Care Plan). The practical laboratory sessions for nursing practice, using scenarios, also incorporated the same nursing assessment and care plan. Using this approach enabled students to focus on the individual as client, the family as clients and the community as clients. This approach to teaching and learning, using the Neuman's Systems Model, provided students with a framework for assessment, implementation of care and preparation of clients to return to their family and the community.

LECTURES

Lectures focused on the client, the family as a system which may be the individual, the family as a client and the community as a client (see Appendix B).

The individual as client

The multiple stressors encountered in the child, adult and elderly age groups, which are often responsible for system disequilibrium and which require nursing interventions at all levels of prevention, provided the focus for this portion of the course content. Discussion centred on how stressors affect the system (individual) as they cross the flexible line of defence and penetrate the normal line of defence (see Figure 10.1) as well as on the various possible reactions and restorative factors. An exploration of alternative nursing interventions at the appropriate level of prevention provided students with knowledge of various strategies they might test out in practice. This approach allowed students to study the model through all phases of the nursing process.

The family as client

This component dealt with nursing the family with an ill member. The impact of the illness and hospitalisation of a member of the family, as well as changes within the family resulting from the member's return home, provided direction for study. A family assessment tool, based on the Neuman Model and incorporating intra-, inter- and extra-family factors, helped students to examine family responses to these stressors. Other nursing interventions were also discussed together with the identification of possible community supports aimed at strengthening the family's lines of defence.

The community as client

Risk reduction provided the emphasis for these lectures, which included discussions of the potential impact on the system (community) of major contemporary community health stressors. Since primary prevention was the focus for intervention, several approaches, aimed at preventing penetration either by strengthening the line of defence or by decreasing the possibility of exposure of the community to stressors, were discussed. An excellent example of this is the study by Procter and Cheek (1995); their study demonstrates the use of the Neuman Systems Model in understanding the experiences of Serbian Australians at the time of civil war in the former Yugoslavia.

TUTORIAL CASE STUDIES

A case study format served to direct student learning by providing all students with the same simulated experiential basis (i.e. client situation) on which to test their assessment and decision-making skills. The students used the Neuman Systems Model given in Appendix A as a framework to assess, plan, implement and evaluate care provision for each case study. Students differentiated relevant from irrelevant data, identified client perceptions, interpreted data in the light of their knowledge base and made decisions about appropriate nursing interventions at the three levels of primary, secondary and tertiary interventions. This format appeared to help students recognise the transferability of these concepts among individuals, families and the community as clients as well as among various categories of health stressors.

TABLE 10.1. RELATIONSHIP OF NURSING STUDIES TO FIELD EXPERIENCE

NURSING STUDIES	FIELD/CLINICAL EXPERIENCE
Year 1—Semester 1 **Nursing Practice 1A** 'Health Promotion/Maintenance across the Lifespan' • Self, family • Person with a disability in the community • Introduction to First Aid **Professional Nursing Studies 1A** 'Historical Development of Nursing and Health Care: Theoretical Basis of Nursing'	Community observations e.g. shopping centres, child care centres, services for people with disabilities, Meals on Wheels, occupational and environmental services
Year 1—Semester 2 **Nursing Practice 1B** 'Health Promotion/Maintenance' • Pregnant woman, mother, infant and family • Elderly person and family community • Activities of daily living, needs of children and adults, including those requiring hospitalisation **Professional Nursing Studies 1B** 'Introduction to the Role of the Nurse and the Process of Nursing'	Community settings and maternity units. Community focus on children and adults in community health care settings
Year 2—Semester 1 **Nursing Practice 2A** 'Nursing and Human Dysfunction 1' • Neurohormonal, sensorimotor musculoskeletal, gastrointestinal and metabolic **Professional Nursing Studies 2A** 'Patterns of Nursing Care and Principles of Therapeutic Communication'	Children and adults in hospital (general), pre- and post- operative care **Specialised areas** • Orthopaedics • Eyes, ears, throat and nose clinics • Community agencies • Long-term care facilities

PRACTICALS

Nursing skills laboratory

The laboratory was designed to simulate the clinical environments in which most nurses would practise the art and science of nursing. It is flexible and able to accommodate a variety of activities, from a full scenario of a 'shift' in an acute or extended care setting to health promotion activities. Video cameras and monitors are installed throughout the laboratory so that students may video their own activities, or a whole class may view an educational or instructional program. The videos assist the students in the process of self-assessment.

Scenarios were constructed using simulated real life experiences. The purpose of the scenarios was to facilitate the process of integrating theory into practice, and they helped students to reinforce their knowledge base by acknowledging their prior learning.

TABLE 10.1. RELATIONSHIP OF NURSING STUDIES TO FIELD EXPERIENCE (CONT'D)

NURSING STUDIES	FIELD/CLINICAL EXPERIENCE
Year 2—Semester 2 **Nursing Practice 2B** 'Nursing and Human Dysfunction 2' • Cardiopulmonary, urinary, integumentary, fluid and electrolyte imbalance • Complex Health Problems 1—requiring accident and emergency, operating theatre/recovery and/or acute care **Professional Nursing Studies 2B** 'Bioethical Dilemmas in Health Care'	Children and adults in hospital requiring acute care Observation • operating room • casualty departments • intensive care suites
Year 3—Semester 1 **Nursing Practice 3A** 'Nursing Practice and Human Dysfunction 3' • Psychological and behavioural dysfunction • Reproduction **Professional Nursing Studies 3A** 'The Management Process in Nursing'	Psychiatric units Maternity units Hospital and community agencies, e.g. Women's Health Centre and the South Australian Mental Health Services
Year 3—Semester 2 **Nursing Practice 3B** 'Nursing Practice and Human Dysfunction 4' • Faulty immunological responses, abnormal cell proliferation • Complex Health Problems—requiring palliative care, rehabilitation, extended care and support from community agencies **Professional Nursing Studies 3B** 'Ensuring the Quality of Nursing Care'	Community agencies, e.g. • Domiciliary care • Community centres • Rehabilitation centres • Long-term care services • Palliative care and oncology units

The learning activities inherent in the scenarios are numerous and diverse. They include discussion, questioning, technical skill performance, case study, self-evaluation and peer evaluation, feedback, documentation of patient care, decision making, priority setting and role playing. During the laboratory sessions students completed nursing assessments and nursing care plans to guide practice, based on the Neuman Systems Model (Manning, Broughton & McConnell 1995).

CLINICAL EXPERIENCE

The Neuman Model was used as a framework for the development of clinical objectives to facilitate student learning, both in the clinical laboratory and the field. Case studies were undertaken as part of the student assessment program and demonstrated the application of the model to nursing practice. Students were also exposed to nursing assessment and care planning, using the Neuman framework. The model provided a framework to guide practice and students were able to discuss with clinicians how models and theories can be used in practice. This opportunity for dialogue between clinical role models and students was invaluable in linking theory to practice and debating issues concerning models.

Clinical experiences were offered in a variety of community and institutional settings such as shopping centres, senior citizens' centres, and occupational and environmental services, and metropolitan and rural hospitals. Community visits enabled students to observe health/maintenance behaviours as they occur in our society. Students shared experiences with children, pregnant women and the elderly. Social studies and the biophysical science units supported the nursing studies by contributing knowledge and skills related to organisational constructs of society and human behaviours. Table 10.1 shows the relationship of field/clinical experience to the nursing studies, and again demonstrates the value of using the Neuman Model as a curriculum organiser.

STUDENT ASSESSMENT

Student assessment was based on both clinical and theoretical components of the course. The clinical assessment was guided by the National Competencies for Registered Nurses. The assessment of students' clinical competency was progressive and developed throughout the course. During any given semester, students were able, in conjunction with their lecturers and clinical facilitators, to identify strengths and weaknesses and jointly set objectives for further learning and skill development. The theoretical assessment further developed the necessary clinical skills and competencies expected of beginning registered nurses. A variety of assessment strategies were employed to enable students to demonstrate their individuality and creativity. One successful method of assessment that enabled students to demonstrate a wide range of knowledge and skills were the Case Studies, which incorporated the Neuman Systems Model. As part of their assessment, students were expected to complete case studies that focused on the individual, family and community. Completion of the nursing assessment (Appendix A) and the nursing care plan (Appendix C) was a required part of the case study.

STAFF DEVELOPMENT

One of the opportunities created by the introduction of the model was the development of workshops and other strategies to enhance the understanding of the model, thus increasing the effectiveness of its use with the nursing program. There were generational differences in both understanding the model and in its application, which provided the opportunity for clarification and further exploration of the model itself and for creative strategies such as the development of case studies.

It was also essential that staff who were involved in clinical facilitation were given staff development sessions on the applicability of the Neuman Model to practice. Once staff became familiar with the model, and were comfortable with its use as well as with its potential adaptations, a decision was made to invite Dr Betty Neuman as a visiting scholar. Her visit in 1991 was regarded as a key point in the development of the curriculum, as it enabled academics, students and clinicians to explore with Dr Neuman the potential for the essential ongoing development of the model in modern nursing. One of the outcomes was the development of a nursing assessment model for use in the nursing laboratory and clinical venues (Appendix A).

The model has also facilitated the development of valuable networks with academics and clinicians nationally and internationally. Some academics have published and presented papers using the Neuman Model as well as undertaken research (Procter & Cheek 1995; McCulloch 1995).

SUMMARY

Through use of the Neuman Systems Model, students became familiar with using models for nursing practice in both the community and institutional setting. This was further reinforced by using the Neuman Model as a framework to facilitate both teaching and learning.

Although the major focus of the Bachelor of Nursing was on the Neuman Systems Model, students were also exposed to other models throughout their course. With an in-depth understanding of one model, students were able to appreciate the use of models generally in nursing practice, education and research.

As a curriculum is dynamic, evolving and everchanging, the Neuman Model was clearly an appropriate choice for a curriculum organiser. Preparing beginning registered nurses for practice in a changing health system is both challenging and daunting. However, if nursing models are used for the purpose of curriculum frameworks, nursing automatically becomes the core and focus of the educational process for the students. By using nursing models to teach nursing, nurses may be better prepared to control their practice, be more autonomous and participate more actively in decision making as it relates to their practice, and the delivery of health care.

QUESTIONS

1   Is one framework or model more useful than another with respect to the particular health problems facing individuals, groups and families?

2   What impact does a nursing model have on guiding students' learning in an undergraduate program?

3   Should nurses be left to select and/or develop their own individual nursing model or framework for practice?

or

Should they adopt the model of the nursing department within the agency?

4   How does a simple model, or model of practice, assist in assessing the quality of care?

5   What are the benefits of adopting a nursing model for teaching and learning?

6   How does adopting one model of nursing facilitate students' understanding of other models and theories?

LEARNING ACTIVITIES

1 Using the Assessment Tool (Appendix A) and sample Nursing Care Plan (Appendix C) develop a Nursing Assessment and Care Plan for a client in a specific setting that you are assigned to—for example, an acute care setting, a community setting, or a mental health setting.

2 Develop a mini-teaching session for your fellow students using the Neuman Model as a framework (refer to Appendix B for a guide). When you are working through your learning activities, refer to some of the further readings for worked examples and some ideas.

3 Go to your library and do a search for other work that may use the Neuman Model or might describe the model in clinical practice.

FURTHER READING

Beckman, S., Boxley-Harges, S., Bruick-Sorge, C., Harris, S., Hermix, Meininger., Steinkeler, S. 1994, 'Betty Neuman Systems Model', in Marriner-Tomey, A. *Nursing Theorists and their Work* , 3rd edn, C.V. Mosby, St Louis, pp. 269–304.

Dohney, M, Cook, C, Stopper, C. 1992, *The Discipline of Nursing: An Introduction*, 3rd edn, Appleton & Lange, Connecticut.

Griffith-Kenney, J.W. & Christensen, P.J. 1986, *Nursing Process: Application of Theories, Frameworks and Models*, 2nd edn, C.V. Mosby, St Louis. pp. 25–27.

Leddy, S, & Pepper, J. M. 1989, *Conceptual Bases of Professional Nursing*, 2nd edn, J.B. Lippincott, Philadelphia.

Neuman, B. (ed.) 1982, *The Neuman Systems Model: Application to Nursing Education and Practice*, Appleton-Century-Crofts, Connecticut.

Neuman, B. (ed.) 1989, *The Neuman Systems Model*, 2nd edn, Appleton-Lange, Connecticut.

Neuman, B. (ed.) 1995, *The Neuman Systems Model*, 3rd edn, Appleton-Lange, Connecticut.

APPENDIX A: ASSESSMENT TOOL

University of South Australia
School of Nursing
(City Campus)

Nursing History
(Adapted from B. Neuman, Nov. 1991)

A. ADMISSION DETAILS

Surname:_____

    Given names:_____

    Date of birth:_____

    Female ❏   Male ❏ (please tick one)

    Next of kin:_____

    Relationship to client: _____   Contact phone:_____

    Significant others: _____   Contact phone:_____

Client's understanding of hospital admission:

_____

_____

_____

_____

Known allergies:

_____

_____

_____

_____

Present medications:

_____

_____

_____

_____

B. IDENTIFICATION OF STRESSORS
(These are answered by the client first, and then by the nurse)

1. Major problem/stress/area of concern

   Client's perception

   _____

   _____

   Nurse's perception

   _____

   _____

2. Effect on lifestyle of this problem/stress/area of concern

   Client's perception

   _____

   _____

   Nurse's perception

   _____

   _____

3. Experience of similar problem/situation

   Client's perception (including coping behaviour/response)

   _____

   _____

   Nurse's perception (including evaluation of situation)

   _____

   _____

4. Future consequence of major problem/stress/area of concern

   Client's perception

   _____

   _____

   Nurse's perception

   _____

   _____

   _____

5. Measures to improve health

Client's perception

_____

_____

Nurse's perception

_____

_____

6. Expectation of assistance from family/friends/caregivers/resources

Client's perception

_____

_____

Nurse's perception

_____

_____

C. INTRAPERSONAL FACTORS

1. Pattern of manifestations (physical)
Client's perception (including usual physiological patterns and/or changes/responses to major problem/stress/area of concern

Nurse's perception (including physical assessment)

_____

_____

2. Communication:

Language spoken _____

Speech pattern _____

Language spoken in home _____

Integument:

_____

_____

Respiratory:

_____

_____

Cardiovascular:

_____

_____

Genitourinary:

_____

_____

Musculoskeletal:

_____

_____

Neurological:

_____

_____

Gastrointestinal:

_____

_____

Nutrition:

_____

_____

Senses:

Sight

_____

Hearing

_____

Activities of daily living:

_____

_____

Sleep/exercise:

_____

_____

Vital signs   TPR _____   BP _____

                     Weight _____   Urinalysis _____

3. Psychological

Presenting behaviours

_____
_____
_____
_____

Expressed attitudes/behaviour

_____
_____
_____
_____
_____

4. Social/cultural factors (including religion)

_____
_____
_____
_____

5. Developmental factors (factors related to present situation and impact of present situation)

_____
_____
_____
_____

Summary of impressions

_____
_____
_____
_____

D. INTERPERSONAL FACTORS (SUMMARY OF IMPRESSIONS):

Resources, relationships of family, friends and caregivers that influence intrapersonal factors

_____
_____
_____
_____
_____

E. EXTRAPERSONAL FACTORS (SUMMARY OF IMPRESSIONS):

Resources, relationships of family, friends and caregivers which influence or could influence discharge planning

_____

_____

_____

_____

Discharge summary

_____

_____

_____

_____

Nurse's signature:_____

Date completed:_____

(Source: Both, A., Ellis, T., Manning, J., Owen, E. A., Paech, M. & Rouse, K. (1991), School of Nursing, City Campus, University of South Australia.)

APPENDIX B: SAMPLE LECTURE FRAMEWORK

GASTROINTESTINAL AND METABOLIC DYSFUNCTION

Infection and inflammation resulting in:

a) gastrointestinal

and

b) metabolic dysfunction

Conditions present as a result of stressor penetration and reaction

Stressors arise from two major sources:

1. **Intrapersonal sources** are those within the individual and result from the individual's physiological processes, reactions, development, emotional/psychological status and genetic structure.

2. **Extrapersonal sources** are those resulting from sources in the environment, such as bacteria, viruses, pollutants and hygiene factors.

Focus: Common health problems across the life span

Source

• Health indices

• Morbidity/mortality statistics from South Australian and Australian health care statistical data, and Social Health Atlas (South Australian Health Commission 1990).

1. Alimentary tract

2. Liver, gall bladder and pancreas (biliary tract)

Scope of the session

The lecture will cover:

• Revision of structure and function

• Pathophysiology (vital in early part of 2nd year to facilitate the integration of science and nursing)

• Health assessment

- Nursing care planning
  - — using the nursing process
  - — Neuman's model for intervention
- Identification of common medical and pharmacological interventions
- Diagnostic tests

Health problems

1. Alimentary tract (mouth, oesophagus, stomach, intestines)
   a) *Extrapersonal sources* (bacteria, viruses and chemicals)
   - gastroenteritis (food poisoning, infectious diarrhoea)
   - oesophagitis (ingestion of chemicals)
   b) *Intrapersonal sources*
   - oesophagitis (ingestion of chemicals)
   - peptic ulceration
   - appendicitis
   - peritonitis
   - inflammatory bowel diseases
     - — ulcerative colitis
     - — Crohn's disease
   - diverticulitis

2. Biliary tract (liver, pancreas and gall bladder)
   a) *Extrapersonal sources*
   - hepatitis (viral & chemical)*
   - cholycystitis (diet, lifestyle)**
   b) *Intrapersonal sources*
   - pancreatitis
   - cholycystitis
     - — genetic predisposition/sex
     - — cholesterol—crystals + bile
     - — pigments + calcium = stones
     - — stones cause inflammation

* Most common   ** Uncertain re. cause

Most frequent responses

Physiological

- pain
- temperature, pulse etc.
- nausea
- vomiting
- diarrhoea
- bleeding
- lethargy
- loss of function

HEALTH STATUS ASSESSMENT
NURSING CARE PLANNING

Information must be collected to determine care required by client/patient

Health status assessment

I. The health history

   The approach to history-taking is influenced by the following factors:

   - age—children, adolescents or elderly adults
   - communication level/ability
   - developmental level
   - conscious state
   - physical condition

   Principles of history-taking:

   a) Listening
   b) Questioning
   c) Observation
   d) Integration (summary)

2. Physical examination—4 techniques

   a) Inspection
   b) Palpation   *Students to refer to Nursing Practice*
   c) Percussion   *subjects in year one for revision*
   d) Auscultation

3. General subjective view, which includes how much a patient weighs etc.

4. General objective view
- height and weight
- appearance
- signs of distress
- vital signs

What are the factors that need to be assessed in people from the following groups suffering gastrointestinal and metabolic dysfunction?

1. Infants
2. Children
3. Adolescents
4. Adults
5. Elderly adults

Describe the condition of the following in people who have gastroenteritis;
- Skin
- Mucous membrane
- Abdomen
  - distention
  - fluid
- Breath
- Vomitus
- Faeces
- Urine
- Pain patterns

Problems associated with gastrointestinal and metabolic dysfunction as a result of infections and inflammatory processes.

1. Disturbances of feeding behaviour
2. Anorexia
3. Nausea and vomiting
4. Diarrhoea and constipation
5. Disturbances of digestion and absorption
6. Disturbances of metabolic processes
7. Vitamin and mineral deficiency
8. Fluid and electrolyte imbalance

Common medical and pharmacological therapies used to treat/manage gastrointestinal and metabolic dysfunction:

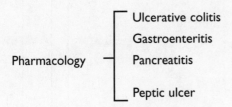

Surgery
- Cholycystitis
- Appendicitis
- Peptic ulcer

Pharmacology
- Ulcerative colitis
- Gastroenteritis
- Pancreatitis
- Peptic ulcer

Lecture notes: Lange, A. (1990) School of Nursing, City Campus, University of South Australia

APPENDIX C: SAMPLE NURSING CARE PLAN

UNIVERSITY OF SOUTH AUSTRALIA
SCHOOL OF NURSING
(CITY CAMPUS)

NURSING CARE PLAN

Summary/general statement of all relevant information re. client's health status (basis for formulating care plan)

PROBLEM	NEGOTIATED GOAL OF CARE	NURSING INTERVENTIONS State whether primary/secondary /tertiary intervention	RATIONALE	EVALUATION/ OUTCOME

Client's signature: _____

Nurse's signature: _____
Date: _____

11

DEVELOPING A PRACTICE-BASED MODEL OF NURSING

BART O'BRIEN

Many people contributed to the understanding behind this chapter and it is impossible to name them all. My particular thanks must go to my PhD supervisor Professor Alan Pearson and to Mr Bernard Mead who supported my study and its application at Julia Farr Centre. Chris Johns of the Burford NDU in the UK provided valuable early critique and encouragement. The staff of the Professorial Nursing Unit (PNU) Grace McKellar Centre, Geelong, and the staff of the Julia Farr Centre Nursing Development Units (NDUs) in Adelaide provided example and inspiration for the theory described in this chapter. My thanks especially go to Pauline Donnelly, Shirley Maloney, Judith Pope and Robyn Kouts. These leaders of the NDUs that I have worked with made this work possible.

LEARNING OBJECTIVES

When you have read this chapter you should be able to:

1 Distinguish between different patterns of knowing in nursing and demonstrate a beginning understanding of different theoretical perspectives that inform nursing.

2 Understand the process of developing a practice-based theory of nursing in a clinical setting.

3 Critically reflect on your own nursing experiences to determine the relevance and applicability of the theory development process, and the theory itself, to your own practice.

Bart O'Brien, RN, DipAppSci, BN, PhD, has worked in acute and aged and extended care settings as a charge nurse, clinical nurse consultant, staff development educator and clinical assistant director of nursing. He is currently senior partner of Australian Nursing Services, Adelaide, a business that offers clinical consultancy and clinical research, with special emphasis on nursing management of continence. His nursing interests include nursing's therapeutic potential, aged and extended care, oral knowing in nursing, nursing development units (NDUs) and the development of practice-based nursing theory.

INTRODUCTION

This chapter describes how a group of nurses began developing a practice-based theory of nursing. It starts with an overview of what theory is and how theory development in nursing has been influenced by the prevailing scientific paradigm—the empiricist method. Following this is an account of practice-based theory development and the reasons for attempting such an exercise is based on the experiences of nurses working in an Australian Nursing Development Unit (NDU). Examples are given of their commitment to the provision of an optimum level of therapeutic nursing and of their experiences in attempting to document and communicate this work to others. The NDU nurses have developed a conceptual framework, or **model**, for a practice-based theory of nursing for aged and extended care. The state of the development of this model and its value and shortcomings are also considered in this chapter. The story of theory generation in an NDU serves to illustrate why and how Australian nurses have set about this task.

WHAT IS THEORY?

In a very broad sense theory can be defined as a *systematic abstraction of reality that serves some purpose*. The phrases 'systematic abstraction' and 'serves some purpose' are the key ideas to understanding theory's multiple meanings.

(*Chinn & Jacobs 1983, pp. 2–3*)

Given the above definition, **theory** is about saying clearly what is being done about something so that others can understand the **concepts** involved and how they relate to each other. Theory is also about ensuring that what is said is useful to others. The rigour of theory development places constraints on the choice of language used to describe practice in theoretical terms. Unfamiliar terms and specific definitions are frequently used, making it necessary for the novice reader to refer constantly to the dictionary. In the interests of holding your attention throughout this chapter, Ann Marriner's book

Nursing Theorists and their Work (Marriner 1986, pp. 3–5) has been used to reduce reliance on a dictionary. Her list of useful **definitions** for terms that appear in this chapter can be found in the glossary at the end of the chapter.

ORIGINS OF THEORY

Science (as a specific body of knowledge) can be traced back to the use of logic, reason and rhetoric by early Greek philosophers such as Aristotle (1976, 1988 translations) and Plato (1987 translation). Greek philosophy survived largely unchallenged until Francis Bacon introduced his scientific method in the late 16th century. There was a real need for such a revision of science at that time. Reason was confused by bodies of **knowledge** derived from existing sciences such as alchemy, magic, mysticism and religious dogma.

These sciences can be categorised as different and separate ways of making sense of reality. **Paradigm** is the term generally used to define separate bodies of thought, grounded on specific sets of beliefs (Kuhn 1970). Kuhn sees paradigms as '. . . universally recognised scientific achievements that for a time provide model problems and solutions to a community of practitioners' (Kuhn 1970, p. viii). Kuhn also points out that a lot of scientific energy is devoted to defining the prevailing paradigm and, consequently, there can be seen to be an extensive vested interest in protecting and maintaining it (Kuhn 1970, p. 24). Bacon set himself the task of establishing a new scientific paradigm from beliefs as diverse as those described above.

THE ESTABLISHMENT AND INFLUENCE OF SCIENTIFIC METHOD

The paradigm that emerged as a result of Bacon's work sought to distinguish a scientific method that would provide valid and reliable results which could be readily duplicated by others (Charlesworth 1982).

Disciplines other than the pure sciences sought to adapt empiricist and positivist methods to their own ends, and methods developed for specific purposes were turned to alternative uses. What was lost in the process was the understanding that science, primarily a means of investigating and understanding the world, was being replaced by empirical Science (capital S), a research paradigm whose parameters were defined by the Scientific method itself. Science (capital S) reflects only one particular branch of investigation, a fact that is all too frequently overlooked.

A look at the prevailing knowledge systems underpinning the health disciplines (including nursing) reveals a strong allegiance to the principles of empirical science introduced by Bacon and further established in the British empiricist tradition by the philosopher, David Hume. The rigour of empirical science emphasises **facts** as black or white, true or false. It creates a perception of humanity as individuals competing against each other, a perception alien to the early Greeks as well as to European philosophy, where society in a collective sense is valued over the worth of individuals. What is frequently hidden or forgotten in the worship of Science is the complementary science of reason: '. . . a prudent understanding of what should be done in practical situations' (Carr & Kemmis 1986, p. 132).

THEORY AND NURSING

Experience of nursing and of being nursed is gained through nurse–client relationships, where nurses' help is sought and/or offered as a result of personal beliefs about the purpose of nursing. The nature and relevance of nursing, to both parties, is explored as the nurse–client relationship progresses.

Pearson (1984b) suggests that the essence of this exploratory approach to nursing is 'being there' in a close relationship with the nursed person, an argument explored in some depth by Salvage (1988) in her Master's thesis on this subject. The nature and importance of being there has also been researched in Australia (Pincombe et al. 1995). When considering the following characteristics of nursing—moral (Benner 1989), ethical (ANF *Standards for Nursing Practice* 1983), scientific (Dunlop 1986), philosophical (Griffin 1980, 1983), political (Clay 1987)—as well as therapeutic (Pearson et al. 1992), it quickly becomes apparent that a conceptual framework is needed to make sure that writer and reader have the same frame of reference and are operating out of the same paradigm.

EMPIRICAL SCIENCE

Empirical science is perhaps the most readily recognisable framework (paradigm) for organising thinking and knowledge generation. Its use of hypotheses, rules and specific, predictable relationships between sets of variables gives rise to research based on 'scientific method'.

In the 1970s, when the nursing process was first introduced as a method for making sense of and directing nursing, research in nursing was also largely based on empirical methods. Both scientific method and nursing process predict that experiment, activity or research will proceed, in an expected fashion, towards specified outcomes (the hypothesis).

The value of this research and knowledge paradigm should not be dismissed lightly. What better way to assess the comparable merits of two types of wound dressing, continence drainage devices, renal dialysers? How else can management evaluate the respective costs of different patterns of practice, variations in skills mix, variables affecting sick leave within an organisation? However, as many of you will have found, there can be a big difference in personal experience when management statistics show a sick leave ratio of 1 per cent for the entire hospital while you are working on a ward where six staff on your shift have reported sick!

INTERPRETIVE SCIENCE

Interpretive science has gained increasing acceptance by nurses during the 1980s and 1990s. It is a useful tool in the face of such experiences as: finding that the perfect wound dressing cannot be reliably supplied; being part of the one ward where sick leave remains unacceptably high for months on end; or trying to introduce new practices in the face of active sabotage by people with vested interests in the status quo. These sorts of issues are more readily addressed by interpretive research.

Interpretive research sets out to understand what is happening in a research setting and what rules guide the behaviours of the group under observation. The aim of the research is to make sense of the behaviours observed and to develop theories of those behaviours that will allow others also to make sense of what is going on.

Grounded theory is an interpretive methodology. It is particularly useful for developing understanding in fields where little research has been undertaken (Chenitz & Swanson 1986). Grounded theory involves collecting clinical data, analysing them and developing a preliminary conceptual framework by clustering together similar concepts, ideas and beliefs. This framework is then checked by further comparison with observed practice, and refinements and alterations made as required. This process—analysis, synthesis, testing and refinement—is repeated until the theory's component parts are 'saturated' with supportive data and no further challenges to its validity can be discovered. At this point a substantive practice-based theory, which describes theory in a specific setting, can be considered to be established. The difference between this 'grounded' theory and the generalisability of formal theories should be noted.

There are clear differences between this methodology and the empirical method, where variables are controlled for and the research proceeds sequentially to test a predetermined hypothesis. Grounded theory accepts what is happening and concentrates on explaining why it happens and to what ends. What better way to identify why it's always your ward that has that high incidence of sick leave, why the postsurgical infection rate is so high in Ward L, or why new graduates tend not to use physical assessment skills once they are employed?

CRITICAL SCIENCE

Critical science (comparable with feminist thinking, postmodernism or critical social theory, for those familiar with these terms) adds a further dimension to the methods of testing and explanation covered by the empirical and interpretive sciences.

> [A] critical social science is one which seeks to uncover those systems of social relationships which determine the actions of individuals and the unanticipated, though not accidental, consequences of those actions.
>
> *(Fay 1975, p. 94)*

In other words, critical science aims to identify (or introduce) and assess the effect of specific activities which are intended to correct perceived problems with current practices. The research looks at what is going on, makes sense of it, identifies the bad bits (in the eyes of those involved) and establishes a program of planned action intended to correct the wrongs and/or overcome deficiencies in practice.

Action research is an example of a methodology that can be used to apply the principles of the critical paradigm. It allows researchers to work with members of a study setting, defining their practice and planning ways in which it can be improved.

There are several approaches to action research (Rappoport 1970) and yet, while it is increasingly being described in the nursing literature, it has only been used to a limited extent in nursing (see Pearson 1985; O'Brien 1992; Gibb et al. 1993), probably because the methodology requires a lot of time. A typical project might last two to three years and funding for projects of this duration is not yet readily available to nurse researchers. Action research has a place in determining how theory developed in other settings can be adapted to your workplace—how to make the best of the erratic supplies of that great wound dressing, or how to turn around the sabotage of your pet project and get your colleagues on side.

PRACTICE-BASED THEORY

> Nursing theory, or at least nursing practice theory, is that which guides the nurse's actions in attaining goals in patient care.
>
> *(Jacox in Nicoll 1986, p. 328)*

For it to be useful, Jacobs and Huether (Nicoll 1986, ch. 37) note that practice-based theory must provide a set, or sets, of interrelated concepts that are sufficiently clearly defined to provide opportunities for testing the theory in practice in order to assess its validity and generalisability. In other words, practice must have been analysed sufficiently to identify and define the concepts and relationships that form the basis of the observed practice. Out of this analysis comes the development of a theory which is clear enough to allow another set of nurses to implement a trial of theory-based practice that will be similar to that of the original practice setting. Practice-based theory serves exactly the same purpose as a cooking recipe. It allows for the transport of ideas from one venue to another, with assurances that following the theory/recipe will produce a consistent result.

The development of theory by the Nursing Development Unit (NDU) nurses, reported in this chapter, is the result of an action research project which started in 1991. A funded component of the study was reported on two years later (O'Brien 1993) and initial publication of the Unit's theory development came in 1994 (O'Brien & Pope 1994). This project involved three stages.

1   Organisational support was gained to establish an NDU and to work with staff of the ward involved to establish as Unit practice the principles of NDU functioning as defined in the literature (Hall 1964; Pearson 1983, 1985; Alfano 1988; Salvage 1988) and in the researcher's experience (O'Brien 1992).

2   A formal evaluation of the process of change in the NDU, and comparison of NDU practice with three other wards offering complementary services, was made. This part of the study involved the use of qualitative and quantitative measures, and funding was obtained to support a research assistant and clinical observers (O'Brien 1993).

3   Theory development resulted from the identified need to be able to share with others the successful advances in NDU practice. Correspondence with Christopher Johns, who was advancing earlier work done in NDUs in the United Kingdom, led to the decision to test a conceptual framework of his design in the Australian NDU (O'Brien & Pope 1994). This chapter, in part, reflects on the outcomes of that exercise and forms the latest contribution to ongoing research in the Unit.

NURSING DEVELOPMENT UNITS: STARTING POINTS FOR THEORY GENERATION

Application of a critical theory-based ideology in nursing practice is recognisable in the pioneering work of Alan Pearson, who developed and applied his theory of clinical nursing (Pearson 1983) by developing Nursing Units at Burford and Oxford in the mid

1980s. His work and that of his successors is well documented (Pearson 1984c, 1985; Wright 1989; Salvage 1988, 1989, 1990; McMahon & Pearson 1991; Pearson et al. 1992), but the originator of the Western belief that nursing was essentially a therapy in its own right was Lydia Hall.

Hall was a nurse theorist educated at Columbia University's Teachers College (Meleis 1985) in the company of many other well-known North American nurse theorists. In respect of the application of her work, Hall's greatest achievement was the establishment of the Loeb Center for Nursing and Rehabilitation in New York, in 1962 (Marriner 1986). Alfano, a former director of the Loeb Center, describes Hall's philosophy as the promotion of healing '. . . through a **holistic** combination of clinical, technical, psychosocial and teaching skills' (Alfano 1988, p. 34). Pearson used the Loeb Center's basic ideas (Pearson 1984a) in his development of NDUs in the United Kingdom, and subsequently his ideas were explored and developed both there (Salvage 1989) and in Australia (Silver 1988; Crane 1989; Donnelly et al. 1990; O'Brien 1992, 1993).

Hall's and Pearson's ideologies have been described (Pearson 1983, 1985; Wright 1989; Salvage 1990) as evolving from a partnership between nurse and patient which, in turn, is conceived in a therapeutic atmosphere conducive and responsive to change. The practice forum in which this vision (ideology, philosophy) developed has been variously described as a clinical nursing unit (Pearson 1984c), a nursing development unit (Pearson 1988; Pearson et al. 1992) and a professorial nursing unit (Donnelly et al. 1990).

The extent of the responsibility assumed by NDU nurses is not lost on Salvage (1988), who cites studies (Buckenham & McGrath 1983; Smith & Redfern 1988) which suggest that nurses tend not to reconcile theory with their practice. Salvage agrees that Hall's and Pearson's vision has been shown to work in practice, but she warns that the establishment and maintenance of such change is not likely to be easy!

Wright (1989 p. 29) defined the phenomena that set NDUs apart from other settings where nursing innovation is taking place. The differences involve:

- the breadth and scope of the nursing innovations they support;
- the way that change is an accepted part of the culture of the nursing setting;
- the clear directions that nursing practice takes, which make care more personal; and
- the way their function is legitimated and funded within the health system.

The NDU under scrutiny in this chapter is part of a large Centre for aged and extended care in South Australia. The Centre provides a State-wide service offering fast- and slow-stream rehabilitation, skills retraining, lifestyle, respite and palliative care, and supported community-based accommodation, primarily to adults with acquired brain damage (ABD). The NDU has 20 commissioned beds whose occupancy levels are regulated by the dependency levels of the people admitted. In 1995, the Unit's population was changed after the transfer to other wards of those with extended care needs. The current population includes people with medical diagnosis of acquired brain damage, including pontine infarction (brain stem CVA) and traumatic brain injury (related mostly to motor vehicle accidents). In late 1995 the NDU was closed as part of Centre restructuring. It is hoped that this philosophy and practice will be re-established elsewhere in the Centre.

The most common presenting medical diagnosis has been pontine infarction, resulting in what is known as 'locked in syndrome'. (A blood clot or abscess in the brain stem causes almost complete loss of physical function.) Clients are cognitively intact but physically almost completely incapacitated, usually presenting with cuffed tracheostomy, gastrostomy feeding and communication limited to eye movements. The person has an active mind trapped in a non-functioning body, giving rise to the description of 'locked in syndrome'. As these people are usually in the 30–50-year-old age bracket and most have been active in society and at work, there is a big incentive to restore sufficient physical independence to allow them to re-enter the community. The development of nursing expertise in slow-stream rehabilitation of this client group (people with ABD) has evolved as the ward adopted the NDU philosophy that nursing is therapeutic in its own right.

In 1991, an action research project to establish two NDUs at the Centre was endorsed by the Nursing Executive—Director of Nursing (DON) and five Assistant Directors of Nursing (ADONs). The ADON responsible for the Clinical Division where the proposed NDUs were located worked with the Clinical Nurse Consultants (CNCs) of the two wards to establish the NDUs. This process was helped by the fact that the Clinical ADON had recently spent two years working with staff to establish one of two Professorial Nursing Units in Geelong, Victoria, under the supervision of Professor Alan Pearson, founder of the UK NDUs (Donnelly et al. 1990).

The initial focus for action was to establish the NDUs as a slow-stream rehabilitation alternative between the existing services of multidisciplinary-based, fast-stream rehabilitation and extended and long-term care. Secondary aims were to establish the effectiveness and efficiency of a primarily nursing rehabilitation service and to evaluate how the NDUs could supplement and complement the limited allied health resources available to the Centre. What follows is the story of how practice and theory evolved in one of these NDUs.

DEVELOPING CLINICAL PRACTICE

In taking the decision to refocus nursing in the NDU from long-term care to slow-stream rehabilitation, nursing staff faced the challenge of redefining their practice. The Clinical ADON and the CNC decided to introduce staff to a loose framework of ideas generated in other NDUs. The idea was to allow NDU nurses to begin identifying the relevant and therapeutic elements of their existing practice, using the introduced concepts as the basis for defining their practice and targeting new skills. The process of action taking was evolutionary, rather than revolutionary, and the reasons for choosing this approach were twofold:

1   There were no extra resources budgeted to assist in the establishment of the new NDU.

2   Experience suggested that staff who contributed to the establishment of a new pattern of practice tended to own it and value it more than staff introduced to a new clinical setting without having contributed to its establishment (O'Brien 1992).

Taking an evolutionary approach involved the NDU in working through the philosophy and practices of other NDUs. The work of Lydia Hall, Alan Pearson and Steve Wright in other NDUs provided a framework that justified staff beliefs in the therapeutic potential of nursing, while a process of reflecting on and evaluating the outcomes of NDU nursing (the NDU Quality Assurance Program) provided feedback to staff on the outcomes of changes made to their practice.

Two **assumptions** about nursing emerged from practical interpretation by the NDU of the pioneering work of Pearson and Wright:

1   NDU nursing is therapeutic in its own right.

2   NDU nursing care is based on an explicit theory of NDU practice where practice and theory inform and challenge each other.

(adapted from Wright 1989, p. 30)

DEVELOPING A THEORETICAL FRAMEWORK

The framework for NDU theory reflects the process of action research which took place as the NDUs established themselves. Five stages of action-taking were used to develop the framework of the NDU theory of practice.

1   Identifying a vision of what NDU practice should be.

2   Reflecting on what elements of practice-in-use were desirable, and why.

3   Identifying and defining concepts that described desirable practice.

4   Developing a conceptual framework that systematically and sensibly linked the various concepts together.

5   Elaborating the principles of nursing (belief system or science) which help justify the selection of concepts and linkages.

The five stages were not attempted in sequence, but initiated as one stage needed to be complemented by another. The left-hand side of Figure 11.1 shows the changes that were initiated by ward staff with the practical intention of establishing guidelines and protocols for NDU practice. As shown on the right hand side, at a more abstract level, reflection and theory development helped staff to say what exactly they were doing, so that others could understand what was going on.

FIGURE 11.1 STAGES OF THEORY DEVELOPMENT

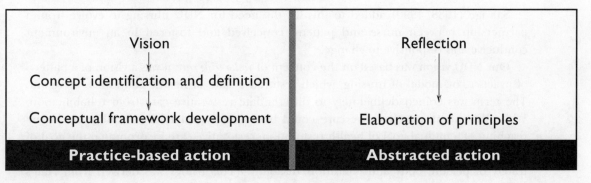

The *five action-taking* stages were connected. NDU staff spent some time reviewing existing NDU philosophies and selecting elements that seemed to be applicable to NDU practice as they *envisioned* it to be. *Reflection* on their own context and practice and how they differed from other settings helped target areas where changes needed to be made. As part of the change process, the language staff used to describe their work came under scrutiny and *concept identification and labelling* became a target for review. Calling something by a different name, especially when the something itself was also changing, required an *elaboration of the principles* necessary to achieve intended outcomes. At the same time, the Unit's pattern of practice was *conceptualised as a framework* to allow for checking of the relationships proposed between concepts in use.

The rest of the chapter develops this summary, using NDU experiences to illustrate the process of theory development through the establishment of nursing **praxis**: 'reflection and action upon the world in order to transform it' (Friere 1972, p. 28).

VISION

Although the situation may be changing, it remains an unfortunate fact in many settings that nurses do not or cannot easily describe the practical nursing philosophy or vision which guides or drives their practice. Yet fundamental to the emergence of nursing as a discipline and profession is the ability of society to recognise and attribute to nursing a unique and valued contribution to social well-being. If nurses find it difficult to summarise their unique and therapeutic contribution, how much harder is it for everyone else to understand what nurses 'do'?

Pearson summarised his vision of nursing in the early NDUs in terms of practice that:

- is based on the belief that the patient is unique, and reflects this belief;

- combines a logical application and unification of caregiving, research, teaching and care management;

- is based on knowledge;

- uses the relationship between the nurse and patient to therapeutic effect;

- is systematic and follows a logical, problem-solving approach;

- is carried out by a nurse who can justify her [sic] actions and, therefore, be accountable for them;

- is seen as equal to the practice of other disciplines.

(Pearson 1984c, p. 22)

Salvage (1988, 1990) added to this list the need for NDU nursing to evolve from a partnership between nurse and patient, conceived and fostered in an environment conducive and responsive to change.

Our NDU vision was based on the concept of *restorative care*; it was a vision of a pattern of practice, or model of nursing, which restored a state of health, soundness or vigour. The term was coined deliberately to differentiate restorative care from rehabilitation. While the intent of restorative care could be equated to that of rehabilitation in the reaching of a mutual goal of health restoration, restorative care incorporated the goal of providing a predominantly nurse-directed therapy which treated with equal respect the trilogy of person, body and condition/disability. (This trilogy was derived from Hall's

---

Example

Brainstorming a vision

The NDU starting point for a vision statement was a brainstorming session which took place at the afternoon nursing shift handover. The session was held early on in the process of establishing the NDU and the brainstorming exercise was suggested by the ward CNC, in response to questioning by staff as to how to begin to understand and define existing practice. The session lasted for 30 minutes (not 5 minutes as planned) and involved 14 registered and enrolled nurses. Three prompt questions were as follows.

1   What do we do here that makes a difference?

2   What would we like to do? and

3   What do we want to change?

In the spirit of brainstorming, all responses were noted uncritically on a whiteboard, listed under three headings suggested by the prompt questions: 'Do Now', 'Want to Do' and 'Want to Change'. The responses were later proposed to other NDU nurses at subsequent ward handovers and a small number of extra items was added. Of relevance to the early vision of the NDU was a 'Want to Do' item called restorative care.

Core (person), Care (body) and Cure (disease) model—Hall 1964.) The essence of restorative care was considered to be its unexplored potential as a therapeutic intervention for individuals who were not best served by existing patterns of care delivery. The vision of the NDU was to develop a practice-based model of restorative care using the combined resources of available lay and professional carers (generally family and NDU nursing staff) with consultative input from the rehabilitation areas of the Centre and the community.

The concept of restorative care was suggested for the purpose of being able to define NDU care as different from, but similar in intent to, rehabilitation care, where the general understanding is that a multidisciplinary, allied health team plans and delivers care to people whose health deficits are likely to respond to such care within a definite time frame (at the Centre this did not usually exceed 3 months). Restorative care was based on nursing therapy delivered over a period of time determined by each resident's potential to progress (in practice, this meant stays of from 6 months to 2–3 years in the NDU). The initial vision statement was framed in terms of NDU nursing's intent to provide restorative care. During this period, the ward was even titled the Restorative Care Development Unit (RCDU).

It seems reasonable to suggest that a simple vision statement such as 'This NDU is about restorative care nursing' can be based around a single concept. Other wards in the Centre have identified vision statements that focus on concepts such as 'self-esteem' or 'creating a homelike environment'. These sorts of vision statements are simple and readily remembered by practising nurses. A carefully chosen vision statement which asserts, for example, that nursing in X ward is about establishing and ensuring self-esteem may form a basic standard against which to measure all clinical nursing activity. Even management activities, such as rostering and patient assignment, can be assessed and challenged by the criterion of whether individuals' self-esteem is maintained as the result of the practice.

In choosing restorative care, however, NDU nurses found themselves faced with the need to define the concept further, so as to be able to state confidently how restorative care differed from rehabilitative care (largely by virtue of who delivered the care and the length of time available), and what would comprise restorative care in the NDU (what was realistic, given the resources of the Unit).

It can be seen already that selection of the concept of restorative care provided the NDU with a number of related concepts. These in turn required definition and incorporation into the emerging vision statement. At the same time, given the philosophical guidelines developed in other units, each new concept and its definition needed to be tested to see if it really fitted three standards:

- the prevailing theory of what NDUs represented;

- the actual and planned practice of the NDU; and, finally,

- the developing vision statement of the Unit.

The NDU's 1995 vision statement is presented in full at this point to illustrate the definition of restorative that was developed and tested against these three standards. Phrases and concepts such as 'lay and professional carers', 'independence', 'lifestyle', 'collaboration', 'trilogy of person, body and disease', 'interaction with community', 'consultation', 'continual monitoring' (quality assurance) and 'reflection' were presented at brainstorming sessions, and subsequently defined in terms of NDU resources and potential and incorporated in the working philosophy given in the box at the top of the facing page.

Examples of the philosophy and some of the associated concepts are given in the boxes on pp. 243–6.

Putting together a vision for the NDU started as a spontaneous brainstorming exercise which threw up the concept of restorative care, a term that appealed to NDU staff and which seemed to depict the rehabilitation alternative that the new unit was setting out to establish. New concepts, or the use of terms to redefine variations on old practices, soon exposed NDU staff to the need to explain and justify their use of new language. Recourse to the nursing literature was quickly seen as a relevant and practical strategy, especially when validation of ideas and descriptions of experienced behaviours (i.e. the adversarial alliance) were needed to explain to others the effect of implementation of ideas (i.e. modified primary team nursing) or the experience of outcomes of newly implemented patterns of care (i.e. nurse–resident/family relationships).

Theory and practice: Gap or dialectic?

As NDU staff came to understand, it is one thing to develop a vision statement and quite another to ensure that NDU practice matched NDU theory. Having developed a vision statement, the challenge for NDU nurses was to see how well it reflected nursing practice in the unit and whether there were gaps (in practice or the vision) that needed to be filled or bridged.

Gap suggests meanings such as divergence, vacant space, interval, disparity, imbalance or contradiction (Macquarie Dictionary 1981, p. 725). The concept of a *gap* promotes separateness and invokes alternative definitions for theory and practice. While practice

Example

NDU Philosophy (vision statement)

Staff assert that care is focused on the individual, and lifestyle and restorative forms of care are offered that reflect the residents' state of independence.

Recognition is given to the rights of NDU residents to a lifestyle and environment that promotes interaction with the general community to the fullest extent possible.

Residents are encouraged to strive for strengthening in areas of weakness and to develop areas of strength, thus enabling them to regain and maintain independence in a safe, caring, homelike environment.

A program of restorative care is provided by the combined resources of lay and professional carers, with consultative input from other rehabilitation areas of the Centre and the community.

A collaborative approach to care is promoted in which professional carers, lay carers and residents are empowered to contribute equally, according to the potential of each group.

Care is best given by those staff who have the necessary skills, experience and knowledge to create a setting where learning occurs through the practical, personal experience of caring, and through reflection on the effects of caring.

Continual monitoring of the cyclical caring process is maintained so that others can benefit from the development, knowledge and expertise gained in this NDU.

Nursing praxis (reflective understanding and purposeful action) is the essential therapeutic agent.

and theory are indeed quite separate in meaning and purpose, at a practical level it makes better sense to check whether it is the practice or the theory that needs changing, rather than assume one or the other is always correct. The process of playing off two apparent opposites against each other to find out what each contributes to a common understanding is known as **dialectic**.

Dialectic is a process of change that starts from a debate over the properties and value of two apparent opposites (Macquarie Dictionary 1981, p. 498). For example, black and white are extremes of colour, and colour (as a concept or phenomenon) combines black and white in a unique fashion. In another sense, black and white complement each other. Nursing is the product (like it or not) of combining nursing practice and nursing theory. The complementary nature of theory and practice and their role in nursing is described by Robinson:

Example

Group, rather than team

The background to the NDU's use of the term 'group' in the philosophy helps to illustrate the underlying beliefs of NDU nurses. 'Group' was chosen to replace team to describe the collection of people involved in the care of an individual. There were two main reasons for this:

1   To hold true to an expressed belief in the individuality of care and the need to regard people in a holistic way, NDU nurses worked to establish a modification of primary nursing care (modified primary team nursing) where the same group of nurses worked with an individual for a period of 3 months at a time. Care delivery was based around individuals and care planning which involved other health disciplines was also individually focused.

2   The NDU also considered lay carers (usually family and/or close relations and friends) to be key partners in care delivery. Part of the rationale for this belief stemmed from the pragmatic understanding that most NDU residents would eventually be discharged into the (at least partial) care of these people, and it made sense to involve them from the start in care planning and education of resident needs.

Team as a concept (at least within the Centre) held connotations of a centralised ward- or unit-focused collection of health professionals who planned and directed care. Indeed, there was little for Enrolled General Nurses or Nurse Attendants to do other than sit in at team meetings. Families and residents also tended to be disempowered by traditional interpretations of team functioning.

Group-based care was conceived as the non-hierarchically defined contributions of lay and professional carers (including self-care from the resident). In the sense that a group represents a collection of people with a common purpose, membership of each care group comprised those people who were delivering care or affected by the care planning for each individual. Drawing on the expectation that resident and lay carers would increasingly become responsible for care delivery, the input and goals set by these people were held to be just as important as goals set by nursing and allied health professionals.

In practice, the new concept worked well, once the modified primary team nursing was established. An interesting and useful side effect of the decision to use group work instead of team work emerged in the process of establishing the new title.

On finding their loved ones were being transferred to the NDU, family members frequently expressed bitterness and frustration at the withdrawal

Example (continued)

of multidisciplinary-based rehabilitation. The general perception of these people was that rehabilitation was associated with physiotherapy and 'lots of it'. The roles of Speech Therapy and Occupational Therapy were also acknowledged, but nursing was considered as scarcely more than assistance to the true rehabilitation provided by 'the physio'. Anger and frustration were repeatedly directed at nursing staff, as the most readily available listeners and as scapegoats for any and every observable deviation from planned care or expected outcomes. The upshot of these outbursts was that nurses or family members would confront the CNC or the Clinical ADON, seeking support, or at least a sounding board.

The concept of group-based care was used on these occasions to point out that members of the group came from diverse backgrounds and understandings, brought together and held there by a common desire or obligation to provide care to an individual. It was explained that the potential for care delivery to produce desired outcomes was best served when group members supported each other and the agreed plan of care. The point was made that working as a group was the best way to bring to an end the need to continue to work together. Obviously each group's life expectancy was based on the individual's need for the care services of members of the group. The notion of group transition through stages of forming, storming, norming, performing and mourning was also used to help identify which stage group members were at, and what strategies might be considered to work in overcoming the presenting source of conflict, anger or frustration.

The counselling process was assisted by reference to the literature. An article entitled 'The adversarial alliance: Developing relationships between families and the team in brain injury rehabilitation' (McLaughlin & Carey 1993) described behaviours and reactions identical to those experienced by NDU staff but focused more on identifying families at risk of developing high stress levels (and resultant outbursts). Other work on the stress experienced by nurses involved in nurse–resident/family relationships (Johns 1991,1994) suggested the potential need for nurses to be competent in personal stress management. Together these articles supported the NDU's decision to continue with a group (rather than team) philosophy, because:

■ the non-hierarchical structure of the group reduced nurses' vulnerability to being 'shot down' (decisions were reached by general agreement or consensus); and

■ the 'work together and we will progress faster' argument was observed to be a successful strategy that reduced blame accruing to individuals, focusing attention instead on the need to develop group cohesion in the interests of helping the resident.

Example

Implementing a theory of primary nursing

The primary nurse holds 24 hour, seven days a week responsibility for planning and administering care, although obviously only providing actual care during her hours on duty. When she is off duty, care is continued by an associate nurse . . . [who] . . . follows the care plan developed by the primary nurse . . . .

(Pearson 1988, p. 28)

To implement individually focused care in the NDU primary nursing, or some variation of it, was considered theoretically desirable but practically difficult to implement. Staff liked the philosophy of continuity of care but shied away from the thought of committing themselves to caring relationships that would last (in some cases) literally for years.

At this point, applying theory developed from other practice, the Clinical ADON suggested a modification that he had observed to work in another NDU where residents were admitted for extended periods. The suggestion was made that NDU nurses be allocated to three groups. Two of the groups were to be responsible for the care of specific groups of residents (the Unit was effectively divided by its geography into two discrete areas), while members of the third group 'floated' between Group A and Group B according to the needs of each group from shift to shift. After 3 months some of the nurses from each of Group A and B rotated to the 'float' group and were replaced by float nurses. This meant that the nurses newly allocated to each group already had some experience of the residents to whom they would now be giving dedicated care, and the nurses rotating into the 'float' team were not totally distanced from the residents they had been caring for. The only nurses not to rotate regularly were two Clinical Nurses (CNs) who led Group A and B. These two senior nurses served as the primary nurse focus for each group (although individual nurses in each group might be allocated specific residents for their 3-month rotation).

NDU nurses agreed to trial this idea for a month and then review it. With some modifications it was eventually adopted on the basis of a 2-month rotation (which lasted for 2 years) and eventually a 3-month rotation. Evaluation suggested that one month was too short a time to implement and evaluate changes to care delivery or to build effective nurse–resident/family relationships. On the other hand, staff considered that after 3 months enthusiasm began to wane, and there emerged the potential to routinise care and miss opportunities to build on changes in residents' health status. For staff in the 'float' team, 3 months of instability provided a rest from day-to-day involvement in intensive care planning, but also introduced some dissatisfaction with being sidelined from this exercise. For the Clinical Nurse 'group leaders', 3 months minimised the need to continually reorient and educate staff, while the ability to negotiate a change of group (usually related to annual leave) provided a potential escape path when the pressures of group maintenance seemed to get out of hand.

Nursing practice then, is not some mindless behaviour. It is related to theory, and theory can be applied to it. All practices have theory embedded in them and all theory is firmly embedded in practice.

(1988, p. 6)

Robinson goes on to make the point that gaps between theory and practice may occur when:

* nursing theory is seen as different to that already in use;

* the language of theory and practice differ, resulting in a communication gap;

* practitioners do not interpret or evaluate nursing theories correctly;

* nurses believe that nursing theory can be produced outside the context in which it is meant to apply.

(Robinson 1988, p. 7)

The process of dialectic helps to unscramble the difficulties which arise when the desire to implement theory (i.e. primary nursing) conflicts with the beliefs of staff about how it will work in practice. The use of reflective evaluation to systematically challenge workplace assumptions empowers nurses to see whether what they say they do actually matches what they are observed to do. In this example, theory was modified to describe a practice which provided improved continuity of care. Modified primary team nursing is a practical application of the theory of primary nursing, applied in a specific context.

REFLECTION

The descriptions and examples provided so far should demonstrate that NDU nurses quickly found themselves having to think very hard about aspects of their practice that had previously been taken largely for granted. Certainly, exercises such as the brainstorming sessions led to staff questioning their practice more spontaneously and, during the first year of establishing the NDU, two activities—reflecting-in-action and reflecting-on-action—became a noticeably acceptable part of staff behaviour. (This is not to say that all staff did it but that it was accepted as a useful behaviour.)

The process of consciously questioning practice is clearly described by Schön:

[P]rofessional practitioners often think about what they are doing, sometimes even while they are doing it. Stimulated by surprise, they turn thought back on action and on the knowing which is implicit in action.

(1983, p. 50)

In these words, Schön captures the philosophies of grounded theory and action research, suggesting that critical reflection is a methodology for implementing change (in practice and in understanding of practice) that any professional can use. Reflection may be used spontaneously (as Schön describes), responding to a surprise side effect of some behaviour, or it may be consciously used as a research tool, to make sense of established practice and to keep track of the effects of introduced change.

The application of reflection to nursing practice is very much in vogue in Australia at present. For example, the Australian Nursing Council Inc. (ANCI 1993) national competencies for entry level registered nurses have 'Reflective Practice' as a discrete domain, with 12 subcompetencies described which apply the use of reflection in and on registered nurse behaviour. Reflection is also widely incorporated into nursing curricula, as a discrete subject, or applied as a learning method. In a number of universities throughout Australia, nursing students are encouraged to keep reflective journals of their observations during clinical placements and to use these reflections in preparation of written work and to stimulate discussion and debate in tutorials and group-based activities. In nursing research, the establishment of methodologies such as **phenomenology** (Taylor 1992), **ethnography** (Gibb et al. 1993) and action research (O'Brien 1992) has involved nurse researchers in keeping and using reflective journals to describe the research process and as a basis for stimulating discussion and debate on observed clinical practice.

The role of reflection in the development of practice-based theory is grounded in the needs of nurses who wish for deeper understanding, or to modify their practice, to comprehend clearly what it is that they currently do, so that outcomes can be matched to nursing activities. Critical reflection is more than saying: 'We follow the procedure manual. We catheterise according to ward protocol.' It involves looking at observed practice to see if procedures and protocols are strictly adhered to *and* what outcomes result. Is it some seemingly innocent short-cut that is leading to an unacceptable level of post-catheterisation infection? Is it the unrecognised personal relationship between specific individuals that makes the difference between one nurse being able to shower a resident while another can't? Critical reflection is a process which tears practices apart, debriefs individuals and groups, defers to the literature—always looking for an in-depth understanding of why nursing practice produces the outcomes it does.

Reflection can be learnt, and I would argue that it is a skill available to all nurses and not just something to be confused with the concept of intuition, as in: 'Some nurses can just do it. It's women's intuition.' 'I just seem to know what to do—it's probably my intuition.' Without entering into a debate on the phenomenon of intuition, I suggest that a lot of what is called 'intuition' is actually tacit or implicit reflection on action—experience calling out to the subconscious. By raising reflection to a conscious level, individuals learn to refine their use of logic and reason to solve problems and improve personal understanding. In nursing, where care delivery is frequently a group activity undertaken by a succession of nurses over 24 hours, reflection has a special role to play. Conscious reflection provides a tool to assist with documentation, handover and assessment.

Schön (1987) suggests that students of the professions (including nursing) learn through practice and through reflection on the effects of their practice.

> The student cannot be *taught* what he needs to know, but he can be *coached*. Nobody can see for him, and he can't see just by being 'told', although the right kind of telling may guide his seeing and thus help him see what he needs to see.
>
> (Schön 1987, p. 17)

Coaching is a teaching–learning activity readily adapted to nursing education. Nurses frequently work together and team allocation is commonly based around a sharing out of the available skills. New nurses are 'buddied up' with more experienced nurses. In this environment, the coaching involves exchanges such as:

- See that . . . that means . . .

- Did you see him . . . that usually leads to . . .

- Did you notice the colour, smell, movement etc. of . . . that means . . .

Regular exposure to reflective coaching of this sort, in an atmosphere where students feel safe to question and experiment, can be a powerful learning medium.

It would be nice to report that NDU nurses accepted and incorporated reflection into all their everyday practices. It is probably more accurate to say that there were sessions and times when reflection was consciously applied to solve special problems or to address and formulate strategies for introducing or evaluating change. The use of conscious, systematic reflection was most consistently observed in senior NDU nursing staff—the Clinical Nurse Consultant (CNC), Clinical Nurses (CNs) and some of the registered nurses. As the people most responsible and accountable for the effectiveness of the model of care in use in the NDU, it is likely that they spent most time refining NDU nursing practice and evaluating its outcomes.

An article by Robert Newell (1993) proved helpful to the NDU's understanding and acceptance of the role of reflection. Newell writes about reflection's incorporation as a key concept in the development and maintenance of nursing expertise in theory and practice (1992, p. 1326), and then explores a number of difficulties associated with establishing it as a workplace tool. While he covers issues such as bias in recall and repression of information, what particularly interested the NDU was the point he made about the effect of work-related stress on reflective ability.

Newell points out that stressful circumstances frequently arise in nursing (e.g. the nurse–resident/family interactions described earlier) and that stress in turn affects or impairs memory and recall. He suggests that, in situations where reflective debriefing may be of greatest assistance, '. . . information available for reflection may become bland and non-problematic, whilst key incidents which are threatening, but offer particular potential for learning, are omitted completely from the nurse's reflective repertoire' (Newell 1993, p. 1329).

CONCEPT IDENTIFICATION AND DEFINITION

In developing a vision statement, it has already been established that a number of concepts, rather than a single one, will be identified. Each concept requires a measure of description and critique to ensure that it helps rather than hinders the development of practice-based theory. NDU nurses found it convenient to start by borrowing concept definitions from a number of nurse theorists whose writing was considered relevant to NDU practice.

The earliest conceptual framework was built around Roper, Logan and Tierney's (1985) description of nursing, Lydia Hall's (1964) care, cure and core concepts, and Virginia Henderson's (1966) Activities of Living. Henderson's Activities of Living more closely suited the NDU's clinical focus and were overlayed on the Roper, Logan and Tierney model. Needs analysis was considered important, and Maslow's hierarchy of needs as applied to nursing (see Murray 1976, pp. 107–8) was incorporated. The NDU's concept of a group (rather than team) approach to care delivery was represented in sociological terms (see Giddens 1989, Chap. 9). Finally, healing, as a concept to replace curing, was defined in terms identified by McGlone (1990). These elements formed the basis of the first NDU practice-based model. At

Example

We work and work and work, and all that happens is we get tired.

Early in the establishment of the NDU, a decision was taken to admit three new residents who met the Unit's criteria of having potential to respond to nursing-based restorative care. The NDU also decided to accept these admissions without any corresponding increase in staffing levels. Prior to this time, the Unit's resident population had been stable for a period of nearly 12 months and most of the residents at that time required nursing assistance to maintain rather than alter lifestyle activity. The effect of admitting three highly dependent residents was quickly demonstrated as NDU nurses found themselves with a revised workload (heavier than before) focused on new and different outcomes (restorative rather than lifestyle care), which in turn led to complaints from the established residents (who found their daily routines disrupted by the changes).

All these issues had been anticipated but, because they had not been experienced before and certainly not in combination, the impact of the introduced changes was found to have been greatly underestimated in the enthusiasm of starting the NDU project. Staff literally reported working their hearts out just to keep the Unit and resident care vaguely under control. Sick leave rose and this made the problem worse, as relieving staff had little background knowledge of the NDU's vision and tended to set about their work in the ways they were used to. This placed an increased strain on staff, who felt the need to orient and supervise relieving nurses closely in order to preserve the changes being implemented.

The situation was stabilised by the CNC, who made time to review and summarise all the decisions made, and changes initiated, in the 3 months prior to admission of the new residents and in the 2 months after their admission. She produced quality assurance results and feedback from allied health staff and presented all her findings to a series of ward meetings. By reflecting back over where the ward had started, and the number of changes that had been successfully implemented towards its establishment as an NDU, she was able to show staff that the NDU initiative was progressing and that changes introduced were having a positive effect on care outcomes. Nurses were encouraged to reflect on the fact that the Unit was certainly busier than before, but that a lot of the stress was related to the fact that staff were still gaining experience of a number of newly introduced procedures, not to the ineffectiveness of those procedures.

Similarly with the new residents, as familiarity and experience of their needs was gained by NDU nurses, so the stresses of interacting with them decreased. These sessions defused a situation that had arisen when staff failed to stand back and reflect on the reasons for the pressures of (self-imposed) change. When the CNC undertook this exercise, the situation was largely defused. Particular trouble spots were targeted for attention, and perceptions of stress relating to all aspects of NDU workload were reduced to an understanding that a, b and c situations were currently stressful, but that x, y and z were being done about them.

this stage, the main aim of NDU nurses was to describe the various elements of their proposed practice and their practice-in-use and how they all fitted together. Less consideration was given to checking that the beliefs underpinning these various contributions were comparable, each with the other and with the Unit's working philosophy.

In other words, where a hole appeared in the model it was 'plugged', using knowledge or literature familiar to the NDU. While there was some review of the relevant literature, it was too early to develop a theoretically and philosophically 'correct' practice-based model when the concepts and their proposed relationships were being tested in (changing) practice. The first model adopted provided a baseline of beliefs about NDU practice, against which nursing could be assessed, amended or refined. There was also an expectation that the model would require refinement, to include aspects of NDU practice not yet described or developed, and to revise (and possibly omit) concepts for which no practice base could be found or justified.

Roper, Logan and Tierney: Nursing model (1985)

The inclusion of elements of this model stemmed from its application in other NDUs, and its incorporation of activities of living (ALs) as a focus for planning nursing interventions, an approach that was common throughout the Centre. The Roper, Logan and Tierney model is one of the few nursing models not to have originated in North America (it was developed in Britain), and similarities between the health systems of Britain and Australia provided a further incentive to consider its potential. The model is:

> . . . based on a model for living, and attempts to describe the reality of nursing to help nurses develop a mode of thinking about the profession which focuses on the processes of living.
>
> *(Pearson 1988, p. 10)*

NDU nurses liked the model's linear continuum concept applied to activities of living—the sense that activities of living and the individual's participation in them vary across the life span and are also affected by fluctuations in personal health. In summary of this concept, and as a starting point for assessment of an individual's nursing needs, Roper, Logan and Tierney's linear continuum concept was modified slightly, away from a straight linear concept applied to specific activities of living, to portray a clock face (representative of time). The upper half of the clock face is shown as an age continuum (from 0–100 years, although this could be modified to suit the potential age group of a ward's admission profile), while the lower half shows a best life–worst life continuum (see Figure 11.2 on p. 255).

Assessment on admission to the NDU starts with mutual identification (by nurse and resident) of the resident's age where, on the best life–worst life continuum, the residents see themselves and where on the continuum they realistically expect to be as a result of NDU-based care. At this point, descriptions of health, lifestyle, needs and wants are recorded in resident-centred language, based on the understanding that NDU nursing is a healing modality that builds on an individual's readiness to progress (McGlone 1990).

Healing

McGlone (1990) describes healing in the following terms:

> . . . healing, to be made whole, is a process of getting in touch with that which is impeding our realisation of wholeness . . . (p. 78)

> The rate of healing is consistent with people's personal readiness to grow and change. (p. 82)

This description fitted the therapeutic intent proposed by NDU nurses. It helped justify the decision to modify Roper, Logan and Tierney's linear continuum concept, because it validated the NDU's perception of each resident as a person first and foremost—a person who might have needs describable in a reductionist sense (such as through the use of activities of living or needs analysis), but who should be accorded the dignity of being treated as an individual greater than the sum of these parts.

Lydia Hall's model: Care, cure and core (1964)

Hall's work underpinned theory development and nursing practice in the earliest NDUs (Pearson 1985) and was found to provide a useful and consistent description of care delivery in one of the first Australian NDUs (O'Brien 1992, pp. 239–48). Hall's model describes three aspects of nursing: care, cure and core activities.

Care. The caring focus considers people as socially interactive individuals, who are also members of socially describable groups (intentionally or otherwise). Seeing people as individuals who could not escape being influenced by the actions of others helped NDU nurses to understand why people behaved the way they did, and how group influences helped or hindered the progress of individual group members.

Figure 11.2 illustrates the concept of a 'group' whose purpose (therapy) and behaviours challenged community norms, with the group deliberately overlaying pre-existing personal, family and social boundaries. The illustration suggests why it is important for a group to work constructively together—so that any negative effects on members can be remedied as quickly as possible. This concept (group processes) also helped to explain to NDU staff why residents and 'loved ones' (lay carers), as well as health professionals, should be considered partners in care planning.

Cure. Needs analysis was used to 'triage' nursing interventions within the model. What this meant in practice was identification of a person's needs and wants (on assessment) followed by the need to prioritise these so as to link nursing and resident/family priorities. NDU nurses found that the contextual nature of nursing meant that priorities could change in the time it takes to walk from a person's room to the treatment bay. The cure concept provides a **taxonomy** (list) for nurses to use in prioritising resident or personal needs so that the appropriateness of planned nursing care can be reviewed accordingly (see box opposite). This concept revised Hall's description of cure (as an activity directed towards cure of disease or physical injury) so that it reflected intent to make each intervention as therapeutic as possible, by ensuring that nursing activity addresses the most urgent or relevant needs of the resident every time the nurse and resident are together.

It will be seen from any reading of Hall's work that her discussion of 'cure' is directed at cure of disease or physical injury. The nature of health care deficits in the NDU

Example

The nursing care plan might identify an individual's morning hygiene, feeding and grooming regime, giving preferences and time frames agreed as part of the plan. From a therapeutic perspective (immediate cure orientation), NDU nurses were asked to assess the appropriateness of such a plan each day, rather than implement it unthinkingly. A sleepless or late night, pain or expressed anxiety are examples of the sorts of stimuli that might reprioritise getting somebody out of bed at 0800.

(requiring extended time frames to remedy) meant that acute illness, disease or injury formed a minor aspect of nursing, and one that interrupted (rather than formed) the main intent of NDU nursing. The decision to revise Hall's description of nursing, cure-focused activity was based on the understanding that NDU restorative care was primarily focused on gradual improvements across the range of activities of daily living rather than on a specific physiological deficit.

Maslow's hierarchy was used as the basis for 'triaging' care, essentially because it was familiar to all nurses in the Unit, having been used as a model for needs analysis in nursing education since the 1970s (see Murray 1976). It was the belief of NDU staff that most nurses could identify with its progression from physiological to esteem needs and actualisation. Belief in the user-friendliness of Maslow's concept was as much behind its selection as any other factor.

Maslow's hierarchy of needs is a good example of a conceptual definition that did not hold up under closer examination and application. With experience, NDU nurses found that what they were really trying to describe was the assessment and prioritisation of presenting resident needs carried out during every nurse–resident interaction. Maslow's hierarchy of needs seemed to be a useful prioritisation taxonomy but its use adds too many other issues to the conceptual definition and these confuse nurses trying to understand the application of the concept. (At present there is no formal taxonomy in use. However, the principle of maximising therapeutic intent by assessing the suitability of planned care to the context in which it is being delivered is still applied.)

Core (Virginia Henderson's Activities of Living model (1966)). Called 'basic nursing care' by NDU nurses, and 'dirty work' by Lawler (1991), the activities of living uniquely undertaken by nurses (washing, feeding, toileting, grooming etc.) came to be called 'essential nursing care' by NDU nurses. An Activities of Living model was widely used at the Centre—for example, to support its computerised nursing dependency and clinical database program (Spry & O'Brien 1993)—but the Centre's list of Activities of Living was not derived from any particular nursing model, nor was it inclusive of all activities of living identified in theoretical models such as Roper, Logan and Tierney's or Henderson's.

Henderson's activities of living were chosen by the NDU, as her list most closely matched the activities identified as relevant to NDU nursing practice. Fairly quickly, the

TABLE 11.1. COMPARISON OF NDU ACTIVITIES OF LIVING WITH HENDERSON'S LIST

THE NDU'S ACTIVITIES OF LIVING	HENDERSON'S ACTIVITIES OF LIVING
Breathing	Breathing
Mobilising	Flexing
Communicating	Communicating
Eating and drinking	Eating and drinking
Eliminating	Eliminating
Level of awareness	Avoiding danger and injury
Maintaining a safe environment	Sleeping and resting
Maintaining body temperature and blood pressure	Maintaining body temperature
Personal cleansing, dressing and grooming	Selecting clothes and dressing
Working/playing	Cleaning and grooming
Expressing sexuality, role/altered body image	Working
Spiritual needs	Playing
Involving family/significant others	Satisfying curiosity
Pain control	Worshipping

list was revised to specify activities of living related to NDU restorative programs, as the comparison in Table 11.1 shows.

The variations between the two lists in Table 11.1 reflect nursing priorities in the NDU related to the specific needs of people with acquired brain injury, resulting in the health deficits susceptible to NDU-based restorative care.

CONCEPTUAL FRAMEWORK DEVELOPMENT

With these concepts as a beginning, the next stage of theory development was a better description of the linkages and relationships that would give them some cohesiveness. The structure of the first NDU model was wonderfully simple. It needed to fit on an A4 page so that it could form part of an NDU brochure. This model had a significant graphical component and the experience of using it endorses the old saying that a picture is worth a thousand words.

Figure 11.2 is a graphic depiction of the NDU practice-based model. Reading of the model starts in the top left-hand corner with a statement of what (NDU) nursing is. Underneath is the age and best life–worst life continuum clock face, illustrating that nursing starts with a holistic assessment of each individual. This initial assessment incorporates early goal-setting, which in turn underpins quality assurance assessment of care outcomes, measured in terms of people's achievements towards desired outcomes,

FIGURE 11.2 A CONCEPTUAL MODEL FOR NURSING IN THE NDU

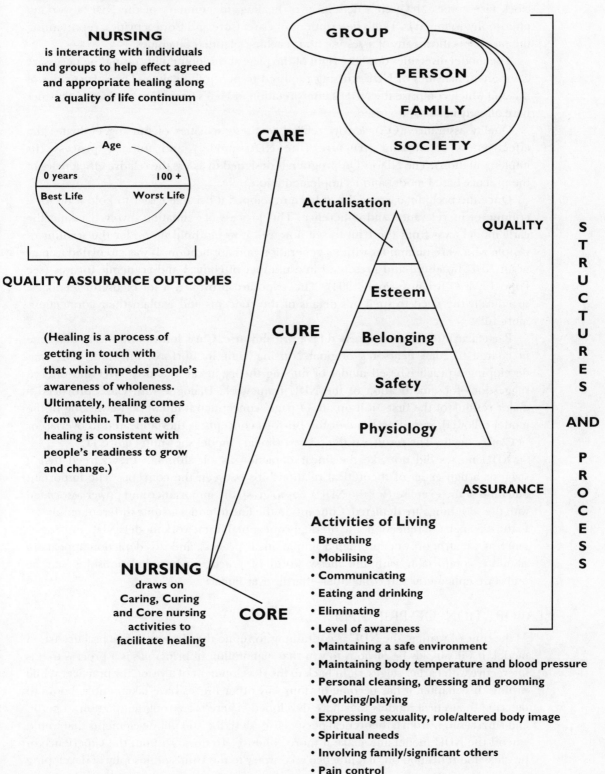

NURSING
is interacting with individuals
and groups to help effect agreed
and appropriate healing along
a quality of life continuum

GROUP

PERSON

FAMILY

SOCIETY

Age

0 years   100 +

Best Life   Worst Life

CARE

Actualisation

QUALITY

QUALITY ASSURANCE OUTCOMES

CURE

Esteem

Belonging

Safety

Physiology

(Healing is a process of
getting in touch with
that which impedes people's
awareness of wholeness.
Ultimately, healing comes
from within. The rate of
healing is consistent with
people's readiness to grow
and change.)

ASSURANCE

Activities of Living
• Breathing
• Mobilising
• Communicating
• Eating and drinking
• Eliminating
• Level of awareness
• Maintaining a safe environment
• Maintaining body temperature and blood pressure
• Personal cleansing, dressing and grooming
• Working/playing
• Expressing sexuality, role/altered body image
• Spiritual needs
• Involving family/significant others
• Pain control

NURSING
draws on
Caring, Curing
and Core nursing
activities to
facilitate healing

CORE

S T R U C T U R E S   A N D   P R O C E S S

away from the best life–worst life continuum point identified on admission. Under the clock face comes McGlone's definition of healing, in summary of the NDU's working philosophy, followed by Hall's descriptions of Care, Cure and Core activities, representing the more specific means of assessing and reaching planned outcomes.

The model diversifies onto the right of the page at this point, illustrating the necessary component activities of NDU nursing required to promote healing. The subactivities of nursing which comprise the NDU's interpretation of Hall's Care, Cure and Core activities have already been summarised.

Quality assurance (QA) activity related to these activities of nursing evaluates the effectiveness of nursing structure (the NDU model) and nursing process (its implementation). The NDU's QA program is designed to assess the relative efficiencies of the practice-based model and its implementation.

Once the preliminary model had been developed it became easier to hold it up for a critique of its relevance and coherence. This process of validation involved taking the early model away from the Unit to see how well it would hold up under the scrutiny of people who were unfamiliar with its generation and application. It was circulated as part of an NDU brochure and presented in a number of clinical and academic forums (see Pope 1993; O'Brien & Pope 1994). This exposure provoked a lot of useful feedback, specifically the need to spell out details of the concepts and explain their connections more fully.

Particular interest was expressed by a British nurse, Chris Johns, who was at that time in charge of Alan Pearson's original Nursing Unit in Burford, England. Chris was developing a practice-based model of nursing theory in the Burford NDU and offered suggestions for modification of the NDU framework. Dialogue with Chris provoked a major rethink of the first 'fit it on an A4 page' conceptual framework. Reworking of the model followed, including some of the Burford concepts as they appeared to overlap or fit Centre needs. The result was the revised (linear) model shown in Figure 11.3.

NDU nurses did not like the linear depiction at all, although they agreed that it suggests a tighter set of theoretical relationships between the concepts. The important outcome of the exercise (for the NDU) was to grasp the importance and power associated with the way things are depicted. Concepts in the linear model assume different emphases to the original. On reflection, the original conceptual framework models NDU nursing as more of a matrix of concepts than a simple linear process, and this depiction appears to sit more comfortably with the messy world of practice, where relationships can be transient, ephemeral and contextual—hardly ever linear!

ELABORATION OF PRINCIPLES

At the time of writing, the NDU is continuing to refine the elements of its practice-based model. It will already be obvious to you that elaboration of principles is a process that is interactive with earlier stages, right back to the development of a vision for practice. While writing this chapter, it has become obvious why other nurses have taken entire books to describe theoretical models they have developed. There is a strong temptation to go on and (increasingly from a theoretical perspective) describe and define elements that would extend the NDU model and make it more cohesive. To do so without the experience of practice and reflection on that practice is contrary to the Unit's philosophy of developing practice-based theory.

FIGURE 11.3 A CONCEPTUAL FRAMEWORK FOR NURSING IN THE NDU

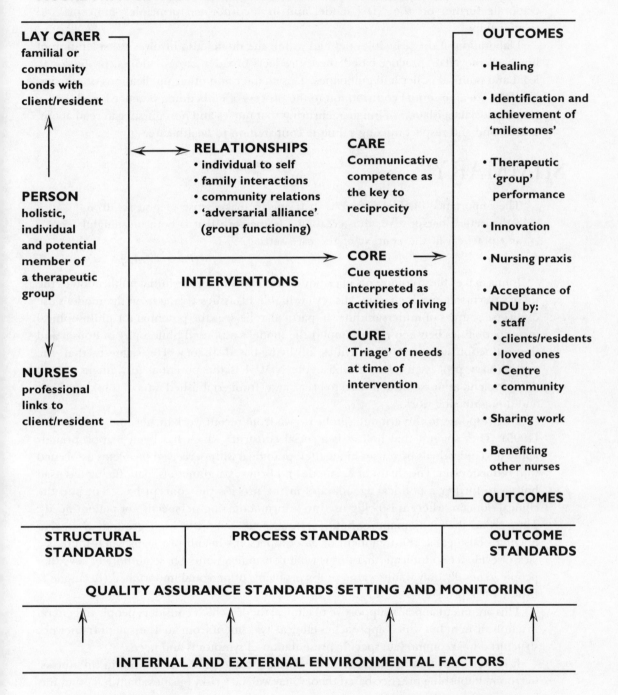

At present, NDU staff suggest that the elements of the model, and the extent to which it has been conceptualised, provide an adequate and sufficient framework to guide their practice. The expression of this belief raises in itself a challenge to the Unit's espoused philosophy of being committed to developing theory that can be used by others. Pragmatically, the CNC suggests that it would take a nurse interested in working with the

NDU at doctoral level to provide the sort of academic and clinical resources necessary to elaborate further on the NDU model and its incorporated principles, concepts and relationships.

Elaboration of the principles defined within the model also involves consideration of how well the NDU practice-based theory reflects broader organisational, professional, legal and political policy and guidelines. This chapter and other publications on nursing in NDUs are an essential contribution to the process of embedding practice-based theory into the social legislation of nursing, ensuring that nurses and non-nurses can read about, understand and respect nursing's unique contribution to health care.

SUMMARY

The importance of this chapter is in trying to make sense of practice from a theoretical perspective, thus creating a framework that is both meaningful and practical in the context of the care setting.

(Johns 1994, p. 207)

Johns makes these comments in critique and reflection of the initial publication of the theory discussed in this chapter. His review highlights issues arising from the model's use of diverse sources of understanding. In particular, he sees the potential for philosophical incompatibilities between (for example) the model's espoused philosophy of holism and the reductionist intent of activities of living-based theory. He suggests that the evolutionary process used to establish the NDU has the potential to limit its theory development, as nurses find it hard to break away from established ways of thinking about and doing nursing work.

One response to this critique can be drawn from recent work by Kermode and Brown (1995). They suggest that holism is a social construct which has been inappropriately applied to individuals by nurses in an attempt to deal with perceived problems associated with **reductionism**. The thrust of Kermode and Brown's argument is that nursing has used holism to further a political agenda and in the process the concept has crept into the clinical domain, where it is being used to inform a nursing perspective of patient needs. They argue that it is inappropriate for nurses to 'seize the high ground' by seeing nursing's business as the treatment of *all* of a person's health problems when there is a lack of evidence to indicate that this is what consumers want. These authors believe that people generally only want treatment for problems of personal importance (Kermode & Brown 1995, p. 14).

This argument appears supportive of clinical theory which considers people in general in a holistic light but which approaches clinical assessment from an assessment framework structured to accommodate specific presentation of symptoms and needs.

It is important that debate such as this occurs in the public arena, not in the nurses' tea room. Publishing practice-based theory may well be a risky business but what other way is there to determine its relevance?

Practice-based theory in the NDU serves the purpose of providing a framework for practice and a set of standards against which the work of the Unit may be judged. Developed 'on site' as it was, it accommodates contextual **phenomena** in a way that more general theory cannot hope to do. Theory review and theory maintenance have become the responsibility of the practitioners who developed it. The issue of ownership of the theory is a driving force behind NDU nurses' desire for further definition of their practice, as a means of continuing to justify their commitment to their own theory of practice. Feedback on this chapter will add to the understanding that they and I have gained in the evolution of this work.

GLOSSARY

Assumptions: statements supposed to be true without proof or demonstration.

Concept: a complex mental formulation of an object, property or event that is derived from individual perceptual experience. Concepts are ideas, mental images, generalisations. Concepts label phenomena.

Definitions: statements of the meaning of a word, phrase or term.

Dialectic: a process of change that starts from a debate over the properties and value of two apparent opposites (*Macquarie Dictionary* 1981).

Ethnography: the 'story' or descriptive activities of interpretative or critical research methodologies.

Fact: something that is known with certainty

Holism: the belief that the whole represents more than the sum of its parts.

Knowledge: awareness or perception of reality acquired through learning or investigation

Model: an idea that explains by using symbolic and physical visualisation. Models may be worded statements, diagrams, drawings, graphs or pictures. They may be mathematical symbols. They may be physical representations (e.g. of body organs) or more abstract representations such as ECG. Models can be used to facilitate thinking about concepts and relationships between them, or to map out a research process.

Paradigm: a conceptual diagram or a large structure used to organise theory.

Phenomena: any occurrences or facts that are directly perceptible by the senses. Phenomena comprise what exists in the real world.

Phenomenology: the study of the meaning or 'essence' of things (phenomena) which attempts to see things as they really are, free from social and cultural bias or belief.

Praxis: purposeful reflection and action with intent to bring about change or transformation (of a ward etc.).

Reductionism: the systematic reduction of one concept or entity to elements or concepts of another kind; for example, reducing the human body to systems and, subsequently, to cellular structures.

Science: a body of knowledge

Taxonomy: a classification system that ranks things according to defined rules or properties.

Theory: a set of concepts, definitions and propositions that project a systematic view of phenomena by designing specific interrelationships among concepts for purposes of describing, explaining, predicting and/or controlling phenomena.

Note. The terms **logic** and **reasoning** (reason) have overlapping definitions and can (generally) be used interchangeably to describe systematic and rigorous ways of establishing what is 'true'. For the purposes of some philosophical discussion, *logic* may be deemed to have more limitations and be more concerned with empirical (objective) facts, while *reason* may draw on social norms and beliefs which do not constitute facts in an empirical sense.

QUESTIONS

1   What are the issues associated with developing a practice-based model of nursing:

    (a)   in a setting where practice is evolving or changing?

    (b)   in a setting where practice is relatively stable?

    (c)   in a new, purpose-built nursing setting (such as some of the step-down or convalescent care units which are being set up in hospitals following the introduction of case mix-based funding)?

2   If theory is developed and described by nurse practitioners, how relevant is it to these same practitioners?

3   Does practice-based theory (once written down) become redundant, oversimplified or overly prescriptive for the nurses who developed it?

4   Can practice-based theory, developed in one setting, be generalised to other contexts? Or does it lose its relevance outside the setting where it was developed?

5   What steps need to be taken to make sure that nursing theory has relevance and application in undergraduate programs?

6   Should nursing theories be used as examples of how clinicians describe their practice?

7   Should methodologies for developing practice-based theory (such as action research) be used to enable undergraduate students to emulate the process of theory development?

8   How can undergraduate students find out where practice-based theory is being developed and used?

LEARNING ACTIVITIES

1   Brainstorm the elements of practice considered important in your current field of practice. Try to reach consensus about what terms should be used to define the concepts you come up with. Reflect on the implications for your practice of the definitions and relationships you have described. (*Note.* Only try this exercise with groups of people who work together, preferably at ward level, but at least in the same institution or close field of nursing. Otherwise, variations in language nuances and context will make the task close to impossible.)

2   Read Brian Fay's book *Social Theory and Political Practice* (Unwin Hyman Books, Sydney, 1975). This short text considers in sequence three philosophical paradigms—empiricorational, interpretative and critical. Fay makes a strong case for each, then moves on to show the limitations of each and, finally, describes how each can contribute a unique understanding of our world. This is a valuable introduction to basic philosophy.

FURTHER READING

Carper, B.A. 1978, 'Fundamental patterns of knowing in nursing', *Advances in Nursing Science*, 1(1), pp. 13–23. Important paper that has been widely used to illustrate different ways of viewing nursing and what it represents.

Fay, B. 1975, *Social Theory and Political Practice*, Unwin Hyman, Sydney. Very good, brief introduction to a number of research and philosophical paradigms. Compares and contrasts the pros and cons of each paradigm.

Holter, I.M. 1988, 'Critical theory: A foundation for the development of nursing theories', *Scholarly Inquiry for Nursing Practice: An International Journal*, 2(3), pp. 223–32. Good introductory paper that justifies consideration of critical theory as a basis for theory development.

Johns, C. (ed.) 1994, *The Burford NDU Model: Caring in Practice*, Blackwell Science, Oxford. Recent, comprehensive publication of the development and application of practice-based theory. Updates work started at Burford by Alan Pearson and shows how the process he started has been continued.

McLaughlin, A.M. & Carey, J.L. 1993, 'The adversarial alliance: Developing therapeutic relationships between families and the team in brain injury rehabilitation', *Brain Injury*, 7(1), pp. 45–59. Not just applicable to brain injury. This article powerfully describes the issues that arise when one party to a caring relationship feels disempowered. The issues are described and problem solving in an adversarial environment is discussed.

Newell, R. 1993, 'Anxiety, accuracy and reflection: The limits of professional development', *Journal of Advanced Nursing*, 17(4), pp. 1326–33. Grounded in psychology more than nursing theory, this article nevertheless raises issues about reflection and its potential when practitioners are under stress. Relevant to nurses, Newell points out that memory under stress can be unreliable.

Pearson, A. 1983, *The Clinical Nursing Unit*, Heinemann Medical, London. The theory of a NDU on which Pearson grounded development of the Burford and Oxford NDUs. Useful coverage of the issues involved in setting up not only a nursing unit but also a climate where change, reflection and research are accepted as part of work culture.

Pearson, A. 1994, 'Reflective practice: Intellectual pursuit of nursing in action', keynote address to the first Nursing Academic International Congress, School of Nursing, University of Canberra, ACT. Describes three uses of reflection by Australian university nursing schools and points out issues arising from each.

12

PRESERVING INTEGRITY
A Theory of Nursing

VERA IRURITA

I wish to acknowledge the support of the Nursing Division of Sir Charles Gairdner Hospital, Perth, Western Australia. It enabled the research, forming the basis of the development of the theory of preserving integrity, to take place.

LEARNING OBJECTIVES

When you have read this chapter you should be able to:

1 Describe grounded theory development, differentiating between substantive and formal theory.

2 Demonstrate an understanding of patient vulnerability and the process of preserving integrity as identified in the presented study.

3 Explain the potential utility of this substantive theory of nursing the hospitalised patient.

Vera Irurita, RN, PhD, FRCNA, is an Associate Professor, and former Head, in the School of Nursing, Curtin University of Technology, Perth. She has had extensive experience in various areas of nursing in both rural and urban settings. Vera gained her Masters degree at the University of Washington, Seattle, under a W.K. Kellogg Foundation Fellowship, and her PhD at the University of Western Australia, in the area of nursing leadership. Her current research interests are in theory development in nursing and caring. Her research also focuses on incorporating the patient/client's perspective using qualitative research methods. She conducts ongoing qualitative analysis seminars (especially in grounded theory) for Masters and PhD students.

INTRODUCTION

This chapter describes the development of a grounded, substantive theory of nursing developed in the area of acute hospital care of the ill individual and focusing predominantly on the patient's perspective. The grounded theory method of theory generation was used to explore the nursing care experience from hospitalised patients' perspective and to discover the underlying problem of **vulnerability**. The core process used to deal with patient vulnerability was identified as **preserving integrity**. The methods of theory development, as well as the proposed theory, are explained in detail. A distinction is made between substantive and formal theory and the theory is compared with other studies and with several frequently cited nursing theories and models. The potential utility of this proposed theory of preserving integrity, in terms of clinical practice, education, management, and further research and theory development, is outlined. Ultimately, the improvement of nursing care should be achieved through a better understanding of the patient's experience gained through this theory. Measures described as effective caregiving strategies could be adopted and those factors increasing patient vulnerability reduced.

GROUNDED THEORY

A **grounded theory** is a theory inductively derived from the study of the phenomenon it represents (Strauss & Corbin 1990)—in this case, the phenomenon of nursing care in an acute-care, hospital setting. The inductive method, as defined by Wilson (1989, p. 726), emphasises data as the source for generating concepts and explanatory relationships. This approach is said to move from the concrete and specific to the general and abstract. Grounded theory was first described by sociologists Glaser and Strauss (1967) and has since proven useful in other fields, including nursing, where generation of theory has been considered important in the furtherance of knowledge development. As described by Glaser and Strauss (1967), and further elaborated by

Glaser (1978, 1992), Strauss (1987), and Strauss and Corbin (1990), grounded theory is a qualitative research method for generating theory from data, rather than generating results to support or test existing theory. This method of building theory is a powerful way of interpreting reality, a reality which cannot actually be known but is always interpreted (Strauss & Corbin 1990, p. 22). Not only is the resulting theoretical formulation said to explain that reality but it also provides a framework for action (practice), thus increasing its utility.

A grounded theory is discovered, developed and provisionally verified through systematic collection and analysis of data pertaining to the phenomenon it represents (Strauss & Corbin 1990, p. 23). The method involves an ongoing process of **constant comparative analysis** (Glaser & Strauss 1967). Data are obtained through **theoretical sampling**, which means that data are purposefully sought from sources likely to provide further clarification of concepts that have proven theoretical relevance to the evolving theory. Ongoing analysis of data and comparing incident with incident reveals concepts of sufficient importance to be given the status of categories. A **category** means a classification of concepts, discovered through constant comparative analysis; it is a grouping together of concepts under a higher-order, more abstract concept (Strauss & Corbin 1990, p. 61). Data collection and analysis are continued until **theoretical saturation** of each category is reached (Glaser 1978, pp. 124–6; Glaser & Strauss 1967, pp. 61, 62, 111, 112). Theoretical saturation means:

> (1) no new or relevant data seem to emerge regarding a category; (2) the category development is dense, insofar as all of the paradigm elements are accounted for, along with variation and process; (3) the relationships between categories are well established and validated.
>
> *(Strauss & Corbin 1990, p. 188)*

Theory has been described by Field and Morse (1985, p. 2) as a conjecture or 'best guess' about reality: a speculation or perception, not an established fact. They suggest that theory, once developed, is tested and retested, becoming more believable or better confirmed but still remaining conjecture. However, according to Field and Morse:

> extensive and important theories may continue to be used for prolonged periods of time (and be 'confirmed' by research) and yet, in essence be totally and completely wrong.
>
> *(1985, p. 2)*

This is more likely to be the case when the theories have not been grounded in systematic research (Glaser 1978). In light of this, and the apparent extensive adoption of some ungrounded nursing theories, it is important to continue to test these theories, but more important is the inductive generation of new theories, grounded in diverse data gathered in nursing practice settings.

SUBSTANTIVE AND FORMAL THEORY

The grounded theory presented in this chapter was developed as a substantive rather than a formal theory. Glaser (1978, p. 144) defined substantive theory as one developed for a substantive or empirical area of enquiry, such as 'organisational careers of scientists', whereas formal theory is developed for a formal or conceptual area of enquiry, such as 'organisational careers'. Both, according to Glaser, may be considered as middle-range theories, falling between the 'minor working hypotheses' of everyday life and the 'all-inclusive' grand theories (p. 144). An analogy may be made by considering a theory of 'nursing' or 'caring' as formal theory and a theory of 'nursing the acutely ill' or 'caring for hospitalised patients' as substantive theory. Typically, substantive theories have important general relevance and become springboards or stepping stones to the development of formal grounded theory (Glaser 1978, p. 146).

It is proposed here that some theories of nursing have assumed the mantle of formal theory without embracing, or being applicable to, the substantive areas within nursing. Hence, there have been frequent expressions of difficulty in applying nursing theory to practice. Nursing is a complex phenomenon undertaken in many diverse settings, situations and contexts, and includes a wide range of roles and differing goals. Therefore, it may be difficult to apply universally some nursing theories that have been developed for one substantive area only. Similarly, it may be inappropriate to use theories that have not been grounded in systematic research, or have not been developed to the formal level by systematic research, or testing in various contexts of nursing.

Glaser (1978) suggested that many formal theories are speculative or ungrounded, deriving from such sources as 'whims and wisdoms of usually deceased great men, conjecture and assumptions about the "oughts" of life, and other extant speculative theory' (p. 143). Some nursing theories appear to be based on ideals about what nursing should be, rather than on what it is, and some have been developed using concepts borrowed from other disciplines (Chenitz & Swanson 1986). Attempts have been made to fit these theories to real-life situations of nursing, to use them to guide practice, curricular or nursing research. When this type of derived (ungrounded) formal theory is applied, it is suggested by Glaser (1978) that it forces the data in many ways, and it may not fit reality. According to Field and Morse (1985), theory derived from reality (as in grounded theory) is unlikely to be the product of the researcher's cultural reality or a distortion of the 'truth' (p. 3), nor is it likely to be completely rejected or replaced by another, although it may require modification as reality changes over time (p. 7).

Grounded theory provides a means to develop theory through the study of real-life situations of nursing practice in natural settings. Using this method, the context in which the phenomenon occurs is considered to be part of the phenomenon itself. As described by Strauss and Corbin (1990, p. 23), a well-constructed grounded theory, faithful to the everyday reality of the substantive area, carefully induced from diverse data, should fit that substantive area and be comprehensible and make sense both to those studied and to those practising in that area. Furthermore, it should be abstract enough and include sufficient variation to make it applicable to a variety of contexts related to that phenomenon. In other words, the theory should fit the real world, work in predictions and explanations, be relevant to the people concerned, and be readily modifiable (Glaser 1978, p.142). An attempt was made to meet these criteria in the theory presented in this chapter.

A GROUNDED THEORY STUDY: NURSING CARE FROM THE PATIENT'S PERSPECTIVE[1]

This grounded theory study (Irurita 1993) was initially undertaken to explore and describe the meaning of quality nursing care from the patient's perspective. It was designed also to discover factors perceived by patients to influence the delivery of nursing care in an acute-care, hospital setting in Western Australia in 1992–93. The main objective was to develop a substantive theory which explains quality nursing care (in an acute-care, hospital setting) from the patient's perspective. A comparison was made with findings of other qualitative studies on aspects of nursing and caring as reported in the literature. These additional sources of data lent support to the theory as presented in this chapter. This theory has potential for further empirical development, ultimately to a mid-range, formal theory of nursing or caring.

In this study, it was not possible to limit the focus solely to nursing care, as patients in their interviews appeared to consider the quality of nursing care to include all aspects of their care while in hospital. Hence, even though the majority of the findings concerned nurses and nursing, they also should be useful to all types of caregivers. In this report, *participant* is replaced by *patient* at times, to emphasise that, even though they were being interviewed as persons not in the patient role, they were presenting their viewpoints as patients. *Client* is deliberately not used as it was apparent in these data that these study participants did not consider themselves legitimate clients. Extracts of the transcribed interviews are included with the findings to demonstrate the development of the categories and their properties as they were identified in the study. Italics are used to highlight key portions of conversation as they related to the findings.

RESEARCH DESIGN

The grounded theory method, as discussed above, was used and provided a way to study human behaviour and interaction in natural settings. It was particularly useful for conceptualising behaviour in complex situations (Chenitz & Swanson 1986). Using this method, all variables relevant to the phenomenon of quality nursing care from the patient's perspective were sought, rather than focusing on specific variables chosen by the researcher as being significant or meaningful. Thus, by using a coding paradigm, it aimed to discover important underlying dimensions and patterns of relationships, as well as influencing factors, involved in this complex, poorly understood phenomenon.

DATA COLLECTION

Data were collected from several sources and collection extended over a 13-month period. The major source of data was recorded, semi-structured interviews with 10 patients, one to two weeks after discharge from four surgical/specialty wards of a large teaching hospital. (Prior approval was obtained from the hospital's research and ethical review

[1]This research was undertaken with the support of the Nursing Division and Nursing Research Department at Sir Charles Gairdner Hospital, Perth. Study participants and their experiences were drawn from a range of hospitals; hence these findings are in no way confined to the above hospital as the primary study site.

committee.) These transcribed interviews, which averaged about an hour in duration, were supplemented by transcripts of 13 interviews with patients discharged (up to three months) from a wide array of hospital settings, these being conducted by postgraduate research students under the author's guidance. Permission was gained to use these patient interviews to supply additional data for variation and to ensure that theoretical saturation of the categories was achieved. Questions guiding both sets of interviews reflected the objectives of the study. Shorter follow-up interviews were conducted with three participants in order to clarify or expand aspects of their experiences. Data obtained from interviews were supplemented by data from literature and other sources relevant to the study, including inpatient surveys administered on patients' discharge as a part of quality assurance, and field notes of observations of clinical practice. Experiences drawn on by these patients included previous experiences in a range of hospitals in addition to the most recent hospitalisation. Two participants, and other secondary informants who had been patients, as well as other researchers, reviewed for credibility the coding and interpretation of the findings during, and on completion of, the study.

SAMPLING

A **purposive sampling** technique was used to select the initial study participants. According to Morse (1989, p. 121) and Hutchinson and Webb (1989, p. 293), purposive sampling requires selecting informants who are knowledgeable about the topic and are experts by virtue of their involvement in specific life events. They must have undergone, or be undergoing, experience of the event being studied, be able to reflect on, and be willing to share, detailed experiential information about the phenomenon. Thus, patients were selected on this basis, a minimum of five days in hospital during the present episode being an additional requirement. As the study progressed, theoretical sampling (Glaser 1978) guided data collection, the researcher seeking informants and other sources of data as directed by the initial findings of data analysis. The aim of theoretical sampling was to look for variation, and to seek data that would shed more light on the developing theory, clarify categories and/or indicate new properties of the categories or processes.

A mix of male and female patients, reflecting a range of ages, as well as booked and emergency admissions, surgical and non-surgical cases, experienced and first-time patients, were sought in order to explore fully the phenomenon under study. The 10 patients from the primary study site, while still in hospital, were approached by the researcher (who was not a caregiver, nor wearing a uniform), and asked whether they would volunteer to participate in this study. A member of the nursing staff from the relevant wards advised the researcher which patients met the inclusion criteria, were soon to be discharged and were well enough to be approached. A convenience sample was used for the additional 13 patients whose interview data supplemented the above.

The researcher explained the study to potential participants and sought their consent to undertake and record one or more interviews with each of them following discharge from hospital. Those who accepted gave the researcher their home telephone number and address, after signing the consent form (a copy of which they retained). Permission was sought from patients for the researcher to visit them in their home, or a mutually agreed upon location, between one and two weeks following discharge from hospital. This was done to remove the perceived threat of divulging sensitive information while still in the 'dependent' patient role, while at the same time allowing time to adjust to home life and allowing for recall of hospital experiences. Being away from the hospital setting, it was hoped that patients would speak more openly of their hospital experiences. This was enhanced by the researcher not being associated with the delivery of care. The appointment was made by telephone after the patient had time to resettle at home (five to seven days). This also gave patients the opportunity to withdraw from the study if they had changed their minds since the initial contact. All the contacted patients confirmed their willingness to participate in the study and all interviews were conducted in the homes of the participants.

Over several weeks towards the end of the study, field notes were made during participant observation of nursing in the study setting. The main purpose of the observations was to confirm findings obtained through interview and to raise any additional aspects to be included in further interviews. These observations were undertaken by a research assistant who was a clinical nurse specialist in the area of study. A sample of inpatient surveys was examined with the same objective. Informal discussion also took place with several practising nurses, as well as other people who had been patients at some time, to clarify emerging categories.

DATA ANALYSIS

The constant comparative method of data analysis was used and involved coding the data for categories, comparing incidents applicable to each category, integrating categories and their properties, delineating the theory, and writing the theory (Glaser & Strauss 1967; Glaser 1978; Strauss 1987; Strauss & Corbin 1990). This required the simultaneous collection, coding and analysis of the data throughout the study period (May 1992 to May 1993). Writing memos and/or the diagramming of schema of ideas about the categories and their relationship was undertaken concurrently with the coding and analysis procedures. The Ethnograph computer software (Seidel 1988) facilitated the organisation and management of the data generated from the transcribed interviews. It enabled the researcher to code, recode and sort the data files into analytic categories. This enhanced the process of constant comparative analysis. Face/cover sheets enabled biographical and other variables to be attached to each data file and codes were sorted by such variables when required.

Initial coding was performed manually on printed copies of the transcribed interviews on which the lines had been numbered and a wide margin left for entering codes. As each code was selected to identify conceptual categories, it was listed, with the definition of its meaning, in a separate folder. The steps in coding included, first, *open coding*, which involved coding each line, sentence or incident for as many codes as might fit the data. This enabled the data to be broken down, examined, compared, conceptualised and categorised. Properties (attributes or characteristics of a category) and dimensions (location of properties along a continuum) were sought. Segments of data were coded and entered on the transcripts using The Ethnograph (Seidel 1988). Retrieval of coded segments facilitated the constant comparative method of analysis.

The second step is called *axial* or *theoretical coding* (Strauss & Corbin 1990; Glaser 1978); this involved putting the data back together in new ways by making connections between a category and its subcategories. A coding paradigm involving conditions (causal and intervening), context, action/interaction strategies and consequences was used to build categories, clarify them and make them persistently more dense until relationships between the categories became apparent. In this way, major categories forming a framework for theory were identified. *Selective coding* is the phase of analysis directed towards discovering the core category—the one which has the most explanatory power and recurs frequently in the data, and which accounts for the most variation in patterns of behaviour. Most of the categories and their properties are related to the core category (or process) which links the various data together. In this case, a core process of *preserving integrity* was found, this being used to deal with the basic social, psychological or core problem experienced by patients, identified as *vulnerability*.

Sampling and analysis continued until theoretical saturation occurred—that is, all levels of codes appeared complete, with no new conceptual information available to indicate new codes or the expansion of existing codes. In this way there was a sense of closure or completeness: all the data were found to fit into the established categories; interactional and organisational patterns were visible; behavioural variation was described; and behaviour in this specific context could be predicted (Hutchinson 1986). This approach avoids premature closure of the study.

FINDINGS

The participants described the experience of making the transition from a person (normal human being) to 'being a patient'. The transition from person to patient can happen to anyone, of either gender, of any age, from any position in society. Being a patient occurs when one is admitted to hospital for any one of a wide range of reasons (minor to serious), either suddenly or planned, for a short duration or an extended period. Some people never experience being a patient, whereas for others it may happen once or repeatedly. Regardless of the circumstances surrounding the experience of being a patient, the admission to hospital and to the care of others was found to affect individuals in various ways. Being a patient can mean experiencing the problems of pain, disturbed sleep, discomfort, lack of privacy, loneliness, fear, being confined or restricted, being in unfamiliar surroundings, and/or being deprived of choice in many aspects of daily living.

VULNERABILITY: THE CORE PROBLEM

On analysis of these data, it became apparent that the basic problem patients had to deal with was vulnerability, due to a loss of control and their integrity being at risk. Whereas some degree of vulnerability in patients seemed inevitable, it was evident that some factors caused or increased this vulnerability and that measures could be taken to reduce it.

Vulnerability, in this study, means being susceptible to physical and/or emotional hurt, harm or injury; defenceless or weak in respect of defence or self-protection, open to assault. Individuals have diminished control over their life and their integrity is at risk.

Integrity refers to having control over one's life; being able to protect oneself; maintaining dignity as a human being; being an individual; remaining 'whole', intact, undiminished (in the course of life events); and being in as good condition or as sound or unimpaired a state as possible.

Vulnerability, as a threat to people's integrity when they become patients, was portrayed in many ways in the interview data, some clearly describing the problem, others alluding to it:

> It was something I'd cope with myself normally but just in that sort of state—you feel so *vulnerable* . . . the big thing was not to make a fool of myself, *breaking down . . . weeping* . . .

Vulnerability was present in varying degrees for all participants. It was found to be influenced by, and vary in relation to, a number of causal, contextual and intervening conditions, as well as the strategies used to deal with this phenomenon. The main attributes of patient vulnerability were found to be:

1 Risk/threat to integrity (the greater the risk or threat, the greater the degree of vulnerability). The risk factor could threaten the life, as in serious illness, or emotional and/or physical aspects of integrity.

2 Reduced control of their life situations (the less control retained, the greater the vulnerability).

VULNERABILITY CONTEXTS

Three vulnerability contexts were identified in this study:

1 high vulnerability (high risk, low control);

2 moderate vulnerability (moderate risk, low to moderate control); and

3 low vulnerability (low risk, high control).

Each context involved different levels of patient vulnerability and different perceptions of types of care (actions and interactions) required to deal effectively with, or reduce, this vulnerability. Patients moved in and out of the different vulnerability contexts during hospitalisation, depending on the causal conditions. Moreover, depending on the context and the management of these conditions, the experience of being a patient could range from a minor disruption to normal life to a devastating experience with long-lasting effects.

CAUSES OF VULNERABILITY

Please note—although the informants emphasised strongly the causal factors of vulnerability, these will be condensed and presented superficially here. This chapter will focus mainly on preserving integrity, the process used to deal with vulnerability.

The various factors that overlapped to influence and vary the degree of risk/threat to integrity, and the amount of control that the patient could retain, included:

1 the illness, injury, impairment or intervention;

2 the level of dependence related to the illness or impairment, or to the diagnostic or therapeutic intervention;

3 the power imbalance between caregiver (nurse) and patient—abuse of power or rough-hand care;

4 the age of the patient—ageism;

5   lack of information or preparation; and

6   loss of identity/individuality related to the transition from person to patient.

Comments inferred changes in normal reactions/behaviour during illness. When there was a serious illness, some patients felt almost disoriented, isolated, and very dependent on others for basic needs: 'I was *too sick* at that time'; '. . . I felt like an *object* lying there . . . '. One described this as follows:

> It was such an *enclosed world* in that little room. You are so *dependent* on everybody else to do anything . . . you can't avoid that if you're sick . . . you feel so *vulnerable*.

> . . . not being able to *see* or *hear* on that side, trying to get through to people . . . *I couldn't really get through to people*, . . . I felt so *vulnerable*.

Fear of death was expressed in various ways by participants who had been seriously ill, reflecting high vulnerability with the perceived threat to their life: 'You might *fall off the edge* and disappear'; 'What do I do now, do *I bury you*, kind of thing'; and 'I was sure I was *going to die.*'

The patients' ability to control their life situation was limited when they suffered any form of restriction to their physical ability or mobility and/or their sensory input. These factors made them dependent, to varying degrees, on the assistance of others. If the required level of assistance was not available, was withheld or delayed (as in answering the call bell), their vulnerability was increased, with heightened risk of physical or emotional harm:

> One time I was vomiting and I had to end up vomiting in the cup I had my cup of tea out of, because *I kept ringing* and *no one came* . . . I *felt pretty bad* about it.

> The *bell was not answered* [promptly]. I don't know if it was because they were *busy*. It *made me feel vulnerable*, because I *couldn't get up*. If you know they're coming in five minutes, that's fine. But you can't do that; *you don't know what's happening down the corridor.*

Because of the nature of the patient role, there is an inbuilt imbalance of power between the caregiver (nurse) and the patient. When this power differential was exploited by the nurse, exerting inappropriate control over patients, vulnerability was increased:

> The *bullying*, that's what it was. *I felt like a child.*

> . . . it's just because *she had the power* . . .

> . . . you feel so *vulnerable*. . . . . The *difference*, I suppose, was the *carers*, the people who really *cared for you as a person* rather than just as a *slab of meat* that had to be done before a certain time.

The despair and frustration following an experience in which it was perceived that nurses had abused their positions of power, using a rough-hand approach, are reflected in the following sentiments:

Instead of making me feel better, like 'I'm sorry about it, Mr . . . , I'll put it right in a couple of minutes' . . . I *felt worse than death*. As far as she was concerned, the fact that I had messed up the whole bed, was that I was a *dirty old man* . . . it was *degrading* . . . and the worst thing was that *it could have been avoided* . . . I had *begged*, almost *argued,* to go to the toilet.

I got a bit emotional . . . I broke down and wept.

A consequence of caregivers' behaviour reflecting ageism was patients' expressions of fear for the future:

. . . they look upon you as more or less *expendable* when it comes to you or the next person who is *younger*.

. . . it's terrible. I felt that *I would hate to ever go into a nursing home*, or a place where I am not in control of my faculties or mind. I think [when you're old] you'd be treated terrible. *You'd be absolutely at people's mercy*.

There was overwhelming consensus among the participants regarding the importance of being well informed about their medical/surgical condition, all aspects of care, the hospital routine, and preparation for discharge; yet there was a general agreement that they had, in most instances, been inadequately informed. Furthermore, not having sufficient information or not being well prepared had reduced their ability to control their situation and hence had increased their vulnerability:

If they can *prepare you* as much as possible *from the start* . . . . When you *don't know what's happening,* it's really *intimidating*.

Being in the dark doesn't help anybody.

A common concern about being a patient was related to feeling depersonalised or dehumanised. This occurred when they were in unfamiliar surroundings and routines, when individual differences were not considered, and when patients were treated like a number or an object. For example:

As a person, a human being, who in my mind I'm quite intelligent, I *can make decisions* in business, run a business and then to have someone *overruling* me, without even listening to what I'm trying to say . . . . The utter *frustration* of *not being listened to*, as though you're *not even there*, or you're *not even a person*; you're just nothing.

DISCUSSION: VULNERABILITY

Lawler (1991) described the relationship that a nurse has with a hospitalised patient in acute care settings as one based on the mutual recognition of the patient's vulnerability, and the patient's partial or complete dependence on the nurse for help with events which, in their everyday lives, people do for themselves (p. 156). She found that nurses help reduce, or make manageable, that vulnerability by creating an 'environment of permission' (p. 158), which in turn gives patients some control. Those findings lend some support to the theory developed from this study.

Several nurse theorists have mentioned or alluded to the concept of patient vulnerability in their theories or conceptual frameworks. Wiedenbach (1964) described the nursing client (or patient) as: 'a person who is under care of some member of health care personnel, who is in a vulnerable position, with a perceived need for help' (Meleis 1985, p. 266). Levine's (1969, 1973) conservation model (Kozier, Erb & Blais 1992; Meleis 1985) promotes wholeness as its goal of nursing and incorporates the concept of integrity, which is presented as structural, personal and social. The fourth conservation principle includes actions to conserve energy. Levine described person as:

> an everchanging organism who is in constant interaction with his environment and who is constantly striving to maintain his integrity. Responses of a human being are a unified whole.
>
> *(Meleis 1985, p. 279)*

Patient (or nursing client) was described by Levine as:

> a total, whole person, a system of systems, in a state of dyssynchronization and in need of assistance to conserve energy, structural, personal, and social integrity; ill clients were said to maintain their integrity through physiologically predetermined protective responses.
>
> *(Meleis 1985, p. 279)*

The nursing problem was given by Levine as 'the internal or external environment as it threatens the total integrity of a whole person . . . '. Other theorists who have included integrity as a concept in their conceptual models include Roy, in the adaptation model, and Rogers' science of unitary human beings (Kozier et al. 1990, pp. 48–50). Virginia Henderson (1966), in her complementary-supplementary model defined the client as 'a whole, complete and independent being . . . ' (Kozier et al. 1990, pp. 48–9).

The concepts as they were presented by the above theorists have some similarities to the integrity and vulnerability concepts identified in this grounded theory. The category of vulnerability described in this chapter requires further study and refinement. The vulnerability contexts will need further development and testing. Some causal conditions for vulnerability were not fully explored—for example, the risks/threats to patients' integrity focused mainly on factors related to their medical or surgical condition and aspects of their hospitalisation. Personal factors, apart from age, were not explored (nor were they strongly evident in the data). Family support as a means of reducing patient vulnerability was addressed superficially, as were spiritual aspects. Physical and emotional aspects of patients' integrity were dealt with in this study, but may need further exploration, together with social and spiritual factors. As well as providing a basis for further research, these findings should increase our understanding of the experience of being a patient. They could also prove to be useful for assessing the nursing needs of patients.

PRESERVING INTEGRITY: THE CORE PROCESS

The process for dealing with patient vulnerability, identified as the core process around which other categories were integrated, was preserving integrity. *Preserving integrity*, based on these findings, means conserving, protecting and restoring the patient's integrity. It included measures to minimise risks, such as keeping safe, protecting, defending, guarding or shielding from injury or harm to the integrity. The term was used to describe protecting patients from physical or emotional harm and enabling them to retain their dignity as human beings; it involved recognising and accommodating, where possible, the patient's individuality as a person. It also entailed actions to facilitate retention and restoration of patients' control and to promote the return to as intact, whole, or as unimpaired, a state as possible.

Preserving integrity was described from the patient's perspective, which included actions and interactions taken to reduce vulnerability under specific sets of contextual conditions, intervening conditions that facilitated or constrained the strategies taken within specific contexts, and the consequences of the actions and interactions. Measures aimed at holding together the patient's integrity, and reducing vulnerability, involved minimising risks or threats to integrity, and maintaining and restoring or increasing patients' control of their situation.

Preserving integrity involved the actions/interactions of the nurse (caregivers), the patients and others in the role of advocates. Depending on the vulnerability context, different levels of preserving integrity were needed to achieve positive outcomes from the patient's perspective. Patients who were at a high level of vulnerability were in greatest need of these strategies; those in the moderate vulnerability context required a different level of intervention; and those in the low vulnerability context were found to be less vulnerable and hence to need less integrity-preserving intervention.

THE PATIENT'S ROLE

Patients, especially experienced patients, perceived that they had certain obligations to contribute to the quality (and amount) of care that they received. Some had learned strategies that helped them receive more or better attention. They included:

1 being a 'good patient', unselfish, uncomplaining, undemanding and not ringing the bell too often;

2 trying to recover (or being seen to be trying to recover);

3 enhancing the development of the nurse–patient (or patient–nurse) relationship.

Examples of these strategies were evident throughout the patient data:

I didn't call because I didn't want to worry them . . . I didn't sound the buzzer that often.

The care you get is *a lot to do with you.* If you *try* and make your stay *as best you can,* and *not expect too much,* you'll come out on top. But if you *expect too much* and *moan and groan* for the least little thing, they're not going to spend time with you . . . *if you're too demanding they're going to back off.*

Nevertheless, for various reasons, these patient strategies were mostly unsuccessful for preserving integrity.

LEVELS OF NURSING CARE

The most significant means of reducing vulnerability was found to be the type of nursing care given. It was revealed that patients perceived different levels of quality in nursing care, and that the words *hands* and *touch* were central to the concepts of both vulnerability and caring. Patients spoke of being *'in her hands'* and *'in good hands'*, inferring both vulnerability and trust. The *'personal touch'*, which referred to doing extra things for patients, and the therapeutic effects of *'human touch'* were interwoven throughout these data. *'Hands-on'* care was contrasted with being *'off-hand'* or *'button-pressing'*.

The study revealed that the highest quality of care was interpreted in terms of *soft-hand care*; mediocre, technically competent, or clinical care was interpreted as *firm-hand care*; *hard-hand care* reflected a failure to be effective in preserving integrity; and compromised care, described in relation to rough handling and the caregivers' abuse of power (inappropriate use of control) was referred to as *rough-hand care*, already given as a cause of vulnerability. One of the patients, who had experienced frequent hospitalisations, explained the difference in caregivers:

> Some people have *soft hands*, some people have *hard hands*. People that you classify as hard hands are people that it is *a job*—this is not a terribly *interesting case*, but Bill Brown down the passage, now that's a *type of illness* I'm interested in . . . . They're in so much of a *hurry* . . . [they are harder] in their approach to you . . . It's [nursing's] a *means to an end*.

TECHNICAL CARE

In general, technical aspects of care were not discussed by these study participants. There was an expectation, or trust, that technical competence would be present and that this should not need to be questioned by patients. Even though they didn't necessarily understand the technical skills required for the delivery of a high quality of nursing care, they assumed that these would automatically be present. It was the *'other things'* that accounted for high-quality care, according to the patients. Nevertheless, to be assured that they were in *'good hands'*, it was considered to be important that nurses were knowledgeable about all aspects of their role and that they 'showed *self-confidence'*. Technical nursing care was said to be 'not something that you think of, you *take it for granted'*. In cases where the patients' expectations of nursing care were exceeded, descriptions of the positive aspects of care did not usually include technical competence. As described in the following sections, the satisfaction was usually expressed in relation to soft-hand care that had a strong expressive component.

These findings contrast with those of previous studies which found patients' perceptions of the most important nurse caring behaviours to be technical, or instrumental, such as 'competent clinical know-how, knows how to give shots, IVs etc., and to manage the equipment like IVs, suction machines, etc.' (Mayer 1986, 1987; Larson 1984, 1987). In those studies, technical aspects were followed by such things as: being cheerful, encouraging the patients to call if they had a problem, putting the patient first, knowing when to call the doctor, frequently checking on patient, sitting down with the patient, etc. In the studies she reviewed, Brown (1986) declared that, even though patients consistently ranked instrumental activities as most important to care, whereas nurses ranked expressive activities more highly, both groups agreed that both these components are necessary for the experience of care.

Morse et al. (1990) suggest that these discrepancies may be related to patients not being aware of all the nurse's intentions underlying nursing actions. It is also possible that those findings which showed patients as valuing instrumental activities more highly than expressive activities, in conveying caring, could be a product of the difference in methods of data collection from those used in this study. It is possible that, if the patients in this study had been asked to rank certain behaviours, they could have chosen technical aspects of care over expressive ones. However, in open-ended interviewing on quality care, these aspects were not given priority. Technical competence was assumed in statements about nurses demonstrating knowledge and confidence in their ability. The major emphasis was put on the dimensions identified as soft-hand care, which was most effective for preserving integrity.

ROUGH-HAND CARE

This causal factor of vulnerability reflected the caregivers' abuse of power. Properties of this category included nurses (and others) threatening, bullying, rough-handling, being impatient, not being dependable, ignoring and treating patients as objects or 'slabs of meat'; collectively, the term *rough-hands* was used to describe these approaches (see Table 12.1). Not only was vulnerability increased under these conditions, but dehumanising, despair, frustration, fear and anger also occurred as a consequence:

> . . . it's just that a couple get a bit rough with you . . . one girl went to sit me up and instead of waiting for me to hold onto something nearly pulled my nightie and *hurt me* and I said 'Hey, you're *very rough* . . . don't be *so rough*'. She sort of pulled me up by the neck . . . I found a couple haven't got *patience* and you need patience badly—you can't be *bullying* people around.

TABLE 12.1 ROUGH-HAND CARE

ABUSE OF POWER
• threatening, bullying
• rough handling
• impatience
• unreliable
• ignoring patients, not listening
• treating as object, 'slab of meat'

The consequences of impatience and '*rushing* and *hurrying*' and '*copping nurses* in a *bad mood*' were explained:

> . . . it's not very nice, because *I get hurt*. But lately I've been bucking back. One time, I would just take it and not say anything—I wouldn't open my mouth. I would allow it to happen. I thought, 'I'm a *human being*; I'm *not a piece of meat*.' So I didn't argue with her, I just said it in a joke, 'Come on—hey, you're *hurting me*'.

Rough-hand care was shown to produce very negative consequences, increasing patients' vulnerability instead of reducing it. In some cases, it had led to 'just *wanting to get out*', or '*feeling as though no one cared*', or '*treating you as though you're either beyond it or too old*'.

Patients' perceptions of non-caring behaviours and attitudes, described by Riemen (1986), matched properties of rough-hand care discovered in this study. These included Riemen's descriptions of 'being rough and belittling patients', 'not responding' and 'treating patients as objects' (p. 32). Riemen also found these non-caring elements had increased patients' vulnerability (as was the case in this study) and had led to similar consequences to those found here—namely, the client (patient) felt devalued, degraded, humiliated, not in control of the situation, frustrated, afraid, depressed, angry and upset.

HARD-HAND CARE

The hard-hand care concept was reflected in this study as the level of care that was not technically adequate and was ineffective in preserving integrity. Some of these aspects have been presented under causes of vulnerability. This level of care reflected nurses (and others) being technically inadequate; being mechanical, doing the minimum; being 'off-hand, unfeeling'; rushing, bustling, appearing 'over efficient', regimenting care; forcing independence prematurely; and treating patients as 'just a patient or a number', not a person or an individual (see Table 12.2).

TABLE 12.2 HARD-HAND CARE

INEFFECTIVE INTEGRITY PRESERVING
• technically inadequate (omissions of care, errors)
• mechanical, doing minimum
• being 'off-hand', 'unfeeling'
• rushing, bustling, 'over-efficient', regimenting
• forcing independence prematurely
• treating as a patient or number, not a person

In spite of the patients' expectation that all nurses would be technically competent, some lack of technical competence (in the form of drug errors, inaccurate information, omissions of care) was commented on, usually with surprise, by the patients:

> The *technical side* . . . that to me is the *day-to-day running of things* . . . . I *trusted* them to do what they had to do . . . . They all seemed to *know less than I expected* them to know.

Failing to provide assistance for dependent patients, or forcing independence prematurely added to their vulnerability:

> Nobody ever asked me whether I wanted them to shower me or bath me, it's *automatically assumed* that you *are capable of it*. And this is not always so; at times *you need the support of somebody*.

. . . if a person is quite *unable* to feed herself or himself, a *little time should be taken*. Now, oddly enough, in hospital *the more you try to help yourself*, you are told, 'well, you can *do it yourself*, we don't have to worry'.

Delays in answering the bell featured prominently in the interview data:

. . . the time it took them, from the time you pressed the button, sometimes *it took a long time for them to come* . . .

Comfort actions were not always taken and their omission was noticed:

After vomiting, unless it's asked for, no *mouth wash* or *flannel* is given. Nor are *lambs wool skins* for bed comfort offered . . . . If you have a pan, and you don't ask for it, they don't bring you anything to *wash your hands* with afterwards.

Lack of information had reduced the patients' ability to control their situation:

You *wonder what's going to happen* . . . *the most important thing is knowledge* . . .

Not enough information is given . . . I had *no idea* what my operation was going to be like . . . at least I would have *known what I was in for.*

Other elements of hard-hand care were represented in the following ways:

Some nurses didn't really give a damn; *putting in the hours,* . . . a couple of the nurses were quite good, but they were very *off-hand* or they *did the minimum*.

. . . the inexperienced nurses were probably more *methodical*, more *mechanical* with whoever they dealt with. It would have been *frustrating* and rather *depressing* if [all] *care* had been given out in a *methodical* and *mechanical* way.

What nurses could do is just *have the time,* so they *don't have to rush off straight away.* Then you know you've got time to talk to them, instead of *feeling that you're keeping them.*

All the study participants commented on the differences in the type of care given by different nurses. They frequently had difficulty expressing these differences, but it was clear that being treated as an individual, a human being, rather than '*just a patient*' was one of these factors:

I *noticed the difference* between various nurses. They were all nice, but some treated you like they had to get you to the shower before ten [o'clock] type of thing . . . Others *treat you as a person*, rather than just as a *slab of meat* that had to be *done before a certain time* . . . I did get the impression with some of them, like with the doctors, *just a slab of meat*.

The lack of individual consideration by nurses, or the nurses being in a hurry, led patients to feel devalued. For example, 'I was treated like a *nuisance*', and 'quite often you *feel* that *you're a number.*' In summary, hard-hand care encompassed ineffective or inadequate preserving integrity. It failed to reduce vulnerability and in most instances it increased it.

Bottorff and Morse (1994), using techniques of qualitative **ethology**, identified four types of attending (structural units of nurse–patient interaction that capture patterns of caring). These were 'doing more', 'doing for', 'doing with', and 'doing tasks'. Their description of 'doing tasks' in part reflects hard-hand care in that it was interpreted as 'using a routinised approach', 'appearing hurried', 'getting the job done' in an 'indifferent or apathetic' way. It did not, however, include technical incompetence as was found in hard-hand care.

Non-caring behaviours and attitudes, described by Riemen (1986), also matched properties of hard-hand care. 'Being in a hurry and efficient' and 'doing a job' reflected hard-hand care described by these participants, whereas Riemen's descriptions of 'being rough and belittling patients' and 'not responding' were more in line with what was identified in this study as rough-hand care. 'Treating patients as objects' was found to overlap with this study's findings of both hard-hand care and rough-hand care.

FIRM-HAND CARE

Firm-hand care was identified as the first level of preserving integrity and was described as *'perfectly adequate, technically'*, but not demonstrating *'feeling'*, *'sensitivity'* or *'compassion'*. Aspects of care included in this first or basic level of preserving integrity involved taking effective protective and restorative nursing measures to reduce threats to life, to physical integrity and, minimally, to emotional integrity. This encompassed demonstrating technical competence; providing adequate, relevant information in a timely manner; attempting to equalise the power imbalance by increasing the control retained by patients; involving patients in decision making (not abusing their position of power and trust); facilitating patient independence without forcing this prematurely; and individualising care, being flexible (see Table 12.3).

TABLE 12.3 FIRM-HAND CARE

FIRST LEVEL OF PRESERVING INTEGRITY

- technical competence
- providing information (adequate, relevant, timely)
- involving patients in decision making
- facilitating patient independence
- individualising care, flexibility

Firm-hand care was described in relation to individualising care and providing adequate assistance when needed. A successful measure for helping patients to maintain some control, some degree of independence, was given as allowing flexibility in their daily routine:

> *High-quality nursing care* means basically getting me back into the home and back into the *normal situation* as quickly as possible . . . to *tailor care* to the *actual patient, getting them back into the mainstream.*

I found they *allowed me* to do my thing in *my own pace* . . . they left my shower till after morning tea and I more or less *did my own thing*. If I wanted to get back to bed, I just rang and they came and got me back into bed . . . it's *not like a sergeant major thing*, regimented; it was sort of *like home*, for such a *big turnover* it was *very homely*.

In order to facilitate patients to regain control, measures were undertaken to restore their independence, without forcing this prematurely:

The nurses would *make me do as much as I could*, shower-wise and dressing-wise. They sort of *pushed me*, which was very good. *And if I couldn't do it*, they were *always there*.

The importance of receiving adequate information was given as an aspect of high-quality care: '. . . making sure that you *fully understand* the treatment that you're having' and:

If you're told, *you know*, there are certain things coming up, whether they're good or bad, it doesn't really make a difference. Except that *you know*, then you *can prepare yourself*.

I was a little bit *nervous* and *didn't know what to expect* . . . and one of the nurses came in and *sat down with me* and sort of got rid of my nerves and *explained* what was going to happen, the whole procedure . . . It really helped. I was *prepared* for it. *Most patients get very nervous when they don't know what to expect*.

The limitation or inadequacy of firm-hand care alone for patients in a high-vulnerability context was explained:

. . . she's probably a very good nurse . . . She's just *totally clinically a nurse*, does it as she sees it or as *she's been taught*. She's *never learned to put a hand on a patient*, just to say 'don't worry, you're in good hands'. She was so *indifferent* . . . *compassion* was just *totally lacking*.

. . . they were just like *robots* . . . They were there, probably monitoring what you were doing, but as far as anything you wanted, they *didn't hear you* . . .

Technical competence was, in the main, described as adequate. However, this was not given a high priority by these participants when evaluating the care they had received:

Even the one I found *threatening*, did her job *perfectly adequately technically*, but she just *didn't feel*, or she didn't give the impression that she felt.

It was evident that some nurses gave only the basic care, without that 'something extra', and that this was clearly felt by these patients, especially for those in high-vulnerability contexts:

The ones that just *stick to the nursing code*, can *leave you very cold* . . . *clinical*, doing exactly as, probably, they are *required to do*.

'Doing for' and 'enabling' were identified by Swanson (1991) as two of the five caring processes in a middle-range theory of caring derived from phenomenological studies in perinatal contexts. Descriptions of these processes contain elements consistent with firm-hand care in the subdimensions of 'protecting', and 'performing competently or skilfully' in 'doing for', and 'providing information or explaining' in 'enabling'.

SOFT-HAND CARE

Soft-hand care entailed the aspects of care included in firm-hand care, as well as additional elements specific to soft-hand care. Strategies which were over and above those of firm-hand care and were central to soft-hand care are displayed in Table 12.4. These included: the personal touch, doing more than the job required or little extras; being there; empathy and compassion; touch; effective nurse–patient relationship; and patient advocacy. This level of care was found to be essential for patients in high-vulnerability contexts where preserving integrity was most needed, and was also very important for those in moderate-vulnerability context. It served to reduce vulnerability and was described as high-quality care. When nurses extended beyond the level of firm-hand care, it was appreciated:

> . . . If you want a civil answer, you won't get it from the nurses who are *strictly nursing*. The *other ones will reassure you*.

> They didn't really talk to you as though they were *only there doing their job* . . . you had the feeling like you were *not just a patient*; I mean that is what you're there for but . . .

The personal touch

Doing the 'little extras', more than the job was perceived to require, enhanced the physical and psychological comfort of the patient:

> *Real nurses did everything* to make you *comfortable* . . . they *went to a lot of trouble*.

> *Little things* to make you *comfortable* . . . just little things like that mean a lot to people like me [dependent] . . . I think everything is important when you're in hospital because you're away from your own environment . . . and sometimes those sort of *little things* are *more important* than the *bigger things*.

Nurses being observant and anticipating comfort needs when they had not been asked by the patients were mentioned:

> . . . others hadn't taken that notice, you know, *little things* like that you'd find one had a *little extra*, would do a little bit extra whereas the other one wouldn't. *Some do just basics* and *others do the lot*.

> *She went above and beyond what she was supposed to do.*

This aspect of doing more than the patients' perceptions of what the job required was in contrast to firm-hand care, where it was perceived that minimum requirements of care were met. The personal touch, doing little things to help reduce patients' discomfort (and vulnerability), was an important aspect of soft-hand care and was supported in the literature. Bottorff and Morse's (1994) descriptions of 'doing more' as a type of nursing

TABLE 12.4 SOFT-HAND CARE

FIRM-HAND CARE PLUS

- the personal touch, doing 'little extras', more than the job required
- being there, available, dependable
- empathy, compassion
- touch
- effective nurse–patient relationship
- patient advocacy

attending were similar to these findings and involved nurses 'doing something beyond what is usually required to complete care' (p. 53). It involved the nurse 'doing extras—doing a lot of little things' for patients that were not necessarily treatment-related (p. 57). Aspects of Swanson's (1991) descriptions of 'comforting', 'anticipating' and 'preserving dignity', as elements of the caring process of 'doing for', also lent some support to these findings. According to Swanson, studies have shown that 'clients perceive caring as those ministrations that are person-centred, protective, anticipatory, physically comforting and go beyond routine care' (p. 161).

Being there

Being there for patients when needed, being available, dependable and trustworthy, enhanced a sense of security or safety and reduced vulnerability. This involved: answering bells promptly (identified as a major problem in this study); 'popping in' or calling by to see the patient regularly—not just when treatments were due; taking time to sit, listen to, and talk with patients; the use of touch (especially in high-vulnerability contexts); showing confidence so that the patient was 'in good hands'; and keeping promises. In this way, the patients could trust the nurses to be there and to protect them from potential harm. It was especially significant for those in a high-vulnerability context and was expressed as:

> That they're *there when you need them*. The nurse *remembers me* and doesn't make me wait around . . . just basically to *be there* for you . . . Always had *time for you*.

Expressions of satisfaction with the quality of care consistently included this aspect of the nurse *being there.*

> When you're not used to being in a hospital and you're *lonely, depressed,* can't get used to being bedridden, it was important to have them *there* to *talk* to you. They were *always there* when I needed something, as in *morale.*

> They put the bell under your pillow and you *know* that *they'll be back* to look at you.

The importance of having the bell answered promptly (as outlined previously) was reiterated throughout these data:

> I would not expect to get my every whim, but if I *rang* and I *needed something urgently*, I'd expect to have it.

Not only was it perceived as being very important to have the bell answered promptly, but the nurse coming to check on the patient regularly, when other treatments were not scheduled, was also valued. This meant that the nurse could be depended on to be there fairly frequently:

> The ones who'll *come back* of their *own accord* and say, 'Are you okay, Mr . . . ?'

> . . . the nurse *popping in for no reason* . . . *when they didn't have to* . . . just to see how you are . . . if you were *comfortable* . . . My impression was that *the carers popped their head around the corner and the non-carers didn't.*

Another aspect of being there for patients was described as the nurse having the time to sit and talk or listen to the patient. The act of the nurse sitting with the patient, for any reason, gave patients the impression that the nurses had time for them, thus increasing their feelings of security. This aspect of soft-hand care was described in various ways by these patients:

> . . . they introduced themselves, and one *sat* with me . . . my feet were sticking out of the traction so she put a sock at the end, just *little things* like that . . .

> They were always friendly, *not just doing their job*, very chatty, *had time* for you.

The willingness and ability of the nurses to spend time with the patients also contributed to the development of the nurse–patient (and patient–nurse) relationship. It was described also as requiring sensitivity or empathy in the nurse. When explaining the meaning of high-quality nursing care these concepts were frequently grouped together:

> Nurses would *come in* on a pretty *frequent* basis . . . . Basically, the sort of *presence* they had . . . you definitely did pick up on the sort of vibrations that you got from those people; they were *sensitive* to your position . . . . The *support* they gave you . . . just to *have a chat*, here and there . . . just *talk to me* . . . give me a bit of *moral support*, just through the *way they interacted* with me.

When this did occur in high-vulnerability contexts, the consequences were given as positive, reassuring. However, when this was withheld, along with other soft-hand strategies, the consequences were perceived to be extremely negative. It was found that when the risk to integrity was very high and the patients' ability to control their situation was very low, the consequence of lack of soft-hand care was serious. The effects of the lack of the presence of nurses were compounded by the perceived lack of compassion in the following example:

Because, in intensive care, of all the times if I was going to *slip over the side*, that was the time and that's when *you want contact* with *another human being*, not . . . like *robots*, ignoring your requests . . . we're all human . . . I was *so sick* in there and in my mind *I didn't give a bugger if I died*, if I could just go home to my family. I didn't care. I just wanted to get out because I felt just *totally alone*. I felt *absolutely, totally* as though I was trying to *fight* whatever I was fighting, *alone*, and I was sick of the pain. And I just wanted to *chuck the towel in and go home*. As long as I got home, I didn't care if I died there; just get me out of there because . . . I was just *totally alone*. And I just *couldn't stand it anymore*. And that's true, that's how I felt then. I just *felt so alone* . . . I felt absolutely *devastated*. I know I was sick, but I also knew I was on my own completely, *totally on my own*.

Riemen (1986, p. 34) described the features of the nurse being too busy and hurried to spend time with the client, and not sitting down and really listening to client's individual concerns, as non-caring interactions. Taking time to sit and talk to patients was also found to be an effective nursing intervention in a study undertaken by English and Morse (1988). Being there could be inferred in Bottorff and Morse's aspects of 'doing for', described as the nurse not being hurried and patients appreciating time given by nurses 'just chatting' (1994, p. 57). 'Being with' was identified by Swanson (1991) as a caring process which involved 'being there', conveying ongoing availability, an emotional presence, and sharing feelings (p. 163).

Jenny and Logan (1992) found that self-presentation, an action of knowing the patient, was the nurses' conscious efforts to gain the patients' trust by displaying professional knowledge, self-confidence, dependability and concern (p. 256). This involved strategies of 'being honest and truthful to the patient, keeping promises made to them, following the care plan closely, and being available and visible to the patient as much as possible'. These strategies, together with others included by Jenny and Logan as part of knowing the patients (especially communicating and showing concern), were found in this study to reflect aspects of soft-hand care, especially being there.

Empathy and compassion

Being sensitive or understanding the patient's situation or feelings was needed in order to show compassion. Demonstrating consideration, respect and understanding of all patients as unique individuals who are not necessarily diminished in intelligence or ability was said to be important:

. . . nurses need a certain amount of *compassion, sympathy, empathy*. They need to be observant, just *caring people*.

. . . *empathising*, just *putting yourself in the person's position* and thinking 'how would I feel if I were like that?' . . . It *makes all the difference* . . . they should really find out what it's like on the other side. I guess the idea of *being a patient for a while*; being a patient for a week would be wonderful.

. . . some of them *knew exactly how I was feeling*.

This aspect of empathy was said to facilitate the protection of both the physical and emotional components of integrity:

> In terms of the physical care, it was wonderful but *emotionally, some were better than others* . . . It would help if they knew how to *take care of me in a physical sense*. But emotionally, just *put yourself in that person's position*, and think, 'Can she reach this, can she smell this, can she see this?'

The way that compassion was demonstrated was explained:

> . . . had the ability to come in with *self-confidence, put a hand on your shoulder* and immediately you felt as though you were *in good hands, compassionate* hands. It *went through you*.

Under conditions of very high vulnerability the positive impact of demonstrated compassion was most marked. According to one participant, '*compassion* is almost as *important as the treatment*'. This was explained further:

> Because if someone's really *pulling with you* . . . like they'd come up to you and just say 'How are you? . . . Is there anything I can do to help you?' People who are *genuine* . . . just *holding my hand* and saying, 'Come on, now, you've got to keep trying.' *You couldn't believe what that meant.* . . . Someone saying, 'don't worry, *we're here.*' Just [being] there and a *hand comes out and just touches you*. It *reassures you* that *you're still alive*; you're *not falling over the side*.

In this study, compassion and empathy were found to be closely related to being there and the personal touch. This aspect also overlapped with the use of touch, outlined in the next section. Swanson's (1991) description of 'knowing' as a process of caring incorporated the concept of empathy. Kozier, Erb and Blais (1992), in their discussions of the helping relationship, described caring as 'sharing deep and genuine concern about the welfare of another person' (p. 326). They suggested that the potential for empathy increases once caring develops. Empathy was described in this study in a way that reflected other aspects of Kozier and associates' (1992) description of the helping relationship. Descriptions of this helping relationship included elements such as demonstrating genuineness, showing respect for the patients and a willingness to be available, being honest, listening actively, and putting yourself in the other person's shoes or being able to empathise—all of which were valued by patients in this study.

These findings suggest that, in order to show empathy and compassion, nurses needed to know their patients. This aspect of knowing patients was inhibited if they did not spend sufficient time with them, or they were not assigned repeatedly to the same patient.

Touch

In addition to taking the time to sit and talk or listen to patients, it was perceived to reduce patient vulnerability when the nurse touched the patient. This seemed most appropriate under high-vulnerability conditions:

Human contact is absolutely essential, as much as medication . . . . *Medicine alone doesn't cure people*, I'm positive of that.

It's very, very obvious. They will come to you and want to know are you all right. They'll *come* and *put their hand on your hand*, just so that you *know that you're not alone*, especially when you're in intensive care.

The use of touch was found to be an additional aspect of 'being there' and providing security. The effect of touch was explained by a patient who had been in a life-threatening situation:

About five nurses just came past and would just *touch your hand*. You couldn't believe that *bond* that came from that person, when they touch your hand, to say 'You're a human being, a fellow human being' or 'I'm with you, I'm helping you, I'm attending to you'. That to me was truly *as important as medication*.

In spite of the perceived therapeutic effects of the human touch, it was suggested in these data that this was less noticeable in nursing than in previous years. One participant attributed this to advances in technology detracting from the human element of caring:

We live in *changing times*. It's a case of *no more hands on*, it's button pressing time . . . but you still *need the human touch*.

Nurses using touch and taking time to listen and talk to patients were found in this study to be components of being there, as well as demonstrating empathy and compassion, and the personal touch, doing the 'little extras'. These were the extra dimensions of preserving integrity found in soft-hand care and were most effective in high-vulnerability contexts, with diminishing need in low-vulnerability contexts.

Bottorff (1993) studied the use and meaning of touch in caring for patients with cancer, identifying five types of touch. These were described as comforting, connecting, working, orienting and social. The therapeutic value of touch, as found in this study, was supported. These five types of touch were further incorporated in Bottorff and Morse's (1994) types of nursing attending. Types of touch, as explained in those reports, were not identified in this study, however—the patients' comments appeared to refer to comforting and connecting touch. Weiss (1988) found support for the propositions that, first, caregivers use task-related touch to a greater extent than expressive or comforting types of touch and, second, the use of touch by nurses may improve the patient's affective response to the nurse–patient interaction (p. 21).

Morse (1992) identified touching, listening and talking as comforting behaviour, and suggested that comfort was an outcome of therapeutic nursing intervention. This notion has been supported in these findings, where comfort was also viewed as an aspect of reduced vulnerability. In Morse's (1983) previous study of patients' perception of comfort, the main components identified were touching and talking, as well as listening, and comfort needs were found to vary in relation to context.

Cameron (1993) suggested that comfort, as a major tenet in nursing, needs clarifying. She undertook a grounded theory study of the patient's experience of comfort and found that this was not a passive process whereby patients waited in hope of receiving comfort. On the contrary, Cameron found comfort to be a dynamic process in which patients actively engaged to increase their personal comfort levels. Nevertheless, it was suggested that nurses had a part to play in assisting patients to advance along the 'comfort continuum'. Elements which were identified in this study as patients seeking to enhance the nurse–patient relationship usually resulted in their comfort needs being more effectively met. Estabrooks and Morse (1992) identified touching as central to the nurse–patient relationship, which they saw as a reciprocal equation. Cueing was described in their study as the process used to determine the need for, and appropriateness of, touch. In this study, touch appeared to be most needed and appropriate for patients in high-vulnerability contexts.

An effective nurse–patient relationship

Several of the participants clearly described quality nursing care as being a two-way responsibility with input from the patient as well as the nurse. In addition to the strategies outlined previously, means for improving or enhancing the nurse–patient relationship and thus the quality of the care received were put forward. These included getting to know the nurse(s), asking them questions, relating to them personally and encouraging the nurse(s) to consider them as human beings, rather than objects or 'just patients'. In this way, it was suggested that they would receive increased attention:

> If a nursing system is going to work for you, you've got to work with the nurse. You've got to be a *team*. The *patient and nurse have to work together*. Each one has to work at it . . . *they're* going to give you medication, *they're* going to give you your treatment, so if you want that to work, you must *work with them* and for them to work with you, to make it a success. You're *both* there to *get you better*.

> . . . if you say, 'Oh, I know your home place' [or a mutual acquaintance], that gives them *a bigger interest in you* . . . you've got a *common interest,* when they come back to do your treatment, *they're not in such a hurry to race off* . . . it means they *will come back. You'll get more attention*.

The fact that the patients didn't have the choice of which nurse was assigned to their care increased the significance of the nurse's attitude in dealing with them:

> You probably have *contact* with the nurses every couple of hours of their shift. So it's important that they come to work in *good moods*, or can *leave their problems home* . . . it's like when you go to a shop [and the shop assistant is rude] you can walk away and leave there, not see them again. But if you're *confined* to that *one spot*, it's *important* that *they're not grumpy*.

Several factors were found to inhibit the development of the nurse–patient relationship in this study. These were said to be related to having too many competing demands on the nurses' time; being short-staffed; shift rotations; patients being moved to other areas; and lack of continuity and consistency in nurses assigned to care for individual patients.

Many of the features of the nurse–patient relationship identified in this study are very similar to the findings of Morse (1991), who described 'negotiating commitment and involvement in the nurse–patient relationship'. These latter descriptions also reflected the aspects described here as being a good patient, which were interpreted by Morse as making overtures towards the nurses so that they would 'willingly become involved in their care' (p. 461). Descriptions, in this study, of good nurse–patient relationships (and parallel patient–nurse relationships) reflected the main types of mutual relationships described by Morse (1991) as:

- clinical (when the contact between the nurse and the patient is relatively brief, professional and impersonal);

- therapeutic (in which the nurse views the patient first as a patient and second as a person with a life outside); and

- connected (in which the nurse, while maintaining a professional perspective, views the patient first as a person and second as a patient).

Evidence of overinvolved relationships, described by Morse as a close personal relationship in which the professional aspect is abandoned, was not found in this study.

Firm-hand care appears to contain elements of Morse's (1991) description of clinical nurse–patient relationships. *Clinical relationships* were described by Morse to be characterised by:

- the time being short/transitory;

- the interaction perfunctory/rote;

- the patient's needs being minor and treatment-oriented;

- the patient trusting the nurse's competence;

- the nurse's perspective of the patient (and the patient's perspective of her or his own role) being only in the patient role—not as a person; and

- the nurse's commitment being only professional.

(1991, p. 457).

Findings of this study also suggest that firm-hand care, reflecting clinical relationships (Morse 1991), may be appropriate in low-vulnerability contexts but is insufficient in high-vulnerability contexts.

Soft-hand care appeared to correspond with some of the elements described by Morse (1991) in relation to both therapeutic and connected nurse–patient relationships. *Therapeutic relationships* were described as having the following characteristics:

- the time being short/average;

- the interaction professional;

- the patient's needs, being minor-moderate, are met;

- the nurse considering the patient first in the patient role and secondly as a person;

- the nurse's commitment being primarily professional with patient concerns being secondary; and

- the patient showing trust in the nurse's competence but testing trustworthiness.

Therapeutic relationships could be related to soft-hand care for patients when in moderate-vulnerability contexts.

However, it would appear that, for high-vulnerability contexts, elements described in soft-hand care reflected more the category described by Morse (1991) as the connected nurse–patient relationship. Characteristics of *connected relationships* were given as:

- lengthy in time;
- intensive/close interaction;
- patients' needs being extensive/critical and nurses 'going the extra mile';
- patients trusting nurses' competence and confiding in them;
- nurses consulting on treatment decisions;
- patients considered first as a person and secondly in the patient role; and
- nurses committed primarily to the patients' concerns and secondarily to treatment concerns.

(Morse 1991, p. 457).

Patients in this study who showed dissatisfaction with firm-hand care were mainly in high- and moderate-vulnerability contexts, and had needs that would have been more appropriately met by soft-hand care, or Morse's description of either therapeutic or connected nurse–patient relationships. Their needs were mainly quite extensive and, in some cases, they were in life-threatening situations.

It was suggested in this study that the shortened length of contact between a patient and any one nurse would tend to preclude the development of connected relationships in most cases. Even though primary nursing was said to be in place at the principal study site, patients were rarely able to identify one specific nurse as their primary caregiver. Most gave five to six nurses that they got to know and one suggested that the physiotherapist was the primary caregiver. Morse (1991) described similar factors which shorten the length of contact between any one patient and a nurse as interfering with the development of nurse–patient relationships, and suggested further that, even when primary nursing care is being implemented, the concept breaks down unless the primary nurse is regularly assigned to the same patients.

Being a patient advocate

This study revealed that vulnerability could be reduced by the interventions of an advocate, especially in contexts where the patient had a high level of vulnerability. **Advocacy**, or advocating—pleading for, supporting or defending another—was identified in this study as an important aspect of preserving integrity, mainly by its absence. Patients felt more confident, more protected (less vulnerable) when advocacy was used (or available) and, conversely, expressed feelings of despair and increased vulnerability when it was absent. It was found that advocacy may be provided by family or other patients, but that this was not always possible or effective; it was most effective if provided by caregivers (e.g. nurses). Patients explained the need for advocacy, as well as failed attempts at advocacy:

> I had one man next to me who was *critically injured* . . . in *terrible pain*
> . . . he was *begging for a nurse*, and I said, 'for Christ's sake, nurse, would

you *please go and attend to that man*. He's begging you.' . . . I *could feel his pain* . . . I knew that poor fellow was going through purgatory. She said, 'Oh, he's always like that, it's just his race.' I said, 'Do you know what the pain's like? . . . You know he's in intensive care, he's getting agitated.' But as far as that nurse was concerned, it was when she was ready. And at that time, there were four of them talking.

An apparent failure of the nurse to intervene on the patient's behalf was described:

One doctor had said I could have the main drip out of my arm in the morning . . . . Well, during the night, it was *getting bad, painful*. The veins were collapsing . . . . So *they got a young doctor to come along*. I said, 'Please, *would you please not put it* [the IV drip] *back* in again. Two doctors, my specialist and the doctor, said to me this is going to come out in the morning. . . . 'But she just *totally refused to listen*. I said, 'If you can't guarantee that my arm won't be damaged', and she said, 'Of course, I can't do that.' It was almost like a *stand up fight*. So in the end, *she put it in* up here, when I said, 'Not there, that's out. I can't even touch it for the pain.'

Disregarding the patient's expressed wishes and denying his rights to refuse treatment was interpreted as an extreme case of abuse of power, in this case by a doctor, and reflected the need for advocacy. The participant explained further:

She was not saying to me, 'Well, Mr . . . is the patient but he also must know his own arm, how bad the pain is.' She would not remove the drip. Even though I had explained it. I said, '*Please ring* and *confirm*, will you? I know it's late but if you can't guarantee me my arm won't be damaged for sure, *please don't put it in again*.' But, no, they *don't listen, they just go on*.

Instead of caregivers reducing patient vulnerability, ignoring patients' rights and failing to take on an advocacy role had increased vulnerability. Incidents in which advocacy had not been available in high-vulnerability contexts had led to 'feeling absolutely *devastated*, totally *alone*'.
Others reiterated the need for advocacy:

. . . if something really *distresses you*, some part of your treatment or something, you could ask to speak to whoever it is. If something *went wrong*, or something that you didn't understand, or weren't happy about, *you've got to have somebody you can go to*.

Nurses were found to be in the best position to be advocates for patients, but apparently did not fulfil this role in most instances in these data. This could explain the need for patients to seek other sources of advocacy.

According to Bandman and Bandman (1990, p. 21), patient advocacy is part of the expanding relationships nurses have in the care of their patients and is essential to patients' health care rights. In order to assume advocacy roles, it was given that the notion of the patient coming first must be accepted that—along with the views that the patient should define what nursing is about—the patient has rights, and that patients depend on significant others to protect and care for their rights when they themselves are unable to do so. These views were supported by the findings of this study.

Advocacy was also linked to the patient's need for information, in that the patient advocate role is one in which patients are informed about the nature of their health problems and the options or choices available for resolving these problems (Arnold & Boggs 1989; Bandman & Bandman 1990). Thus, making informed decisions, which should then be supported by caregivers, would be the desired outcome for patients. It appeared that, in many instances in this study, the lack of information given to patients had compounded their problems of lack of support for their wishes or rights. The lack of sufficient, relevant and timely information was found to be a factor contributing to patient vulnerability. Furthermore, basic respect for the worth and dignity of individuals, and accepting people as they are, are necessary components of advocacy and may help reduce the threat of illness, facilitating the reduction of stress (Bandman & Bandman 1990). These views were given support by the findings of this study.

Phases in the process of preserving integrity

Further analysis of the data revealed phases which subsume the identified levels of care and the patient's perceived role. These phases have been identified as *knowing what to expect, contributing to care* and *eliciting a nursing presence*.

(a)   *Knowing what to expect.* This initial phase of preserving integrity involved, first, the patients knowing what to expect and what was expected of them—being well informed or prepared in relation to all aspects of hospitalisation and their care. Second, knowing the nurses (and the nurses knowing the patients) contributed to the establishment of an effective nurse–patient relationship. Third, knowing they were in good hands encompassed technical competence and the nurses appearing self-confident.

(b)   *Contributing to care.* This phase included the aspects of preserving integrity in which patients were able to contribute to their care and depended on the caregivers listening or attending to them, facilitating independence without forcing, including them in decision-making, and acknowledging that patients 'know their own bodies' and have a role in their care. The availability of an effective patient advocate in cases where the above were not possible or not allowed was emphasised. Patients' efforts to contribute included trying to recover and contributing to the establishment of the nurse–patient relationship.

(c)   *Eliciting a nursing presence.* The category of being a good patient was included in this phase, as was being seen to be trying to recover. These aspects were intended to attract the favour of nurses, ensuring a quicker response to the call bell and less impatience shown by the nurses. Strategies described as contributing to the development of an effective nurse–patient relationship also aimed at attracting more attention in that nurses would stay at the bedside longer to talk, not rushing away, or they would return more often. Sustaining presence, especially in high vulnerability contexts, was crucial to preserving integrity and encompassed the categories of being there, the personal touch, empathy and compassion, the use of touch and the presence of a patient advocate when necessary—all aspects of soft-hand care.

These phases show some similarities to those identified by Price (1993) in her study of the process of receiving quality nursing care in which she focused on the perspective of parents of hospitalised children.

COMPARING PATIENTS' AND NURSES' PERCEPTIONS

A comparison of nurses' and patients' perceptions of high-quality care (Irurita, Williams & Reeves 1994) found considerable consistency between the findings of the study described here and those of a similar study, undertaken during the same period and using the same setting and methods, but focusing on the nurse's perspective of care (Williams 1994). In the latter study, the core problem of vulnerability was not specifically identified. Nevertheless, the notion of patients being vulnerable was inferred in the nurses' descriptions of 'being there' and 'providing a protective responsibility for patients' (Irurita et al. 1994). Furthermore, hospitalisation was described as 'threatening' and 'frightening' to patients. Ageism, strongly identified by patients as a cause of vulnerability, was not apparent as such in the nurses' data. This aspect will require further study.

Four types of nursing care were described by Williams (1994). Low-quality care reflected the delivery of minimal physical care, with some omissions of care. Basic care focused on providing adequate physical care, whereas high-quality care was described as incorporating both physical and psychological elements of nursing care. The highest level of care was called exemplary care, which was said to consist of high-quality care with the additional dimensions of 'extra care'. These levels partly correspond with the levels of care identified in this study.

Rough-hand care, involving threatening, bullying, rough handling and treating patients as objects or 'slabs of meat', was not evident in Williams' study of nurses. However, some aspects, such as ignoring and not listening to patients, and being impatient and unreliable, overlapped with low-quality care. Descriptions of low-quality care were more consistent with hard-hand care, while basic care was similar to firm-hand care.

Similarities with the category of soft-hand care were found in the nurses' descriptions of both high-quality and exemplary care. High-quality care was partly consistent with firm-hand care, although some of the psychological aspects of care overlapped with those in soft-hand care. The 'extra care' incorporated in exemplary care reflected the elements of the personal touch, doing more than the job required and the 'little extras' for comfort found in soft-hand care. Being there was identified in Williams' study as part of high-quality care. Nurses' accounts of the caring role included touch, empathy and compassion; an effective nurse–patient relationship was given emphasis in both studies. Patient advocacy was described by Williams as part of the protective responsibility in the nurse's role.

In contexts of limited time, nurses were found to prioritise nursing care, to ensure that the needs of each patient were met within the parameters of safety (Williams 1994). Nurses assessed the needs of individual patients and placed these in the context of the needs of other patients in their care. Nursing care was then prioritised in the ascending order of physical care (especially comfort/pain relief), psychological care and then extra care. Based on this process, the level of nursing care that time allowed was delivered, either immediately, or delayed, or left to be handed over to the next shift. It appeared also that some care was omitted.

By comparing the findings of these two studies, it appeared that nurses prioritised nursing care delivery based on the patient's physical needs in the first instance, with emotional or psychological needs being given secondary consideration. Vulnerability in relation to these needs was not identified. On the other hand, the theory of preserving integrity, based on the patient's perspective, proposes that, when determining the most effective nursing care approach, vulnerability should be assessed, incorporating all aspects of the patient's integrity. By identifying the major causal factors of vulnerability, and determining the individual patient's vulnerability level on an ongoing basis, prioritisation of care in contexts of limited time should be more effective in terms of preserving integrity than using the approaches described by nurses in Williams' (1994) study.

DISCUSSION: PRESERVING INTEGRITY

Elements of the theory of nursing developed from this study have been supported by several studies which also used qualitative research methods. Furthermore, the theory reflects some of the aspects contained in Levine's Conservation Model (1973). Levine described nursing as a human interaction, the goal of which is the promotion of adaptation and the maintenance of wholeness. The conservation principles may be used by nurses to identify interventions that will maintain wholeness, or integrity, for the patient (Schaefer & Pond 1994, p. 53).

Ludwig-Beymer et al. (1993) used unsolicited letters, patient satisfaction questionnaires and quality care surveys to study patients' perceptions of care. Their findings include aspects as described in this theory of preserving integrity. These categorised nurses as: capable (competence, knowledgeable); communicative (providing information); caring (acceptance, compassion, empathy, 'giving of self'); respectful (treats with consideration, patience, courtesy, dignity, treated like a person or 'treated as someone special'); enthusiastic, encouraging (support, reassuring, promoting independence, and using social humour); and 'going the extra mile' (flexibility, responding quickly, 'taking time to be with me').

Morse et al. (1990) identified five epistemological perspectives in their examination of the concept of care as reported in the nursing literature. Aspects of preserving integrity, as described in this chapter, were found to be similar to some of the views of caring put forth by those authors. Their category of 'caring as a moral imperative or ideal' described caring as the adherence to the commitment of maintaining the individual's dignity or integrity (p. 5). 'Caring as an affect' emphasised that the nature of caring extends from '... an empathetic feeling for the patient experience' (p. 5); or, as described by McFarlane (1976, p. 189), caring 'signifies a feeling of concern, of interest, of oversight with the view of protection'. Caring was also categorised by Morse et al. (1990) as a human trait (which included compassion, competence and confidence), as the nurse–patient relationship and as a therapeutic intervention. This latter linked caring more directly than other views to the work of nurses and included caring actions such as attentive listening, patient teaching, patient advocacy, touch, 'being there' and technical competence—in other words, all nursing actions that enable or assist patients.

Brown (1986) studied 50 patients' descriptions of their experience of being cared for by a nurse, and the themes identified in that study are given some support in these findings. The major themes identified by Brown included 'recognition of individual qualities and needs'. This was described by Brown as the nurse doing something 'extra' that was not required in the ordinary provision of service. Care was seen as being personalised rather than routine, and this reflects the aspect of soft-hand care identified as the personal touch—doing 'little extras' to ensure comfort. Another major theme identified in Brown's study was the 'reassuring presence' of the nurse, described as the nursing quality most important to the patient's experience of care. That theme is similar to the soft-hand care component of being there, being available and dependable. Being there was also reflected in Brown's description of 'amount of time spent', in which the nurse took more time than was actually needed to do something for the patient. Similarly, in this study, patients had described actions to enhance the nurse–patient relationship, with the view of the nurse spending longer with the patient, 'not rushing, taking longer with procedures' and 'coming back' more often. This emphasised further the importance that patients placed on the nurse being there. 'Surveillance', described by Brown as interactions which involved nurses keeping the patients under watch, with emphasis on their physical condition or safety, could equate also to the category of being there.

Aspects described by Brown which could constitute firm-hand care identified in this study included 'provision of information', 'demonstration of professional knowledge and skills', 'assistance with pain' and 'promotion of autonomy' (making the patient an active decision-making participant). All these themes, identified by Brown, could be considered as fitting into the theory of preserving integrity. Furthermore, the notion of firm-hand care forming the first level of preserving integrity, with the second level of soft-hand care being built on, is supported in Brown's (1986) contention that:

> Fundamental to the experience of care is the patient's confidence in the ability of the nurse to provide the necessary physical care and treatment. As this professional competency is demonstrated, the more expressive activities become important.
>
> *(p. 62)*

Gardner and Wheeler (1987) undertook an exploratory study (using interviews and the Supportive Nursing Behaviour Checklist) to ascertain patients' perceptions of support, and they found categories of support which are compatible with categories identified in this study as forming the process of preserving integrity. One hundred and ten patients described an incident in which they received support; more than 50 per cent of the behaviours were determined by Gardner and Wheeler to comprise the category of the nurse being available, and another 20 per cent were placed in the promoting comfort category (including reducing anxiety). These behaviours, highly valued by patients in that study, match this study's participants' descriptions of the soft-hand care elements of being there and the personal touch, the little extras to ensure comfort.

Another strong category of patients' perceptions of support identified in Gardner and Wheeler's (1987) study was giving information to patients, also supported as an important first-level integrity-preserving action in this study. The other categories of support were found to be assisting in expressing feeling, performing specific nursing tasks, helping to solve problems, having a friendly and pleasant attitude, relieving pain, giving reassurance, individual care and touching. Most of these fit in with the categories forming the process of preserving integrity in this study.

The most frequently mentioned non-supportive behaviour was lack of availability of the nurse; other non-supportive behaviours included lack of comfort and information, negative attitudes (aggressive or rejective) of the nurse, lack of treatment by the nurses and lack of reassurance (Gardner & Wheeler 1987). These correspond with aspects of hard-hand and rough-hand care found in this study. These findings of Gardner and Wheeler's study highlighted the importance of the availability of the nurse to the patient, and the attitude of the nurse towards the patient (p. 129). Furthermore, as was the case in this study, availability (or being there) was said to imply physical and psychological presence.

According to Jenny and Logan (1992, p. 254), 'knowing the patient' signified a cognitive and relational process whereby nurses identified salient aspects of a particular patient situation, while at the same time demonstrating their credibility and eliciting patient trust. In their qualitative study of how expert nurses wean patients from mechanical ventilation, Jenny and Logan found that 'knowing the patient' meant that nursing interventions were directed to personalising the patients' care, which encouraged patient collaboration in their care. When nurses demonstrated their commitment to the patient's concerns and comfort through knowing activities, they gained the patient's trust. These views mirror aspects identified in this study as soft-hand care.

In this study, the way that the delivery of nursing care was organised affected the nurses' ability to give soft-hand care (and thus affected the level of patients' vulnerability). This related particularly to consistency in caregivers: where a patient had multiple caregivers (nurses) during a hospital stay, many of the aspects of soft-hand care could not be effectively enacted. Difficulty in establishing a good nurse–patient relationship was an obvious outcome of this. In addition, there was an increased risk of mistakes or omissions of care, and a lack of individualised care, due to nurses not knowing the patient well. Moreover, Morse et al. (1990) have suggested that constraints on nursing time may inhibit the development of a caring feeling towards the patient (pp. 5, 6).

THE PROPOSED THEORY OF NURSING

As discussed in this chapter, effective or quality nursing care was interpreted as a process of preserving integrity. Preserving integrity had two levels called firm-hand care and soft-hand care. When a person became a patient, individuality and some control were lost and the integrity was threatened, leading to vulnerability. A certain amount of vulnerability in the patient role was found to be inevitable. Nevertheless, it was discovered that appropriate caring interventions could ward off, or reduce, some of the threats to integrity; vulnerability could be reduced and integrity restored.

Vulnerability contexts were apparent with three different levels, each requiring adjustments to the nursing interventions. Firm-hand care is proposed as the first level of preserving integrity and may be sufficient for patients in low-vulnerability contexts. However, for moderate and high levels of vulnerability, it is suggested that firm-hand care alone does not deal adequately with some of the threats to integrity and may actually increase the patient's vulnerability (and dissatisfaction with care).

Soft-hand care represents the most effective level of preserving integrity, and is built on to the basic elements of firm-hand care. In other words, it extends beyond the technically competent firm-hand care and provides the additional dimensions of protection, conservation and restoration needed to restore integrity and reduce the vulnerability of patients, especially those in moderate- and high-vulnerability contexts.

Hard-hand care, or failure to preserve integrity, contributes to vulnerability, especially in moderate- and high-vulnerability contexts. Rough-hand care more accurately represents non-caring, as it is used to describe poor care, and abuse of the caregivers' position of power. Rough-hand care is portrayed as a threat to integrity and is shown as increasing patient vulnerability in any context.

Using the proposed theory of nursing, it is suggested that nurses could assess patients' vulnerability contexts and institute appropriate measures to preserve their integrity, and thus to reduce the level of vulnerability. Moreover, patients' vulnerability levels fluctuate during a period of hospitalisation, and so the need for soft-hand care approaches will vary for the same patients over time and between patients at any one time. In contexts of limited resources, by adjusting the care in relation to the vulnerability level, it is proposed that preserving integrity will be more effective. Furthermore, patient comfort, as well as patient satisfaction with the care, should increase, and negative consequences such as fear, frustration, anger, and feeling humiliated and dehumanised may be avoided or reduced.

Whereas it was evident in this study that soft-hand care was considered to be high-quality nursing care, it was acknowledged that patients could not always expect this level of care, due to the demands being made on what were perceived to be limited resources (especially nursing time). Nevertheless, it was found that the added dimensions of soft-hand care should not be withheld from patients in high-vulnerability contexts, and should also be available for those in moderate-vulnerability contexts. It is proposed that these soft-hand care actions/interactions need not take much extra time; minor adjustments to approaches to nursing care delivery could enable this care to be more readily available to all patients. Adjustments to the degree that these strategies are used could be made for individual patients, depending on their needs in terms of vulnerability level.

The proposed theory will need further refinement and testing in different contexts. Some causal conditions for vulnerability may need further exploration. Nevertheless, this theory should increase our understanding of the experience of being a patient and provide a basis for further research. Furthermore, it should make a valuable contribution to theory development in nursing and caring.

SUMMARY

This chapter has described the development of a grounded theory of nursing in the substantive area of acutely ill, hospitalised patients. When admitted to hospital and to the care of others, individuals experience some loss of control and a degree of risk or threat to their integrity. This was described in terms of vulnerability contexts, which varied for individual patients as well as fluctuating during the hospitalised experience. Specific causes of vulnerability were identified and explained from the patient's perspective. These included the illness, injury or intervention; dependence, abuse of power or rough-hand care; age/ageism; lack of information or preparation; and loss of identity/individuality.

Preserving integrity was described as the process for dealing with vulnerability and for conserving, protecting and restoring the patient's integrity. Patients perceived their role to include being a good patient, trying to recover and developing a patient–nurse relationship. Levels of nursing care were identified in relation to preserving integrity.

These were:

- *rough-hand care*, which reflected abuse of power and non-caring, and was a cause of vulnerability;

- *hard-hand care*, found to be technically inadequate and ineffective in preserving integrity;

- *firm-hand care*, the first level of preserving integrity, and constituting technically competent care; and

- *soft-hand care*, which incorporated technical competence in addition to more expressive, caring components (including the personal touch, doing more than the job required, the 'little extras' for comfort, being there, empathy and compassion, touch, an effective nurse–patient relationship and patient advocacy).

Phases in the process of preserving integrity, incorporating the above aspects, were identified as knowing what to expect, contributing to care and eliciting a nursing presence. Relationships between the levels of care and vulnerability contexts were proposed, and the proposed theory was discussed in relation to similar findings or nursing theories.

GLOSSARY

Advocacy: pleading for, supporting or defending another.

Category: a classification of concepts, discovered through constant comparative analysis; a grouping together of concepts under a higher-order, more abstract concept (Strauss & Corbin 1990, p. 61).

Constant comparative analysis: this involves coding the data for categories, comparing incidents applicable to each category, integrating categories and their properties, delineating the theory and writing the theory (Glaser & Strauss 1967; Glaser 1978; Strauss 1987; Strauss & Corbin 1990). It requires the simultaneous collection, coding and analysis of the data. Writing memos and/or the diagramming of the schema of ideas about the categories and their relationship is undertaken concurrently with the coding and analysis procedures.

Ethology: a method using techniques to identify complex behavioural patterns through systematic (non-participant) observation and description of behaviours under natural conditions.

Grounded theory: theory inductively derived from the study of the phenomenon it represents (Strauss & Corbin 1990, p. 23). It is discovered, developed and provisionally verified through systematic collection and analysis of data pertaining to that phenomenon. The method involves theoretical sampling and an ongoing process of constant comparative analysis until theoretical saturation occurs.

Integrity: having control over your life; being able to protect yourself; maintaining dignity as a human being; being an individual; remaining 'whole', intact, undiminished (in the course of life events); and being in as good condition or as sound or unimpaired a state as possible.

Preserving integrity: conserving, protecting and restoring the patient's integrity. This includes measures to minimise risks, such as keeping safe, protecting, defending, guarding or shielding from injury or harm to the integrity. It means protecting patients from physical or emotional harm and enabling them to retain their dignity as human beings. It involves recognising and accommodating, where possible, the patient's individuality as a person. It also entails actions to facilitate retention and restoration of patients' control and to promote the return to as intact, whole, or as unimpaired, a state as possible.

Purposive sampling: selecting participants who are knowledgeable about the topic and are experts by virtue of their involvement in specific life events (Morse 1989; Hutchinson & Webb 1989). They must have undergone, or be undergoing, experience of the event being studied, be able to reflect on, and be willing to share, detailed experiential information about the phenomenon.

Theoretical sampling: the researcher seeks informants and other sources of data as directed by the initial findings of data analysis. The aim of theoretical sampling is to look for variation, and to seek data that sheds more light on the developing theory, clarify categories and/or indicate new properties of the categories or processes (Glaser & Strauss 1967).

Theoretical saturation: all levels of codes appear complete with no new conceptual information available to indicate new codes or the expansion of existing codes. There is a sense of closure; all the data fit into the established categories, interactional and organisational patterns are visible, behavioural variation can be described, and behaviour in this specific context can be predicted (Hutchinson 1986). This approach avoids premature closure of the study.

Vulnerability: being susceptible to physical and/or emotional hurt, harm or injury; defenceless or weak in respect of defence or self-protection, open to assault. Individuals have diminished control over their lives and their integrity is at risk.

QUESTIONS

1 How does the theory of preserving integrity differ from some of the well-known theories of nursing, such as those of Orem, King, Roy, Rogers and Newman?

2 What does vulnerability mean in the theory of preserving integrity?

3 In what ways is the notion of protection incorporated in preserving integrity?

4 Why does the nurse have a central role in the process of preserving integrity?

LEARNING ACTIVITIES

1 The next time you are on duty, categorise the nurses you are working with as having 'hard hands', 'firm hands' or 'soft hands'. How do patients interact with these nurses?

2 Based on your experience and the proposed theory, describe several examples of the different levels of vulnerability experienced by patients, and the situations in which these may have occurred.

13

NURSING THEORY AND PRACTICE MODEL OF PUBLIC PARTICIPATION

ROBIN WATTS

LEARNING OBJECTIVES

When you have read this chapter you should be able to:

1 Identify the essential elements of critical enquiry.

2 Generate questions to apply to your own area of clinical learning or nursing practice.

3 Reflect on and improve your learning/practice accordingly.

Robin Watts, RN, DipNED, BA, MHSc, PhD, FRCNA, is Professor of Nursing at the Curtin University of Technology, Perth. Her nursing training was undertaken in the hospital system—she combined paediatric and adult nursing to obtain registration as a general nurse. Robin also has a midwifery certificate which she gained at the Royal North Shore Hospital in Sydney.

To her nursing qualifications Robin added a Bachelor of Arts degree, a Canadian Masters degree in Health Science with a specialisation in health care practice, and finally a PhD from the University of Colorado, USA. The knowledge that she gained from these qualifications has been applied to practice in northern Queensland, the rural areas of British Columbia in Canada and the mountains of Honduras in Central America, as well as in Western Australia.

As a result of this experience in very different parts of the world, Robin's areas of professional interest are primary health care, nursing in rural and remote areas and reflective practice, with a particular focus on related aspects of nursing education.

INTRODUCTION

To achieve the learning objectives of this chapter I will draw on knowledge and insights I have gained from my own practice and from conducting a specific research study. The model of practice that developed from these personal experiences will serve both as an illustration of the process that occurred and as the vehicle for raising questions about nursing models. The content of this chapter should generate questions, and aims to provide you with some answers to issues such as what does and does not constitute a 'nursing model', what stimulates the development of such models, and what use they are in the real world. These answers should not be considered final and complete but rather, should act as a stimulus or springboard to specific questions about your own nursing practice and the way you go about that practice.

PRACTICE MODEL

The model focused on in this chapter is concerned with public involvement in health care. It is based on a particular vision of what we should be aiming for in health care delivery, together with a number of presuppositions or assumptions. The model addresses the contributions of the public to health care, their roles and the means whereby that involvement can occur. It is designed for application in the Australian context—that is, it has been developed within a specific historical, socioeconomic, cultural and political context.

One question that immediately comes to mind is: What does this have to do with nursing? If a narrow definition of 'nursing model' is adopted—that is, if only theories and models related to 'hands-on' nursing are included and therefore are exclusive to nursing—the answer would be: Very little, if anything. My response is that a model of this type has everything to do with nursing. This model provides a framework for nurses to put nursing philosophy into action, to operationalise concepts such as **empowerment** at all levels of nursing care, including policy formulation. It is not, however, a model that is for the exclusive use of nurses but is available to all involved in health, including clients. Given the current emphasis on interdisciplinary cooperation, teamwork, and refocusing on best practice and the client rather than on professional territorial boundaries in the delivery of health care, this model is one tool for achieving those goals. As the content of the chapter develops, you will be able to draw your own conclusions about the relevance or otherwise of this model to nursing.

Another criticism that could be made is that the model is based on 'borrowed' theory, that is, political theory. To some nurse scholars this is anathema, and precludes a model from nursing. The concept of 'borrowed' theory is one I have always been uncomfortable with, as it is based on the assumption that certain disciplines 'own' certain types and aspects of knowledge. Once knowledge is 'discovered', it is there for all to use and apply to their particular situation. To subscribe to the idea of owning knowledge would, in fact, to be at odds with the theme of this chapter.

MODEL DEVELOPMENT

There are several major approaches to constructing a model. Some work from theory to practice, others work in reverse—practice to theory. A third way is to gather information about how things actually work in practice, compare that to existing theory, and revise that theory if indicated by the information you have obtained. The next stage uses the knowledge gained from the first three stages to construct a model that is appropriate to the environment in which it is to function. This practical form is then implemented and new knowledge is generated from the model being used in the real world of practice. What results is a continuing process of practice interacting with theory and both being improved in the process, or what is referred to as **praxis**.

I chose this third method. I collected information about democratic practices in health care (or lack of them), compared that information to theories of democracy, and then designed a model that would facilitate more meaningful involvement of people in health care delivery.

What follows is a detailed discussion of that process and the theoretical concepts that relate to the process.

MAJOR CONCEPTS

The model I am developing has its origins in the concept of community participation, one of the watchwords of primary health care and a concept characterised by attention in word rather than action in the Australian health care system. In this model, however, the term 'public involvement' has been substituted for community participation. In the initial stages of the research study, out of which this model emerged, I was using this latter term.

Both the literature and data from the participants in the study, however, illustrated the variety of meanings associated with 'community'. This posed problems, both in interpretation and putting the model into practice. Also, data from the study indicated very clearly that involvement in the health care system occurs on a continuum from individual decision making right through to high-level policy formulation. Using the term 'community' restricted the levels of health care delivery in which this model could be used.

Underlying community participation, as the primary health care movement envisages its actualisation, is a specific form of democracy: what Pateman (1970) refers to as participatory democracy. This form contrasts with the contemporary model (Bachrach 1967), which is confined to a set of representative institutions at the national, State and local levels—for example, parliament and local councils. The involvement of citizens is restricted to periodic sets of voting, with decision making the responsibility of the elected representatives. In contrast, in true participatory democracy there is equality of power in determining the outcome of decisions. People are viewed very positively as being able and aware.

Several other concepts are referred to in this chapter but they will be defined later in the discussion in the context in which they are used.

GENESIS OF THE MODEL

Every model or theory has its own life history. The process I am working through is no doubt unique in some or many ways, but there are probably similarities to the experience of others. What starts someone off on the path of developing a model or theory? This is, I suspect, always a retrospective question, as you are already some way down the path before you realise where it is leading.

Although I cannot claim to have started out with the intention of developing a model, that is what eventuated from the process. In fact, it is very difficult to identify exactly where and when the idea was born. Reflecting on why I became interested in the concept of democracy as it relates to health care systems, several historical and contextual factors, as well as individuals, stand out as being influential.

I was not aware of it at the time, but the seeds of my belief in the necessity of democracy in health care were sown during the two years I worked in a rural area in Honduras, Central America. The effects of the lack of democratic principles, in terms of the community's ill-health, were all too evident. The system was characterised by an extreme imbalance of power, a failure to link priorities of care with people's health needs, lack of community knowledge on which to base self-care, the lack of any mechanism or knowledge by which the community could have input into health care decisions, the belief on the part of those with power that the majority of the community had neither the ability nor the right to have this input, and a pervasive lack of concern for the community's welfare. These problems were illustrated by the popular description of the country as 'The land of 70%: 70% malnutrition, 70% illiteracy, 70% illegitimacy and 70% infant mortality'.

My experience on returning to practise in Australia, a country regarded as democratic and developed, increased my awareness that the rhetoric of democracy often did not match the actuality of practice. The pattern began to crystallise for me when, in the early 1980s, I read an article by Mahler (1977), then the Director of the World Health

Organization. In this article, he clearly emphasised the need to focus on an integrated social approach, rather than exclusively on medical services, in order to assist communities and nations move towards health. One of the three foundational principles of primary health care that Mahler identified as being essential to achieving this aim was community involvement.

This process of pattern recognition on my part was supported by my ongoing studies in the social sciences. Dry and dusty studies in politics came alive as I delved into an analysis of the forces that were at work in the overthrow of the democratically elected government of Chile in the early 1970s. My naive assumptions that the actions of those in power would be congruent with their stated beliefs in democratic principles were finally laid to rest.

My first personal experience with the implementation of the democratic principle of community involvement in health care came in 1986. While on a three-week visit to the Faculty of Nursing at Prince of Sangkla University in southern Thailand, I had the opportunity to observe a student group working with a rural community during their public health nursing experience. I was particularly impressed by the degree of consultation with, and feedback to, the village health committee at all stages of the assessment and implementation of the project the villagers had selected.

I returned from this stimulating experience to continue working in a management position in nursing education. The associated responsibilities brought me into close contact with people at all levels of the health care system. As a result, I became increasingly aware of barriers to the democratisation of health care, and the overt and covert forces that continue to prevent authentic involvement occurring.

At what point my interest was transformed into engagement with the idea of democracy in health care, I cannot identify, but there is no doubt that this engagement occurred. The opportunity to demonstrate that engagement in a tangible way presented itself in the form of a PhD degree. As my research topic was refined, it became apparent that the critical enquiry approach was the most appropriate for investigating the apparent gap between the rhetoric and the reality of public involvement in health care in Australia.

THEORETICAL FRAMEWORK

The theoretical framework of the model can best be described as *critical enquiry*. Critical enquiry is guided by the tenets of critical social theory and the critical, praxis-oriented paradigm (refer back to the section on model development for an explanation of praxis). The best known philosopher associated with this theory is Jurgen Habermas. His view of the essential nature of critical social theory is that it is 'a theory of the centrality of non-constrained, democratic decision making within a community' (Allen 1988, p. 95). 'Critical' is not used in the negative sense of finding fault with something but is constructive and rational, being guided by the goal of improvement (Grundy & Kemmis 1988, p. 324).

CHARACTERISTICS

Critical enquiry has a number of essential characteristics. These characteristics include:

- a particular view of society;
- the goal;

- the approach taken to the development of knowledge; and
- specific values.

View of society

The view of society that drives critical enquiry is that of *inequality*. This inequality may exist between individuals or social groups. Not only are people unequal in status but sections of society are also alienated from the social processes of which they are part. These groups are not conscious, or only partially conscious, of the social forces that maintain this state of affairs (Comstock 1982).

A number of examples of this inequality can be found in our own society and health care system. The most obvious example involves the Aboriginal and Torres Strait Islander people. Individuals from non-English speaking backgrounds are another group. The vast majority of recipients of health care could also be considered at best to be only partially conscious of the processes and forces that operate in the system which provides that care, a system in which professionals and bureaucrats have the power.

As providers within the health care system, nurses are themselves often perceived as being a prime example of a group affected by inequality.

Goal

The goal of critical enquiry is to move beyond describing a particular situation of inequality to a critique of the situation and the building of a more just society. This goal is achieved by assisting disempowered groups, such as those identified above, to gain a better understanding of the social relationships that are operating. This is done by helping these groups to become aware of how the system works and how their behaviour helps to maintain the current unequal relationships. Through this process, the potential for change and the reason for action can be identified. Critical enquiry therefore is 'not about a social process but rather is for particular social groups' (Comstock 1982, p. 379).

Development of knowledge

The knowledge developed from the process of critical enquiry is generated in a *dialectical* manner. 'Dialectic' is defined by the Macquarie Dictionary as 'a process of change that results from an interplay between opposite tendencies' (1981, p. 506). Although theory and practice are the 'opposite tendencies' when applying the definition in this context, a division between theory and practice is not implied. In contrast, theory and practice are linked and, as a result of using one to reflect on the other, both knowledge and practice are developed and improved. Existing theory informs the enquiry but is then re-examined/reflected on in the light of what is found in the process of enquiry. For example, the common experience of nurses implementing a particular nursing theory may indicate the need to modify some aspect of that theory. Practice is changed on the basis of that knowledge, which in turn generates new knowledge. Knowledge development does not stand still—that is, knowledge is not fixed. Emerging knowledge is further revised by implementation in practice and changing contexts. In the process, those who are involved also develop and change (Heydebrand 1983).

Values

The values associated with critical enquiry are those of *social justice*. These values are equity, autonomy, a mutually supportive society and support for the process of participatory democracy. Respect for fellow human beings is central; in particular, respect for the intellectual and political capacities of those who lack power (Lather 1986).

FRAMEWORK FOR MODEL DEVELOPMENT

The framework adopted for data collection and analysis was based on Comstock's (1982) model. This model consists of four phases:

1   empirical–analytical
2   interpretive
3   critical–dialectical
4   practical.

To clarify these terms, a brief description of each phase as it applied to the study will be provided and then illustrated by the data that were collected.

The first step was to collect and analyse information about the context in which public involvement in the Australian health care system has to operate (the *empirical–analytic phase*). Then information was obtained from both providers and client groups in order to gain an understanding of their definition, views and experiences of involvement of individuals and groups in health care (the *interpretive phase*). As information from these first two phases was generated, it was used to reflect on existing theory to see how well the experience of these people fitted with the theory. Where common experience and theory did not fit, changes to the theory were indicated (the *critical–dialectical* phase). The final phase was the *practical phase*, where insights gained from the process of reflecting on existing theory in the light of common experience were used to inform the development of a model that could be implemented in the real world of health care.

THE CONTEXT (EMPIRICAL–ANALYTIC PHASE)

As health care is influenced by the context in which it is provided, the process of developing a model of care must take this context into consideration. Three major contextual elements were identified from the analysis of the information obtained from various sources:

1   historical
2   structural
3   political.

Each of these elements was examined for factors that might influence public involvement in health care.

The relevant context in this case is the Australian health care system. The division of responsibilities for health care among national, State and local governments results in some variations at the State level. These variations are, however, relatively minor as the various bureaucracies tend to adopt changes being implemented in other States.

Historical context

An analysis of developments in public involvement in health care over the last 25 years in Australia indicated some activity in this sphere. There has been political support for the concept both at national and State level. Translation of this support into the establishment of formal participatory structures is relatively recent (Kearney 1993) and to date has been dependent on a particular political party being in power. Getting these structures to work has been even more of a problem. There are several reasons for these problems: strong opposition from the medical profession, lack of commitment from bureaucrats, inadequate resources and lack of required skills on the part of community representatives.

Structural context

The effect on public involvement of the restructuring of the health care system at State level, whereby regions become responsible and accountable for the health care services provided, is still to be assessed. In most States, community health advisory boards have been recently established or are planned. Only time will evidence the actual role they play and the extent of involvement achieved.

Political context

Public involvement in the political sense is not considered a notable characteristic of the Australian people. In situations where voting is not compulsory (e.g. local council elections) voter turnout is very low. This perceived apathy is explained by the *laissez-faire* attitudes of most citizens and their expectation that the elected government will provide for their needs and deal with their problems. These attitudes and expectations serve to render the bureaucracy more powerful. The continuation of this apathy is also encouraged by other groups who see more public involvement in decisions related to health care as a threat to their professional power base.

The contextual information obtained from both documents and informants identified a number of factors that either facilitate or hinder meaningful involvement of the public in their own health care, in that of the community in which they live, or of groups in the wider society (e.g. Aboriginal people and Torres Strait Islanders). Among the facilitating factors are the requirements at national and State levels of community advisory boards, and the development of consumer organisations. Negative factors include the disbanding of effective representative community structures (e.g. the Victorian District Health Councils), public attitudes typified by the expression 'She'll be right, mate', and the failure of health professionals to encourage involvement.

LIVED EXPERIENCE (INTERPRETIVE PHASE)

Based on their experiences with the health care system, the participants in the study identified the purpose and benefits of public involvement, and the factors that affected it (Table 13.1). Analysis of the experiences and views they shared also uncovered a more significant level of discourse. This level contained a single theme, which connected the relatively discrete topics focused on at the more superficial level of discussion. This theme was the distribution of power in relation to public involvement in the health care system,

TABLE 13.1 DISCOURSE THEMES: COMMUNITY INVOLVEMENT

LEVEL 2

Deterrent Power Strategies
Erection of barriers
• communication
• structural
Discouragement
Defeat
Tokenism
Diversion

Reasons for Disempowerment
Alienation
Negative self-perception
Lack of resources
Lack of perceived benefits
Problems with representation

LEVEL 1

Definition of Community
Location
Commonality
• need
• problem
• interest
• issue
• type of service
• demographic characteristic

Functions
Ideal—empowerment
Instrumental
• communication
• provision of care
• management

Benefits
Economic
Cooperation
Accountability

Factors affecting Public Involvement
Moral basis
Characteristics of participatory mechanisms
Resources
Demonstrated support
Scope
Preparedness of the community
Provider–community relationship
Source of initiative

expressed as the strategies to retain or gain power, and the problems experienced by those without power.

Purpose

This was seen as the achievement of two outcomes: ideal and instrumental. The ideal purpose of involvement was empowerment at both the individual and community level ('community' being defined as a group of people having something in common, be it location, need, problem, interest, issue, type of service or demographic characteristic). Several factors were identified as contributing to this empowerment process. One factor was the gaining of knowledge and the development of new skills as a result of involvement. Another positive outcome of being involved was the development of networks, which in turn provided support and a sense of cohesion in the group or community. The development of a community sense of ownership was another contributing factor, as well as an indicator of empowerment. The dual nature of this sense of ownership, as both a contributing factor and an indicator, supports the idea of empowerment as an ongoing, spiralling process.

The instrumental functions that public involvement can fulfil cluster into three linked categories.

1   Communication: establishment of two-way channels between providers and the community and also between community groups.

2   Provision of care in a complementary role to providers.

3   Management of services, ranging from feedback to improve services, through involvement in decision making, to control of services.

Benefits

The benefits the participants identified as flowing from these functions were financial savings, improved cooperation between the public and providers and increased provider accountability to the community. Participants indicated, however, that the ideal and instrumental functions, and the benefits of public involvement, could not be realised within the present power structure. To make the necessary changes, the strategies used by those individuals and groups presently in control to maintain this power structure must first be identified.

Power strategies

The strategies that had been experienced or observed can be grouped into five categories.

1   Erection of barriers to involvement (e.g. control of information; organisational structures that do not allow for community input).

2   Discouragement of people's interest in being involved (e.g. devaluing their input).

3   Defeat of moves to involve people (e.g. removal of effective community workers).

4   Tokenism (e.g. token representatives on committees; requesting input but not using it).

5   Diversion of people's attention or energies (e.g. by overwhelming them with information—or the 'Yes, Minister' approach, so called after the strategy adopted by bureaucrats on the English television series of the same name).

Whichever strategy was used to maintain control, the end result was the same—disempowered individuals and communities.

Disempowerment

This disempowerment manifests itself in several ways. Many individuals and communities have a negative perception of their abilities and contributions. An example of this perception was one participant who admitted that for many months, on a committee, she prefaced the few remarks she did make with the statement: 'I'm just the community representative.' Others become totally alienated from the system as a result of earlier negative experiences. As a result of this alienation, those affected feel devalued and distrust any individual, group or structure associated with the system.

The disempowered lack knowledge and skills. They have limited or no knowledge of how to access the system, they lack assertiveness skills when dealing with bureaucrats and health professionals, their verbal and written communication skills are poor and they lack information on the extent of health problems in the community. Energy and enthusiasm are not evident and leadership skills are lacking. They have also lost hope, or have never had hopes, that solutions to their problems will result from their involvement.

REFLECTION ON EXISTING THEORY (CRITICAL–DIALECTICAL PHASE)

This next phase of the model's development consisted of comparing the information obtained from the first two phases with existing theory. Where did the contextual information and experience related to this particular issue fit with relevant theoretical concepts? If contradictions appeared, these indicated that the theory might need to be modified.

Analysis of the data indicated three major groupings of themes and counter-themes (Table 13.2). These three groupings were:

1 ideology

2 provider–community relations

3 goals and process.

To illustrate the reflective process, illustrations from two of the groupings will be discussed.

TABLE 13.2   MAJOR GROUPINGS OF THEMES AND COUNTER-THEMES

THEMES	COUNTER-THEMES
Group 1 Ideology	
Individualism • self-interest	Communitarianism • caring for the community and its members Social justice and equity
Group 2 Provider-community Relations	
Dependence Alienation Control Conflict Professionalism	Partnership Valued Role Empowerment Cooperation Humnaness
Group 3 Goal and Process	
3.1 Management	
Corporate—top-down Centralised control Specialisation and professional decision-making Established objectives, priorities and strategies	Community—'bottom-up Decentralised Combination of community and provider expertise Negotiated local variation
3.2 Primacy of Goals	
Short-term Quantitative Economics, efficiency	Long-term Qualitative Human development
3.3 Guided by	
Medical model of health	Social model of health

Provider–community relationships

A number of subthemes and counter-themes relating to provider–community relationships emerged from the data. The partnership relationship espoused by the self-help groups and other participants in the study indicated interdependence between the community and the providers. This partnership model incorporates both the health planning and community development approaches to public involvement in the health care system, as developed by Rifkin (1981).

Rifkin characterised the health planning approach as one in which the professionals act as team leaders, the public is motivated to become involved by the opportunity to influence resource allocation, and the organisational structure adopted is a modification of the existing delivery system. The involvement of influential community leaders is sought to act as a communication channel between professionals and the community for consultative and education purposes. The role of the public is defined by professionals. This limited role involves providing input into planning, management and evaluation aspects of the delivery of care. The professionally defined goals are oriented towards the achievement of tasks in an efficient and effective manner.

In the community development approach, the emphasis is not on the delivery of services but on health as a human condition. The community has the major power in decision making, with the professional acting as a resource. This approach therefore involves a significant shift of power from the expert to the people, and a major restructuring of the system. The emphasis is on education and community-based health care, not on creating new institutions that are community-oriented.

Neither of these two approaches is entirely congruent with the approach advocated by participants in the study. The participants generally agreed on a division of power and a role for the community that falls between the division of power and the roles adopted in Rifkin's two approaches. From the data available, those in control of the current health care system were, at best, prepared to allow the health planning approach.

The emergence of the counter-theme of partnership rather than independence is of interest in relation to self-help groups. In Rifkin's model, the self-care approach is typified as regarding professional influence as peripheral. This was not the case for the self-help groups who participated in the study. These groups acknowledged that the professional was necessary. This acknowledgment was balanced by an insistence that both parties contribute jointly to the provision of care, with each party's contribution based on its particular area of expertise. In effect, both providers and community members become part of the health team. This group of participants agreed with Rifkin's view that self-care groups identify the major function of community involvement to be the meeting of needs for which professionals are unwilling or unable to provide care. In the view of the self-help groups, this instrumental function did not, however, result in professionals being regarded as peripheral. In contrast, the self-help groups' contribution to the provision of holistic care forms the basis of the groups' demand to be treated by professionals as partners.

Goals and process

The goal of empowerment is considered a long-term objective of the public involvement process. The long-term, qualitative nature of this goal is in direct contrast to the goals of the current corporate model of management (Considine 1988). The corporate management approach to evaluation of productivity demands short-term, quantitative objectives, and outcomes that are specific and measurable. This management model is driven by economics rather than a concern for human development.

These differing goals are reflected in the contrasting definitions of health. The present Australian health care system is based on the restrictive medical model definition of health. The focus is still on disease, as is illustrated by one State's health goals and targets document (Dobson & Penman 1994). For empowerment of individuals and communities to be a possibility, the social model of health must be the guiding principle. Nowhere is this principle more clearly illustrated than in relation to Aboriginal health.

The means by which these goals are achieved are also markedly different. The emphasis in the corporate management approach is on central control. The organisation is directed by the upper levels of the management hierarchy to ensure that all sections work in a methodical, streamlined manner towards centrally determined goals and strategies. In order to achieve maximum efficiency and effectiveness, specialised division of labour is adopted; hence, professional skills are sought and rewarded.

In contrast, a management structure and means of functioning that maximises public involvement requires decentralisation of management and a reversal in operational orientation—that is, from the bottom up. In this structure, community members are regarded as a source of expertise. Community input is sought on the identification of objectives, priorities and strategies. Although efficiency is still regarded as desirable, it is not of central importance and is not the only factor taken into consideration when optional means of working towards goals are being considered. Management acknowledges that there may well be more than one strategy that is appropriate to achieve a desired outcome, and variation is encouraged. Although the democratic process may at times be 'slow, cumbersome, halting and beset by backeddies' (Lindeman 1921, cited by Jones & Smith 1981, p. xiv), the long-term benefits are regarded as making the process worthwhile.

PRACTICAL PHASE

The final phase of the model's development required me to take the insights and information gained from the preceding three phases (analysis of the context, exploration of lived experiences, and critical reflection on these data in light of existing theory) and construct a model which was of use in the real world of health care practice.

As a preliminary step in this phase, a number of aspects had to be addressed. These aspects included identification of the vision that was to guide the model and the presuppositions on which the model was to be based.

Vision

'Every successful plan begins with a commitment to a preferred future' (Commission on Catholic Health Care 1988, p. 15). As Cauthen asserted:

> . . . visions of an ideal future can be powerful and effective in shaping the actual future when enough of the right people are grasped by them.
>
> *(1985, p. 338)*

McKnight (1987) identified three visions of society that dominate current debate: therapeutic, advocacy and community. The first two visions are the ones that have guided Australian health and welfare practice. The *therapeutic vision* sees the well-being of individuals as dependent on professional services provided to meet all needs. The *advocacy approach* conceives of a defensive wall of helpers protecting the labelled individual from an alien world. The third approach of *community* is the vision on which this model of public involvement is based.

The application of this vision of society as community to public involvement in the health care system generates a model in which the public and the providers work together as partners. The partnership needs to work to develop a health care system that is egalitarian, effective, efficient and democratic; one that is responsive and accountable to the community that it serves. Although both the ideal and instrumental purposes for public involvement are acknowledged, the emphasis is on the development of citizens and the developmental process, not the outcomes. The model for involvement is a community development rather than a managerial model.

To achieve this aim, public involvement must be an integral component of the structure and function of the health care system, not a marginal feature added for the sake of appearances or merely to collect management information. In other words, the involvement of the public is of a substantive nature. The means and mechanisms developed to facilitate involvement and partnership need to be sustainable in the long term. The primary characteristic of the partnership must be open, undistorted communication between the providers and the public.

Presuppositions

Based on this vision of community and the information obtained from the preceding phases of the model's development, nine presuppositions on which the model would be based were identified.

1   Health is the expansion of consciousness (or awareness of self and one's environment and what affects oneself and others) and is therefore a dynamic process (Newman 1986).

2   Change is necessary in the present technocratically oriented health care system.

3   In a democracy, the public has both rights and responsibilities. A balance exists between the responsibilities of the individual and the State.

4   Representative democracy, although necessary in many aspects of the governing of large industrialised societies, is not sufficient to facilitate empowerment.

5   Empowerment of individuals and communities requires opportunities to be involved in decision making, indicating a sharing of power between providers and the public.

6   Meaningful involvement of the public has positive outcomes, both for the individuals and communities involved, and the health care system.

7   To achieve these outcomes, involvement must be active and long-term in nature.

8   Motivation to participate requires incentives. Members of the public are primarily motivated to become involved by issues that affect them personally. Individuals will participate only when they see the need and receive rewards for becoming involved.

9   The public has both the potential ability and the practical wisdom to contribute to the improvement of health care.

The model

The conclusion I have arrived at, after all this data collection, analysis and critical reflection, is a model of public involvement that encompasses the following essential elements:

▪   purposes that are both ideal and instrumental, while emphasising the empowerment of individuals and communities (however defined);

▪   mechanisms that cover the many dimensions of public involvement, allow for authentic involvement in decision making, and are applicable at the various organisational levels of the health care system.

To meet these requirements, a combination of representative and participatory democratic forms was identified as appropriate (see Figure 13.1). The resulting framework will, of necessity, be complex and needs to be coherent while allowing for flexibility. At the various organisational levels of the health care system, permanent structures based on representation are required to deal with long-term policy and planning issues. Given the nature of representative structures, the achievement of the instrumental purposes of involvement is more appropriately assigned to this mechanism.

Direct involvement by individuals and groups is more appropriate for local and personal issues. Empowerment is emphasised as the purpose of this type of involvement. As involvement in these situations tends to be issue-specific, the form of involvement is temporary in the sense that it is limited to the life of the issue. The form of direct involvement also varies with the nature of the issue—for example, public meetings, formation of political action groups or direct negotiation with providers.

IMPLICATIONS FOR NURSING PRACTICE

For nurses to be able to facilitate the empowerment of the individuals and communities they work with, to become involved in decision-making about health and the health care system, nurses need to be empowered themselves. The old hierarchical nature of both the nursing and health care systems, which still influences many nurses, forms a barrier to this empowerment. Until nurses become aware of the obstacles to unconstrained communication, they will not be able to help the public raise its awareness. Raising the awareness of individual nurses and, in turn, the profession will enable nurses to become conscious of constraints and to name the barriers that stand in the way of open, undistorted communication. Only then will nurses be able to assist the public to identify the barriers to achieving a more balanced power relationship.

FIGURE 13.1 MODEL OF PUBLIC INVOLVEMENT

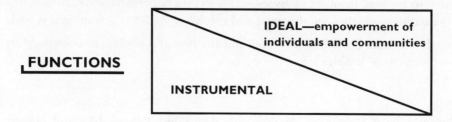

FUNCTIONS

IDEAL—empowerment of individuals and communities

INSTRUMENTAL

DEMOCRATIC MECHANISMS

	Representative	Participatory
Role	Authentic involvement in decision-making	
	Long-term policy and planning	Specific personal, group or community issues
	Input—quality assurance	
Means	Management levels in Health Dept structure • State • regional • district	Direct involvement of individuals and groups Varied means, e.g. • political action groups • public meetings • negotiation with providers

Keen (1991) suggested that one barrier to nurses' empowerment is their failure to recognise that they are an oppressed group. To assist both herself and other nurses explore the extent of this oppression, Keen developed a checklist entitled 'Is your oppression showing?'. Several of the characteristics of oppressed groups that Chinn, Wheeler and Roy (1988) identified are particularly pertinent to this discussion. These characteristics are:

- little or no desire to affiliate themselves with another powerless group (in this case, the recipients of care);

- a fear of freedom and viewing themselves as incapable of taking risks.

Freedom from past patterns will allow a new model of professional nursing practice, focusing on the development of individuals, groups and communities to be implemented. This model of professional practice must be based on a philosophy of development, rather than on the use of development merely as a strategy (Jackson,

Mitchell & Wright 1989). In contrast to a model of practice that encourages dependency, this model nurtures abilities and confidence in those abilities. The model also encourages the valuing of the public's contribution to its own health care and that of the community.

Nurses will need to adopt a critical attitude to professional practice in order to identify which aspects of their current practice are consistent with a participatory model of caring and which aspects maintain dependency, alienation and disempowerment. Many practices and the theoretical foundations on which these practices are based need to be examined.

A refocusing, for example, on contextual factors that act as barriers to an individual's or community's movement towards health brings into question the relevance of using adaptation theory as the exclusive basis for practice. Is it appropriate for the client and nurse to be putting their energies into adapting to the environment, or should those energies be redirected into changing some aspect of the client's environment (Chopoorian 1986)?

Another aspect of practice that requires critical assessment is whether certain nursing activities constitute advocacy—that is, empowerment—or, alternatively, serve only to maintain dependency. We need to examine our contacts with others for actions, however unintentional, that alienate people. Failure to listen actively to what people are trying to tell us, actions that are perceived as disinterest or lack of caring, comments that can be interpreted as disparaging of people's efforts to care for themselves or their family can all lead to alienation over a period of time.

Access to information is essential for individuals or communities to become empowered. The issue of access involves understanding the information. This requires nurses to reflect on whether their modes of communication, both spoken and written, facilitate client access to the information they require. For example, is nursing diagnosis terminology understandable to the average patient or client? Or is nursing, in using the negative strategy of controlling information to achieve professional status, setting up structural and communication barriers and denying people the means to start taking control of their own health?

There are also implications for nurses' involvement in policy formulation and implementation. This is an area, particularly given the massive changes currently under way in the health care system in this country, in which nurses have a professional obligation to become involved and to influence. In becoming involved in this process, the principles underlying this model should be applied. The principles are in line with the three essential features of public policy that Schultz and Schultz (1987) identified, based on Nodding's ethic of caring. These features are as follows.

1   The clear reflection of humans valued as persons.

2   The fostering of self-initiative, and personal and community growth, including empowerment and self-realisation (that is health enhancement).

3   A policy open to change if, in its implementation, interpersonal caring and engagement with the community is made more difficult or impossible.

Reflection on practice needs to be ongoing. Some activities, for example, may initially appear emancipatory but in time prove otherwise. The process of continuing reflection can be facilitated by involvement in action research that focuses on the nurse's own practice, by participating in a self-reflective professional group, or by becoming a member of an extended 'critical community' (McTaggart & Garbutcheon-Singh 1988).

This change in nursing practice requires an equally radical change in nursing education programs. The emancipatory and empowering goals and principles of practice, and the means of achieving these, need to be applied to both the content and the process of programs. If, for example, students experience asymmetrical communication, domination, non-involvement in decisions that affect them, and alienation, they are likely to transfer those behaviours into practice.

USE IN PRACTICE

If development of models is to be more than just an intellectual exercise, they must be disseminated and trialled, then either rejected, or modified and refined in the light of actual practice. This model is still essentially in the dissemination phase. Following presentations in several forums, enquiries have come from a variety of different quarters—local, national and international. To date, I am aware of only one situation where application of the model has been documented. As part of a submission to the Western Australian (WA) Health Department, on community participation in regional management, the WA Health Consumers Council used the model as a framework for their recommendations on the new regional structures. Unfortunately, another restructure occurred before their suggestions could be implemented. Individuals have indicated to me that aspects of the model have provided a stimulus to rethink certain elements of their practice. Others have indicated that the model has acted as a reinforcement of their practice—to keep persevering in the face of apathy and resistance.

SUMMARY

The material in this chapter has focused on illustrating the use of the critical enquiry approach in developing a framework for practice. The aim, however, was not just to present this process but also to stimulate you to think about aspects of your care. At this stage of your nursing career, this care may be confined to direct, one-to-one interaction. For others, involvement with communities, however defined, is the focus or a component of your nursing role. Yet others may have input into policy at various levels of health care delivery. At whatever level of the system you are, however, the same principles of involvement apply.

GLOSSARY

Empowerment: enabling people to make decisions about their own health, be it at the individual, family or community level. It is important to remember Labonte's (1989) reminder that 'empower' is a reflexive verb. Frequently people talk of 'empowering' others, but only individuals and groups can empower themselves. However, health care providers can facilitate the process.

Praxis: practice or action informed by theory.

QUESTIONS

1   Identify several experiences and/or individuals in your life who have influenced your approach to nursing. In what way have these experiences or individuals influenced you?

2   Can you identify any commonalities in the development process of this and other models of nursing discussed in this book?

3   Do you consider nurses are fully aware of the social forces that operate in the health care system and influence the provision of nursing care? If not, why not?

4   Is there any validity in Keen's claim that nurses are an oppressed group?

5   What stimulates your involvement in some issue that might affect your health?

6   Some people don't want to be involved in decisions related to their health. What should a nurse's approach be in these situations?

7   What implications do the points made in this chapter have for your nursing practice?

LEARNING ACTIVITY

Complete Keen's oppression checklist individually, then discuss in a group. (The checklist can be found in Keen's (1991) chapter in Caring and Nursing—see References.)

FURTHER READING

Watts, R. 1994 'Community participation', in *Primary Health Care: The Way to the Future*, ed. C. Cooney, Prentice Hall, New York, pp. 61–72. This chapter provides a step-by-step approach to examining some of the issues surrounding community involvement in the planning, provision and evaluation of health care services. Relevant theory is linked to discussion of the practical issues.

14

THEORY GENERATION THROUGH REFLECTIVE PRACTICE

JUDY LUMBY

With acknowledgment to the contribution made by the RNs who told their stories
of care and developed a Collaborative Model of Advanced Nursing Care.

LEARNING OBJECTIVES

When you have read this chapter you should be able to:

1 Discuss reflective practice and its place within nursing.

2 Compare and discuss the terms 'profession', 'discipline', 'practice' as they relate to nursing.

3 Consider ways of becoming reflective in your practice.

Judy Lumby, RN, PhD (Deakin), MHPEd, BA, Assoc DNE, currently holds the EM Lane Chair of Surgical Nursing, a joint clinical chair of the University of Sydney and Concord Hospital. She has 16 years of clinical experience, primarily in intensive care, and has been involved in nursing curriculum development and in the coordination of post basic nursing courses for several major hospitals and the NSW College of Nursing.

Since 1984 Judy has been involved at a senior teaching and management level in NSW universities, including six years as Head of the School of Nursing at the University of Technology, Sydney. She has been a member of several Australian university external advisory committees, a consultant nationally and, over the last two years, has played an important role in the development of curriculum for New Zealand Polytechnics in preparation for the transition to bachelor degrees in nursing.

Judy has written extensively in the area of teaching and learning, reflective practice and nursing knowledge. Her primary research interests include explicating the meaning of illness for individuals and their families in order to provide more effective health care congruent with individual needs and choices, as well as exploring feminist and critical methodologies for nursing research.

INTRODUCTION

This chapter will address the way in which theory (academic knowledge) can be generated from thinking and talking about the way in which people approach and attend to their daily work—that is, their practice. Because this is a nursing text, the chapter focuses on nursing as the daily work but the same principles could apply to any type of work.

Because we normally think that theory is developed first by the thinkers and then applied to practice by the workers, this chapter examines the reasons why this is not necessarily the only way or even the most valid way of developing theories. It does address some of the reasons for these traditional views and the changes which have enabled new views to challenge the old. A real situation involving advanced registered nurses will be used to illustrate how a strategy of reflective enquiry into practice enabled the generation of a theory of advanced nursing practice.

THEORY GENERATION

As you will have gathered from the previous chapters, when we speak of theory we may mean a variety of different things, although in general we are all speaking of some form of knowledge. The way in which the word 'theory' is used depends on the context and author of the **discourse** in which the word is being used. For example, theory can be used when referring to the knowledge underpinning a concept or a practice, such as the way in which bedwetting in children is managed. In such cases the theory has usually been developed out of, or based on, previously discovered scientific knowledge within disciplines such as anatomy or psychology. At other times, the term can be used very loosely, referring to anything that is not categorised as practice. This dichotomising of, or division between, theory and practice, which has occurred through language, has not been accidental but has a long history philosophically and politically and is based on traditional power. It is this historical, traditional, scientific power which has determined the way in which knowledges have been viewed and categorised in our society. Thus, while certain knowledge (e.g. theoretical knowledge) is viewed as real, trustworthy and to be revered, other knowledge is suspect and not to be trusted (e.g. practice knowledge).

PROFESSION/DISCIPLINE/PRACTICE?

The terms 'profession', 'discipline' and 'practice' are often used interchangeably when talking about areas of knowledge and theories. Are they the same? And if not, why not? What is the difference? We need an understanding of this before we can explore how theory may be generated from reflective practice.

A PROFESSION

An increasing number of groups in the community are claiming the right to be viewed as professions because of their unique service and expertise which includes a specialised body of knowledge. The increased awareness of the need to be socially accountable when delivering a service to a community contributes to this plea for recognition. Nursing has spent much time and effort in the past debating whether it is a profession, often to the detriment of other important issues. The traits of a profession that are identified in the literature include:

- a unique body of knowledge (if this is ever possible);

- self-regulating practices, such as codes of ethics and conduct;

- autonomy of practice; and

- a positive contribution to the social structure.

(Friedson 1983)

The only criteria that nursing may not be able to substantiate at this stage of our development is that of a unique body of knowledge (although we certainly have an accumulation of knowledge internationally). Some would argue that much of nursing knowledge is borrowed but this could be said about most professions.

Part of the development of a profession is in sorting out what body of knowledge is unique to it. Some would claim that debates about professionalism are 'to do with establishing and maintaining occupational territory and credibility with the public (as valuable consumers of professional services) whose "needs" must be confidently served by professionals' (Evans 1991, p. 314). Perhaps it is time for a redefinition of the notion of 'professional'.

In discussing nursing's growth as a discipline and a profession, Gray and Pratt (1991, p. 7) assert the importance of recognising the difference between a discipline and a profession:

> Failure to recognise the existence of the discipline as a body of knowledge that is separated from the activities of practitioners has contributed to the fact that nursing has been viewed as a vocation rather than a profession. In turn, this has led to confusion as to whether the discipline of nursing exists.

A DISCIPLINE

A discipline is defined by McWhinney (1966) as:

1 a unique field of action;

2 a defined body of knowledge;

3 an active area of research;

4 a training that is intellectually rigorous.

Disciplines have in the past been defined through university departments, professional societies, textbooks and research funding. Although some disciplines are involved in practical work, they are disciplines traditionally because of their links with an academic institution. However, this defining of knowledge has come under scrutiny recently, together with the way in which disciplines have been categorised. One definition outlined by Lenoir (1993) encompasses many of the notions inherent in the term 'discipline':

> Disciplines are dynamic structures for assembling, channelling and replicating the social and technical practices essential to the functioning of the political economy and the system of power relations that actualises it.
>
> *(p. 72)*

Both Pierre Bordieu and Michel Foucault (Lenoir 1993), contemporary French theorists concerned with the relationship between knowledge and power, emphasise the way in which disciplines control knowledge and power in society by defining the status of groups and individuals, the distribution of wealth and the continuing production and reproduction of knowledge. Indeed, Michel Foucault understood truth in society as being mediated through certain bodies of practice and their discourses. For nurses this has been particularly evident from the way in which medicine appears to have been granted the role of guru in health care, a situation which, in turn, appears to devalue the role of nursing. Feminist theorists such as Carol Gilligan (1982) argue that this is because the discourse of women has been invisible, dealing as it does with the ordinary everyday things of life such as nurturing, caring, domestic organisation and relationships, to name a few. On the other hand, men have been associated with creating the cultural products—in broad terms, 'society'—concerned with matters of the brain as opposed to the heart.

Since nurses are mainly women and doctors in the past have mainly been men, the parallel for health care discourse is clear. Doctors cure (think) and nurses care (do).

Since discourse is the medium through which disciplines tell (and sell) their stories to the public, it is no wonder that nursing practice has not gained a high profile and registered nurses are not always identified as essential. It is only recently that some medical roles have been identified as able to be done by others (mainly registered nurses) and this has caused the medical professional body to react with some concern. Their reaction involves what has been termed 'boundary work' (Klein 1993, p. 185), which is the set of characteristics that differentiates one discipline from another in terms of types of knowledge, methods and organisation styles. 'Boundary work' occurs when disciplines focus on expanding, monopolising or protecting their professional boundaries in terms of accountability, skills and autonomy, often because another discipline appears to be encroaching on their territory.

Increasingly, however, disciplinary boundaries have begun to blur and in some cases collapse (this has been identified as one of the signs of the 'postmodern' condition). This is particularly so in disciplines and professions that include divergent academic groups and more open epistemological structures, such as the social sciences. But even within the so-called 'hard' sciences there are 'softer' subdisciplines, and vice versa, such as optics in physical science and jurisprudence in law (Klein 1993, p. 188). Nursing has been seriously examining its disciplinary boundaries for the last decade in Australia, although professionally it has been involved in the exercise for much longer under the guise of work practices. As nursing focuses on its boundary work, other disciplines such as medicine, physiotherapy and social work are naturally going to mark out their boundaries even more distinctly and clearly than before. This has the potential to be a very positive situation for consumers of health care, since professional groups are being forced to re-examine their knowledge bases, their practices and their accountability as well as the way they all interact. Such quality reviews are important for all practices but are essential when it comes to the health of society, particularly a society that is as divergent as ours in Australia.

Nursing in Australia is now at a point where its practices and knowledges are being examined, re-examined, reviewed and revised through the diverse range of nursing research undertaken by nurses in graduate nursing programs. Nurses are at last theorising about what it means to 'nurse', what it is like to be a person being 'nursed', what makes up that act we call 'nursing' and is it effective? To do this they are going to the places where nursing takes place—the bedside, the home, the community, the school, the clinic and the village, to name only a few of the places where nurses 'nurse'—and to the ones who know—the nurses, the patients, the people, the clients, the consumers. While nurses have undertaken research in the past, they have not necessarily done it within the discipline of nursing but have approached it through the eyes of other disciplines, such as sociology or psychology. A primary reason for this was a lack of access to graduate nursing programs in this country until very recently. And with this move to the higher education sector, nurses began to see their own practice through others' eyes. To theorise about nursing one needs to enquire through the senses, the sciences and the aesthetics of a nurse. Time to reflect and ponder on the findings of any enquiry is also an essential element prior to theorising.

But 'the pressure for the nurse to act—not to stop and think—is very real' (Wald & Leonard 1986, p. 23). The role of nurses locates them as the cog in the wheel of patient care, since it is the nurses who coordinate and carry out the orders of others, as well as making nursing decisions. This is one of the compounding factors that have retarded theory development in nursing, according to Wald and Leonard. Other factors that have been widely debated include the previously subservient nature of nursing work, the female gender of the major percentage of the nursing workforce, the lack of graduate or postgraduate nursing programs in this country prior to 1985, and the social construction of nursing as an applied and passive discipline (and therefore a 'borrower' of theories rather than a creator).

The notion of being an *applied* discipline rather than the preferred *pure* discipline has been used in a variety of ways to disempower many practices. Traditionally, this disempowerment can be seen in the form of withheld entry to research degrees and reduced funding for research for applied disciplines, thus compounding the view that such practices were not really disciplines. So-called 'real' disciplines were those which historically had rite of passage into universities, were generally accessible only to white, upper and middle class males who, on graduation, received salaries to match their appropriate social status. Such disciplines included medicine and law and were extended to include engineering and even architecture. Of course, there were also the pure disciplines, which made up the cornerstones of traditional universities, and these included philosophy, maths and science. Such knowledges are now referred to as 'source' disciplines, since they are used to draw knowledge for other disciplines.

A good example of this in modern-day universities is accounting, which was originally included as part of business studies but now claims its own discipline (although this would be debated by the very traditional and original disciplines). According to Hoskin and Maeve (1993), accounting is a discipline in a double sense: not only is it a modern form of knowledge but it has also enabled the development of modern business organisation and the academic disciplines, economy and psychology. So gradually the myth of the 'real' discipline (as opposed to those that are merely pretenders) has been debunked, although the trappings remain in many institutions, mainly in the form of expansive and exclusive infrastructures. Standing in the community also remains, in terms of status and preferential treatment, although this is gradually being eroded through structures espousing the principles of equity and access.

A PRACTICE

The practice of a discipline should be guided by its body of knowledge, which has been developed out of research into the practice. It is not necessarily regarded as a profession unless it fulfils the criteria outlined; if it does, then these criteria would guide its actions and its organisation. Some disciplines do not necessarily have a professional practice arm (e.g. philosophy, mathematics and sociology), although each of these disciplines could argue that their knowledge is often applied to solve matters of social concern. Moral philosophy, for example, has been drawn on by bioethicists when debating the ethical dilemmas that occur in health care (often as the result of technological advances), such as in-vitro fertilisation. Sociological theories may be used to think through the way in which change may be facilitated, or to understand changes in social structures—an example is the change in the meaning of what constitutes a family which is currently being debated in Australia.

It seems that there are very few (if any) disciplines which can now claim that they are 'pure', in the sense that they develop knowledge but do not apply it. While the actual producers of the knowledge may not be the ones who develop or apply it, a subdiscipline of the main discipline usually emerges in order to transform the knowledge into a form that can be used in society. These subdisciplines often become established practices with practitioners applying theories from a wide range of disciplines. But in speaking and thinking this way, it appears that what we do is take theory from a pure academic discipline and base our practice on it. This is exactly how society has viewed knowledge development and application in the past, as a linear relationship within a hierarchical framework. Thinkers (academics) pass down the knowing to the doers (practitioners), who then practise according to the word from above. Hence the devaluing of practice and practitioners who rely on the thinkers to develop their knowledge base for them, and who apparently work by rote with little reflection on what it is they do.

Implicit in this understanding of the relationship between theory and practice is an assumption of a static practice base until new theories are developed. But, as nurses certainly know, their practice rarely stays the same, changing as experience and context dictate.

PRACTICE KNOWLEDGE

There has been a growing recognition that the knowledge practitioners use to solve the daily problems of practice comes from a variety of sources, but particularly from their practice. This has been called practical knowledge, practical know-how, personal knowledge and even intuition (Kennedy 1983), and is different from the knowledge gained from books and lectures, which is often identified as 'book knowledge'. More recently, there has been a claim for recognising practice as a discipline in its own right, with its own body of knowledge and unique field of action (Cox, Lumby & White 1995). It has become an important area of research for practice-based disciplines such as medicine and nursing, where researchers are interested in how practitioners develop their body of knowledge from practice. The outcomes of such research have already assisted in identifying the best methods of training future practitioners to think about what they do in their daily work in a way that informs their future practice. Cox et al. (1995) identify two essential requirements if we are to move to a recognition of practice as a discipline in its own right—the development of an **epistemology** (or epistemologies) of practice, and a more disciplined enquiry by the practice disciplines into their activities.

Donald Schön (1983) has perhaps been the most influential thinker in the area of professional action. He blames the worldwide emphasis on technical rationality for the view that the relationship of theory and practice is merely applicative and asserts that, when practising in the real world, the practitioner deals with situations that are far from clear-cut.

Certainly, much of nursing practice is messy with, usually, no clearly identifiable steps to be taken, except in prescribed procedures and protocols. Nursing practice, therefore, defies scientific study in the traditional sense, although this does not mean that research into practice should not be carried out in a scholarly way. What it does mean, however, is that we need to adopt methods which allow for the chaos of practice rather than those which are appropriate only for use in a controllable laboratory. The phenomena nurses deal with daily are multifaceted and wide-ranging; our communications are interactive and often individual; the illness experience is not the same for everyone; our practice is context-driven; and the way in which we satisfy the needs of patients requires a variety of approaches, with the option of changing paths during the process. Rather than taking the knowledge taught in the classroom and applying it in the practice arena, practitioners 'need to know "what to do" with the sick human being in front of them' (Cox et al. 1995).

Patricia Benner (1984), who has researched the practice of nurses in their real world of mess and uncertainty, confirms that clinical knowledge comes from living with the actualities of practice and transforming or refining previously learned theories, rather than applying them directly. She explored the development of expert practice by working with real nurses in their worlds of practice and this is recorded in her now widely cited book, *From Novice to Expert: Excellence and Power in Clinical Nursing Practice.* Benner found that experienced nurses learnt from paradigm cases by recalling past clinical situations when confronted with new but similar situations. She thus showed the way in which experience contributes to a body of clinical knowledge, and urged clinical teachers to use their own personal clinical stories in their teaching sessions in addition to, or as a replacement for, abstract principles. Such teaching relies on the practice of **reflection**, and reflection 'in' and 'on' practice (Schön 1983) has been adopted as a learning process by many nursing programs at both undergraduate and graduate level. The strategy of keeping a reflective diary has been widely adopted, with little critical review of how well it encourages students to adopt a reflective approach. So what is meant by adopting a reflective approach?

REFLECTIVE PRACTICE

Cox, Hickson and Taylor (1992), three nurses involved in an undergraduate nursing program which encouraged students to keep reflective journals, describe the process of reflection:

> The reflective process begins with the capturing of experience as it is lived—a gold mine of raw data, which is recorded so that it can be analysed. It requires writing in great detail about what happened, when, where, who was involved, how the situation unfolded.
>
> *(p. 379)*

Nurse academic Carol Emden (1991) suggests that observation and reflection by practitioners require the ability to think creatively and to be open to new ways of thinking about old ideas, concepts, theories and practices. Educational theorist Paulo Freire (1994), in his recently published text, *Education for Critical Consciousness,* speaks of the fact that human beings relate to the world in a critical and reflective way because they are 'not only *in* the world but *with* the world' (p. 3). He points out the difference between *integration* and *adaptation* where human beings are concerned. Integration takes place when individuals not only adapt to their reality but move towards changing it, whereas adaptation occurs when individuals are controlled by others. Freire's focus in his literacy programs in Brazil was the process of *conscientizacao*, which 'represents the development of the awakening of critical awareness' (p. 18) and ultimately a move to critical action. His aim was not merely to teach people how to read but to help them move to a critical awareness of the roles they played in creating their own culture. This was achieved through 'an active, dialogical, critical and criticism-stimulating method' (p. 45), together with other techniques. This new level of awareness meant that individuals began to imagine and plan how they could act to take control of certain parts of their lives.

This move to a level of critical awareness has also been called **praxis**, because of the level of insight we have developed, enabling us to unite the things we do (our actions) with the knowing that we have accumulated from books and experience (our knowing). In this way we are informed in our actions. Thus we know what we do, and do what we know, which encourages a reflexive (rather than linear) relationship between theory and practice and between thinking and doing. As Wheeler and Chinn (1991) explain when speaking of praxis in their text on feminist process, 'as actions are informed by awareness of values, reasons and ethics, our thinking and our ideas are being shaped and changed by our experience with those actions' (p. 2). This is similar to Freire's notion of praxis as transforming the world, as people reflect and act on the world, and to German philosopher Jurgen Habermas's (1965) notion of praxis as central to human activity.

The terms 'reflective practitioner' and 'critical thinker' are often used as though they are interchangeable. But, while not identical, they maintain a reflexive relationship. After all, to adopt a critical approach to the world, it is necessary to reflect on the world and one's experiences in it. This process includes the knowledge gained from experience (said to be practice-based), from observation (said to be empirical), from formal learning (said to be theoretical) and from being in the world as a participant (**ontological**). Brookfield (1991) says of critical thinking:

> Trying to force people to analyse critically the assumptions under which they have been thinking and living is likely to serve no function other than intimidating them to the point where resistance builds up against this process. We can, however, try to awaken, prompt, nurture and encourage the process without making people feel threatened or patronised.
>
> *(p. 11)*

Reflective practice is part of the process of critical thinking, since the term 'critical' is derived from a Greek word meaning 'to question, to discern, to choose, to evaluate, to make judgement' (Brookfield 1991). This derivation means that critical thinking is a multidimensional cognitive process. Critical thinking requires a skilful interplay between knowledge, experience and evaluation. But interplay in itself entails many parts of an interactive process, including both **incidental** and **sustained regulated reflection**. This interactive process was identified by educational theorist John Dewey (1958) as vital to encourage *sustained regulated enquiry* as part of one's daily practices. Incidental reflections form the embryonic phase, involving the primary experience of meeting gross crude material for the first time. Dewey contrasts this phase with the refined and derived phase of sustained reflection, which occurs through the intervention of systematic thinking. Thus it is important to layer reflections and not to stay merely at the level of incidental reflection.

Michael Polanyi (1975), a philosopher interested in forms of knowledge, asserts that it is by thinking about what we are doing (reflection-in-action) and thinking about what we have done (reflection-on-action) that we acquire skills which are internalised in what he describes as our 'tacit knowing'. It is through this tacit knowing, or intuitive judgement, that we evaluate and appreciate situations, particularly those we have some competence in. Interestingly, the notions of **tacit knowing** or intuitive judgement are undervalued in the scientific world and passed off as invalid, subjective and not to be trusted. As more research into reflective practice, critical thinking and practice-based knowledge is pursued, we are beginning to understand the complexity of this whole area. It is not surprising that it has been neglected, since methods to research such a multidimensional area still need to be developed. So, what has been traditionally viewed as 'soft' research is turning out to be very 'hard' research, requiring complex methodologies and analytical tools.

Identifying the lack of research undertaken into the effectiveness of reflective practice strategies used in education, Smith and Hatton (1993) followed students in a Bachelor of Education degree for three years. Preliminary findings of the study demonstrated that the two strategies identified as being most reflective were:

■   the use of critical friend interviews; and

■   peer group discussion during videotaped micro teaching episodes.

Other issues reinforced in this study include the multiple meanings of reflection, the lack of congruent assessment methods within programs claiming to be using a reflective process, and the influence of historical and sociopolitical contexts on actions. While students in many programs were shown to be reflective, they were reflecting only at the level of descriptive reflection (which is the least complex). Not only do students need to be able to document a particular experience, they also need to be aware of the emotional responses engendered by the activity and, as a result, need to be able to describe the outcomes of reflecting on the experience, such as a new awareness. Reflective practitioners need to take that new awareness and use it in a positive way in their practice. Interestingly, Smith and Hatton also found there were no studies showing that students who engage in reflective activities necessarily become reflective practitioners—usually the aim in practice-based undergraduate programs such as education, medicine and nursing.

This research validated for me the technique I had been using for some time with registered nurses undertaking a postgraduate nursing program. The technique was storytelling, which has many of the elements of critical friend interviews. These elements include capturing the emotions, the thinking, the actions, the mystery, the metaphors of an incident so that it lives for the other person who is the attentive listener. While storytelling is not necessarily used to raise the critical consciousness of another, it is effective when used as a strategy for reflective practice. To take this process further for the storyteller, it is then necessary to pursue critical dialogue with a 'critical friend' or 'critical friends'. These dialogues require the use of criticism-stimulating methods to enable the storytellers to become more critically aware of their past and present situations, and the part they play in those situations (their cultures). It is this critical awareness which opens up the imagination. Since I cannot imagine any other world if I have no insight into or awareness of my present reality.

STORYTELLING AS REFLECTIVE PRACTICE

The art of telling a good story is well documented in many cultures and, indeed, is identified as the main means of communicating the norms, traditions and history of a cultural group. Storytelling can be interpreted and named in many ways. It has been named a 'spatial trajectory' by cultural theorist Michel de Certeau (1984), who suggests that stories cross space and time and connect them in a particular way. Gossip can be seen as a form of storytelling and certainly fulfils many of the functions of storytelling (Fine & Rosnow 1978; Rysman 1977; Spacks 1982). My personal experience of storytelling as a powerful tool and a therapeutic process emerged out of my doctoral work, in which I journeyed with one woman through a life-threatening illness. In order to make meaning of our experience together as women, nurses and mothers, as well as her experience as a woman facing life and death, we told stories to each other and eventually made meaning of those stories through a multilayered technique that we named 'critical conversation'. The method which emerged out of the study illuminated meaning for us both about our lives. And, for the woman herself, the medium of storytelling released her from her experience to become the knower as well as the known. She moved back into her world, knowing she could change her culture if she so desired because she no longer viewed herself as the object of others.

Having trialled many strategies purported to encourage reflective practice, and having been involved in much storytelling with registered nurses, I wondered about the two being linked to encourage a critical reflection on practice. The difficulty was to import informal storytelling into a formal academic setting and to have it accepted as a valid and valuable tool for learning. While nurses are particularly good at telling stories in the tea room, how could storytelling be encouraged among a group of registered nurses who were brought up on the 'case study' and scientific method? Since the unit of study in which this storytelling was to take place was called Advanced Patient Care Management, my aim was for the two groups of advanced practitioners to develop their own models or theories of care out of their collective stories. The group structure chosen for the storytelling was the feminist process described by Charlene Wheeler and Peggy Chinn (1989) in *Peace and Power*. This process has been developed over time and in several countries and cultures, involving groups of women who have come together to communicate their experiences and understandings in an atmosphere of trust.

Each evening that we met as a group, two students would tell a story of care of their own choosing. There were no parameters of time or context except that the story had to be about their work as nurses at some time. Each story took only five minutes at the most and, after the story, the rest of the group chatted with the storytellers about their stories, asking questions and comparing similar incidents. These discussions were always carried out in an environment of support and this encouraged the storytellers to critique their care and talk of how they might have done it differently; this subsequently opened up a forum for debate on the type and level of care. Many situations reflected a oneness of experience which members of the group acknowledged they had not realised, given their different contexts. Within such a group process, for two years storytelling was used to explore and critique each registered nurse's practice.

The process of critical dialogue is difficult for many of us because we rarely involve ourselves at this level. It is understood and applied within the world of fine arts, where the aesthetic part of knowing is demonstrated not only to be credible but also to be valuable and valid. In the act of criticism, those involved engage in a sociopolitical interaction in which a work of art is judged or evaluated. In order to carry this out, it is important to attempt to understand the artist's reality, together with other perspectives necessary at the time. This requires an intuitive grasp of the situation, and a knowledge of the historical, ethical, technical and political perspectives. When integrating the act of criticism into the dialogue following the storytelling, it was necessary to involve empathy for the individual, who was often telling a story of loss, indifference, incompetence, unethical behaviour, emotional abuse and/or intimate feelings. With an art critic, the process is far more removed and not necessarily done within a group, or even face to face with the artist. Thus, the critical dialogue used in this student group was approached sensitively.

Increasingly, individuals and the group learned to work with critical dialogue in a way that was constructive and transforming. Each week the stories told were transcribed for reflection and authentication by the storyteller. The written word provided another level of awareness for the storytellers, many of whom expressed amazement when they saw their story in print. 'Did I really say that?' was the usual response.

THEORY FROM REFLECTIVE PRACTICE

The next hurdle was working through the dilemma of generating a theory out of the stories of practice. Theory development has been seen, traditionally, as the work of academics, and theories are developed over long periods of time with the ultimate testing done 'in the field' to see if they match the reality. But the explosion of literature in eclectic ways of knowing, and the acknowledgement of practical knowing as valid and important for the development of theories, have opened up new possibilities. The other part of the equation was the use of storytelling as a tool for gathering data. What was to be said about that?

Orthodox science has given scant regard to the expression of experience, and certainly storytelling as a method of research has been seen as 'subjective' and, therefore, 'soft data' (presumably not real knowledge or truth). The one area of practice in which storytelling has developed credibility is psychotherapy, perhaps because it grew out of medicine and scientific enquiry.

While storytelling has been used in such a positive way for centuries for the transfer of information and knowledge in many cultures, such as Aboriginal Dreamtime and Micronesian Navigators, it is interesting to note that, within the Western world, written knowledge has been valued above oral knowledge. This may have been because of the way in which written knowledge can be accumulated and added to rather than changed. So we have developed the notions of knowledge as accumulative rather than available for sharing, critique and debate, and even for making meaning of our world and our lives.

Within the world of literature, the oral narrative has been recognised as the truth, because it is more lifelike and thus has a plausibility which scientific truth lacks. In discussing the oral narrative, Echartsberg (1981) explains this through the concepts of denotative and connotative thinking. Denotative thinking involves explanations, while connotative thinking involves emotion, expression and intuition. Thus connotative thinking is related more to the world of the Arts, and denotative thinking to the world of Science. Together, they form a coherent picture of the whole when discussing certain truths or knowledges. Educational researchers Reason and Hawkins (1988) discovered the multidimensional aspect of using storytelling as enquiry—it can be used to explain or express, to analyse or to understand. In this way, it crosses methodologies and unites participants. Storytelling enables the meaning of experience to be brought forth, since in telling the story we partake of the experience rather than standing back and analysing it, as is done in experimental or observational methods.

One of the frameworks used in therapy for women who have been abused is that being developed by psychotherapist Michael White (cited in Kamsler 1990), which incorporates the notion of retelling the dominant story so that another story emerges, offering an alternative perspective for the storyteller. This is also known as 're-authoring' and enables the individual to step outside the story and see it differently. White's approach involves the understanding that problems become consolidated for individuals when they are restrained from taking alternative courses. This position places individuals in the position of continuing the dominant story which is 'problem-saturated'. It also creates a situation in which people are blind to alternative solutions or explanations, and often continue to respond in inappropriate ways well into adulthood.

From my experience, storytelling also appears to work particularly well as a method of encouraging nurses to adopt a critical reflective approach to their practice. This may be explained by the fact that they have been exposed (through storytelling) to a level of awareness which enables them to make sense of the context in which they work, and this heightened awareness remains with them as they move back into their environments and see them with new eyes. Nurses who have been involved with me in storytelling have spoken of, and written to me about, the change in the way they approach their practice. This is understandable when we consider the way in which nursing is embedded in stories that are full of descriptions of emotions and sensations which remain with us subconsciously and are brought forward when we encounter them again.

It appears that rich description is stored in the right brain and facts are stored in the left brain; this means that our stories enable us to add to our theoretical knowledge the personal knowledge that can only develop out of experience. Nurses listen to patients' stories throughout their care; they document some of those stories in order to plan care, and the chapters that do not lend themselves to written medicalised notes are often transferred orally to other nurses, in order to ensure continuity of care in a very individualised way. They 'hand over' through a critical dialogue, where they tell and retell the stories of patients and their families to ensure the best care based on the most relevant information, some of which cannot be written down because of confidentiality.

While the process of storytelling in itself was enjoyable, illuminating and at times quite demanding, I believed it was important that the stories and the experience were able to inform future practice. For this reason, I proposed to bring the stories together in a way that might be meaningful, without destroying the richness and individuality of each story. It was decided to use the stories to provide a grounded construct for the development and publication of a model of advanced patient care which reflected the collective experience of the group. This was done at the end of the semester when the storytelling was over. Student evaluations of the process of storytelling at this time showed that one of the most important outcomes was the recognition by participants that what they were doing in their daily nursing work was contributing to the practice and culture of health care in that context. One participant said: 'I had no idea that I made such a difference in a person's life.' Another commented on the fact that she had never realised the importance of her contribution in the ward where she worked.

In this way, participants had already developed a reflective consciousness about individual and collective nursing practice, as demonstrated by their remarks both during the semester and at the end.

The next step was to attempt to develop a model or theory of advanced nursing care out of the stories. This was intended to reflect the collective awareness of the participants. Students were asked to identify one or two main concepts or themes which stood out in their story and to bring those to the final session of the semester. The final session was the one in which we mapped the concepts of care that arose for this particular group of advanced nurse practitioners. The steps we took included:

- negotiation of the kind of language used to describe the concepts;
- negotiation of the categories of concepts; and
- negotiation of the way in which the concepts made meaning within the model of practice.

Concepts in this context included ideas, images and phrases which came out of the stories and which represented meanings. An example might be those times when the stories spoke of relating to another, experiencing conflict, standing up for another, or even the debate between curing and caring. Because these concepts had been expressed using different phrasing in different stories, we needed to gather them together to identify the likenesses and differences and so form categories, as a beginning way of sorting them out. We also needed to find the most appropriate language to use when describing them.

This method has been called 'collaborative research', a term congruent with the reciprocal nature of our group relationship and the intent of the process. **Collaborative theorising** involves moving forward from the *articulation* of what we know to *theorising* about what we know (and for registered nurses in practice this step is vital if they are to move back to practice with a critically reflective focus). In this way, we developed a model of care which made sense for us as a group and may illuminate the practice of others. Certainly, the models of the two years of storytelling were very similar in the concepts that came forward.

The final step was to involve participants in the authentication of the final document, thus giving them ownership of the text. This step is essential if the group and/or individuals are to remain the authors of their stories.

The transcripts offered a wonderfully rich tapestry of stories of care, as well as insight into the dominant discourse of science which has overpowered many nurses in the past and rendered them without speech. To add to the meaning of our stories, a further layer was added. A research assistant who had graduated with an honours degree in communication was asked to look at the transcripts and identify themes which told the story of nursing from the 'outsider's' view. This added another perspective to that of the 'inside' view of the group who owned the stories as a collective whole. The nurses could then move back into practice with a model of care which was the collective wisdom of their group. Students had also been offered other perspectives about their practice which encouraged the development of a critical consciousness when approaching future nursing care. In this way, their knowing and doing might be linked through praxis.

A MODEL OF ADVANCED NURSING CARE

The model of care that was developed by the two groups emerged from linked themes/concepts and was illustrated by a modified concept map. The advantage of designing the model using a concept map was that it provided a flexible map that would enable others to identify their practice through the concepts, even though they may perceive their reality as differently linked. The themes/concepts used as the basis for the concept map are listed in the box below.

Example

Identified themes/concepts

1 Relationship between the nurse, the individual and the family.*
2 Advocacy for the individual being nursed.
3 Understanding and focusing on the individual, not the disease.
4 Doing 'with' not doing 'to'.
5 Developing insights into how the person 'is in the world'.
6 Personal satisfaction by 'seeing it through' with the person.
7 Conflict due to role confusion (care versus cure), leading to frustration, anger, guilt and questioning of practice/s.

*'family' in this text is not prescriptive and includes all those who are an important part of the world of the person being cared for

---

USING CONCEPT MAPPING AS A PROCESS

These concepts were then linked by phrases in an attempt to make meaning of the concept of 'advanced nursing care', a term used quite often without clarification. The students were all working at what they believed was an 'advanced level of practice'. This was exemplified by their stories, their analysis and their insights into the outcomes of their care. Construction of a concept map was seen as the ideal time to clarify the advanced care they had spoken of when telling their story. Advanced nursing care involved the specific behaviours, feelings and attitudes that were emerging from their knowledge and experience as registered nurses, combined with their life knowledge of being in the world.

The concept map placed Advanced Nursing Care as its central focus. The map began with the development of a relationship between nurse and patient/family in which the nurse played an advocacy role which entailed understanding and focusing on the individual, not the disease. This understanding and focusing developed out of a sense of 'being with', not 'doing to', and this enabled the nurse to develop insights into the patient's world. There were two potential outcomes as a result of this type of care and the stressors and structures that often worked against it. The first, and ideal, outcome was *personal satisfaction* for the nurse by 'seeing it through' with the patient and family. Very often, however, the outcome was *conflict* due to role confusion (often because of conflict of foci), which led to frustration, anger, guilt and questioning about the practice itself. Conflict often leads to advanced nurse practitioners leaving nursing.

By mapping their world of work, the registered nurses involved were able to identify more clearly the positive and negative aspects of their role. They were then able to move to a level of critical consciousness concerning the negotiation of their world in order to make it a more positive working environment.

THE SUBTEXT OF THE STORIES OF CARE

The texts of the stories were then searched for underlying themes from an 'outsider' viewpoint. The themes and subthemes that were identified are shown in the box below. They were then illustrated by reference to one or more sections of the stories. When the stories were produced within the final text the anonymity of nurses and patients was ensured.

Example

Themes from the stories of care

1 The myth of the good nurse.
2 Overcoming ingrained (trained) concepts of the 'good' nurse.
3 The team relationship and the issue of accountability.
4 Questioning roles in the nurse–doctor relationship: a conflict of models?
5 Care versus cure: ethical dimensions of nursing practice?

Subthemes

Patient advocacy

Including the family

Seeing the person in the patient

Coming to terms with death

Cultural context and nursing practice

Finally, the model became a tangible outcome for participants which they could carry forward into practice. Many of them commented on how it made them more aware of the person in the bed and of their colleagues, as well as of their personal value as a practitioner. This parallels White's comments (cited in Kamsler 1990) about the externalisation of the problem from the person that occurs through storytelling:

> From this new perspective persons are able to locate 'facts' about their lives and relationships that could not even be dimly perceived in the problem-saturated account . . . facts that provided the nuclei for the generation of new stories.

The comments also demonstrated that individuals in the group had developed a critical awareness of the way in which they contributed to the creation of the health care culture in which they were involved. Positioning themselves as *subjects* who could transform society, rather than *objects* who are manipulated, is a very important step for a professional group such as nurses, who appear to have passively adapted to the social construction of themselves as objects.

SUMMARY

This chapter provides a real-life example of the way in which nurses are able to generate theory out of their everyday practices by a process of critical reflection. Storytelling is only one of many ways in which this process can be done and is already being done. It is a positive process in which individuals gain an understanding of themselves as nurses, and of the similarities and differences in practices across contexts. Central issues of concern provide bonding elements when discussed in groups which provide a trusting environment.

Other issues raised in this chapter, such as the differences between a profession, a discipline and a practice, should provide a framework in which to place your own reflective practice.

GLOSSARY

Collaborative theorising: theorising (developing a theory or making sense of something) with a group of individuals rather than alone. Implicit in this is the notion of theorising in a way which involves everybody and not just a few more dominant members of the group.

Discourse: a 'series of utterances, speech or conversation' (Concise Oxford Dictionary, Clarendon Press). The modern philosopher, Foucault, used the term 'discourse' in a wider sense to encompass the political and social environment in which the speech was being made. This is the sense in which the term is often used in academic writings. As Foucault (1984) said, 'It is in discourse that power and knowledge are joined together'.

Epistemology: 'Enquiry into the nature and ground of experience, belief and knowledge' (Lacey 1986).

Incidental reflection: reflecting or thinking about an event once. It is a glance at what happened rather than a prolonged or critical examination.

Ontological: Ontology is the study of being and, in particular, what there is—for example, material objects, minds, persons (Lacey 1986). Originally the notion of an ontological argument in philosophy was an argument for God's existence. Any argument can be called ontological when it shows how the relationship of certain things in certain ways ensures the real existence of something. Ontology is a central part of metaphysics and borders on the philosophy of religion.

Praxis: This term has been defined in many ways. The transformational educationalist Paulo Freire (1972) states that praxis is 'reflection and action upon the world in order to transform it'. Meanwhile, Aristotle defines the term as 'those sciences and activities concerned with knowing for its own sake' (cited by Pearson 1988, p. 210).

Reflection: is a way of thinking about and looking at something. In reflection as a process one is able to look back to an image which has gone before and think about it in a new way. The image can be an incident which has occurred or a painting, a story, a conversation or even a piece of music.

Sustained regulated reflection: the process of thinking about an event over a prolonged period of time after the incidental reflection. During sustained reflection it is possible to move to another level of heightened awareness because of the layering which occurs as a result of thinking about something over a long period of time.

Tacit knowing: a knowing which is implicit, embedded or assumed because of the world one lives in personally or professionally—for example, knowing that the sun comes up and goes down each day (in certain countries). It involves the knowing that occurs incidentally rather than that gained through formal or informal learning. This type of knowing is also called intuitive or practical knowledge.

QUESTIONS

1 How could you go about identifying a theory for your practice?

2 What strategies could you put in place in your practice which would encourage an attitude of critical reflection?

3 Do you think that nursing is identified as a profession? If not, why not? If so, what criteria is it measured by?

4 What are the advantages and disadvantages of being identified as a discipline?

LEARNING ACTIVITY

Use this chapter as a preparation for a workshop session. You should:

(a) read the chapter;

(b) reflect on your experience as either a nurse/student/patient/daughter/woman/son/father or other relevant person;

(c) come to the workshop prepared to tell a story approximately five minutes long which describes your experience and relates some of your reactions to this experience;

(d) break into small groups of 3–4 and relate the stories to each other. Each member of the group should take part in the storytelling;

(e) take time after each story for the group to provide positive feedback to the storyteller; and

(f) reconvene into the large group and relate what it was like to reflect on an experience and to share it with others in a small group.

FURTHER READING

Deveson, A. 1991, *Tell Me I'm Here*, Penguin, Ringwood, Victoria.

15

FEMINISM FOR NURSING

JAN HORSFALL

LEARNING OBJECTIVES

When you have read this chapter, and some additional material, you should be able to:

1 Articulate an understanding of general feminist principles.

2 Develop a personal position on the relevance of feminist theories to one aspect of nursing.

3 Define power, oppression and gender.

Jan Horsfall, RPN, BA (Hons), MA (Hons), PhD, has been Associate Professor of Nursing in the Faculty of Nursing, University of Sydney since February 1994. Jan has qualifications in mental health nursing and has an undergraduate major and Masters degree in Sociology. She gained a doctoral degree in Women's Studies in 1995.

INTRODUCTION

The aim of this chapter is to introduce you to principles and practices that are important within feminisms. In the first half of the chapter I outline these, and endeavour to explain the circumstances of nurses in the context of power inequalities in the workplace. Having established the conceptual foundations relevant to consciousness-raising, and the connections between the political and the personal, I draw on feminist ideas and processes and relate them to some aspects of clinical nursing, education in nursing and nursing researches.

WHAT ARE FEMINISMS?

Before you can discuss any aspect of feminism, every person included in the discussion needs to be aware of every other person's definition of feminism. Just as the word 'nurse' has a different meaning for different people, including registered nurses, so, too, 'feminism' has different meanings even for those who consider themselves to be feminists.

If students in a classroom do not declare their understanding of the word 'feminism', a conversation may occur without anyone necessarily understanding anyone else. It is essential to establish some definition, yet problematic because of the diversities likely to emerge. Even though there are different feminisms, most feminisms overlap to some extent.

Shulamit Reinharz has written a comprehensive text entitled *Feminist Methods in Social Research* (1992) and she faces the issue of definition early in her book. She records a few brief understandings of feminism articulated by a small group of American Christian feminist theologians in discussion with each other. These include the validation of experience, reclaiming women's personal power, the inclusion of diversity, mutual support and caring, establishing equal rights for women and men, and struggling against sexism. One woman participant declared that 'it doesn't have anything to do with women; it's the commitment to end white supremacy, male domination, economic exploitation' (Reinharz 1992, p. 6). The fact that these women are united by Christian and feminist ideologies, yet can articulate such a range of possibilities, indicates the breadth of the term even from the perspectives of those who describe themselves as feminists.

Feminism is not alone in being unable to state one incontrovertible definition which applies to its own knowledges. How does one define art? For some people art is associated with beauty, others equate it with ideas. Is it possible to draw a definitive line between art and crafts, art and architecture, or art and cultural artefacts?

Where have young adults gleaned their beginning understandings of feminisms from? As a sociologist as well as a nurse, I assume that ideas about feminism have derived from family members, newspapers, television, school teachers and others. When you see the term printed in the media, is the message simple or complex? When you hear the word spoken is it associated with positive or negative overtones, strong or mild emotions?

Many students bring antagonistic preconceptions to bear on the term 'feminism', rather than personal introspection or thoughtful reading. Educationally this is difficult, because views on feminism are often imbued with negative stereotyping of feminists (as people, and of their purported ideas) and/or fears about women and their place in our society. Often, before feminisms can be discussed seriously, the people involved in the discussion need to demystify stereotypes in an attempt to begin to pass through such unidimensional positions. Similarly, emotions such as fear and hostility may require working through before a rational exchange of ideas can take place in the classroom or elsewhere. As a consequence of this, it is usually impossible to explore feminist ideas, theories or perspectives in one two-hour tutorial session.

In the next section of this chapter I will provide a brief overview of common feminist criticisms of mainstream thinking across academic disciplines.

FEMINIST CRITICISMS

First, feminist theorists frequently question the notion that there is one truth (Flax 1992). Second, feminists and other thinkers have come to recognise that many academic disciplines are underpinned by assumptions which are not declared. These assumptions then determine the nature of the objects of enquiry in that discipline, the type of questions asked, the exclusion of certain methods or ways of interpreting information. Such assumptions derive from the fact that the people who developed today's established academic disciplines were European men who came from the economically privileged class, and wrote in particular historical periods when specific ideologies were considered to be of interest.

For example, in the discipline of philosophy, Descartes' 17th-century recognition that 'I think, therefore I am' (see Lloyd 1984) cannot be relocated into the second half of the 20th century as an acceptable interpretation of the way contemporary human beings function. Descartes was an esteemed thinker before he made this pronouncement, his work embedded, even then, in an established discipline. He was a European man. An oriental philosopher would have been unlikely to focus on cognition as a significant determinant of the (supposedly universal) human condition. Descartes spent the latter part of his life in Protestant Holland after the Reformation. Christianity was a powerful force in people's lives and intensely held Protestant belief systems were spread throughout north-west Europe.

All of these socially structured circumstances, as well as others, provide a context in which Descartes' ideas could be articulated and published, and become important in ensuing centuries. This analysis does not deny the truth of his experience but it allows the contemporary critic to examine and analyse these theoretical positions from historical, anthropological, gender, political, economic, religious and other perspectives.

Feminists are particularly interested in the relationships between gender and the belief systems and interests of given disciplines but gender issues often overlap with political, economic and social factors. Feminists may be suspicious of a belief in 'one' truth, or the notion that 'human nature' is universal and singular, or that human qualities, especially those relating to sexual differences, are simply biological rather than the outcome of complex interactions between bodily process and social practices.

Third, because the close study of many disciplines has unearthed the importance of contextual factors on the development of knowledges, some feminists believe that writers and speakers should declare their social positioning. To adhere to this principle, I would say that I am a middle class, Anglo-Australian woman nurse academic of a certain age and sexual orientation. My ideas could be evaluated by taking such information into account and my approach could be seen to be intellectually honest. For some readers, though, this may fuel pre-existing stereotypes, and the ideas I express may not be considered because of the sexist perception that they are 'only written by a woman', or because of anti-intellectual prejudices where 'academics can only think about things, they can't do anything'.

Fourth, as well as being sceptical of universal truth claims, scrutinising texts for undeclared assumptions, and placing writers in their social context, feminists commonly do not consider language to be neutral. At a simple level this is evident in the formal use, over many centuries, of the term 'man' to mean human being. Defenders of this tradition may claim that 'man' is inclusive and means woman as well. Given that—from a grammatical perspective—'woman' has never included man, it seems that some assumptions about gender superiority and inferiority are revealed by the fact that 'woman' has been subsumed by 'man' in many languages.

Jane Flax discusses the significance of language in the following way.

> Each of us is born into an ongoing set of language games that we must learn in order to be understood by and to understand others. Since human beings are 'speaking animals' our personhood is (at least partially) constructed by language. Language speaks us as much as we speak it.
>
> *(Flax 1992, p. 453)*

From this perspective, words are not merely words; they are the medium whereby we exchange and develop knowledges. They constitute part of the social transactions whereby we gain a sense of our self and of those we are communicating with.

A fifth feminist criticism of mainstream belief systems is the separation of theory from practice. As well as taking up critical perspectives and questioning what is given or assumed, feminists also put forward various ideas and are involved in diverse activities. In the next section I will outline some characteristics of feminist projects.

CONTEMPORARY FEMINIST THEORETICAL CONSIDERATIONS

In the 1960s, feminist theorists directed much attention to disciplines which demeaned or omitted women from their discourse. At that stage the primary objectives were to critique negative representations, ideas and assumptions about women, as well as the inclusion of women where they had been excluded (Gross 1986, p. 190). The ultimate aim of these projects was to develop economic and political equality for women, like that available to men as a group, in the domains of law, social security, health and well-being (Allan 1993, pp. 1548–50).

As Elizabeth Gross points out, this orientation 'meant that women's *sameness to men*, only women's *humanity* and not their *womanliness* could be discussed' (1986, p. 191). Consequently, the general directions of feminism moved away from hypothetical and technical equality, towards the rights of women to determine their social, political, economic and intellectual interests (Gross 1986, p. 193).

After close scrutiny of a range of disciplines by women academics and researchers within those disciplines, it became increasingly clear that some knowledges are **androcentric** (see Emden 1995, p. 30)—that is, they could only have been developed by people whose lives excluded women's experiences of work, personhood, family life and reproduction. Western knowledges are in part produced as a consequence of the taken-for-granted political and social status quo. This recognition has meant that many feminist thinkers were working at the **epistemological** level, that is, they were investigating how we know what we know. Feminist projects then included the possibility of women as producers of legitimate knowledges, in the same way that European men had been the unquestioned producers of knowledges in all disciplines for centuries.

These directions indicate that 'feminist theory changed both the content and the frameworks of discourses, disciplines and institutions, attempting to present alternatives . . .' (Gross 1986, p. 194). The audacity of these projects partially explains why some established academics and researchers feel threatened and are hostile towards the questions, the ideas and the women who put them forward.

FEMINIST PRINCIPLES

In this section I will discuss five principles that many feminists aim to adhere to in theoretical and practical works. A common first principle for feminist enquirers, writers and researchers is to acknowledge their own assumptions. This is considered desirable in that mainstream theory and research are built on an infrastructure of assumptions or premises which traditionally have not been declared in an attempt to appear 'objective'. One false assumption behind the notion of objectivity is that no person or organisation is going to benefit more than others. This assumption depends on the belief that everybody in our society is politically and socially equal to all others (see Benhabib 1990, p. 123).

A second principle which feminist projects are likely to articulate is that knowledges emerge from interactions between the subject (writer) and object (person, things, processes studied). Furthermore, knowledge does not emanate from the solitary expert knower but from dialogues between the writer or researcher and others with an interest in the particular field. This is in stark contrast to the idea that a scientist can understand, observe or measure a phenomenon under study—especially sentient beings—without influencing the situation in any way. Such wishful thinking relates to ideas developed around the study of distant and/or apparently inanimate objects which have then been transferred to the study of both humans and animals in various disciplines.

Third, feminist projects are oriented towards the contributions of theory to practice and the contributions of practice to theory. Neither domain is conceived as being superior to the other. The separation of the two into apparently discrete domains is understood to be artificial and is implicated in the distance of past grand theories in all disciplines from the concrete practical experiences of ordinary women and men.

This problem of the separation of superior abstract theory from the inferior concrete detail of people's lives is also challenged by the fourth feminist principle of acknowledging women's lived experiences as valid starting points for critique, theory, research or political action. Such a position is a critique of the notion that reason is untouched by the bodily, social and emotional components of human existence. This belief in **transcendental reason** is particularly androcentric in the discipline of philosophy, where women (if they were acknowledged) were associated with the body, the emotions and other factors that impeded the thinker's capacity to think. The belief that philosophers and scientists can wilfully stand apart from their feelings and life circumstances is commonly questioned by feminists. Feminists consider all theorists to be embodied persons, who work in specific locations in particular historical periods.

An important aspect of the life circumstances of writers and researchers is their value system. Political values can often be discerned when theories are read closely. A fifth feminist principle relates to the recognition that the world view directly or indirectly expressed by economists, nurses, psychologists or biologists will depend on their basic assumptions about people and the proper state of the world. Theorists who endorse hierarchies of power and inequalities will only propose theories that reinforce or strengthen such tendencies. Theorists who believe that men are superior to women and/or should be superior to women will (intentionally or unintentionally) carry out intellectual work that will not contradict or question such a position.

Such beliefs, and the value systems in which they are embedded, are not simple ideas that individuals have plucked from the air; they are, rather, facets of an **ideological hegemony**. Aafke Komter (1991) identifies three characteristics of ideological hegemony: the ideas are 'part of everyday thought'; the belief systems are 'organising' or systematic; and the ideas intrinsic to this hegemony are 'experienced as general interests' rather than viewpoints which bolster dominant groups (p. 58). Ideologies are sets of ideas that are often intertwined and the fact that they are hegemonic means that they commonly prevail over other, minority or socially inferior ideas. Many ideas and beliefs articulated within our society (especially those we have not reflected on as adults) are part of mainstream, or hegemonic, ideologies which pass as the commonsense view of the world.

The notion of ideological hegemony changes the level of argument from that of individual beliefs to that of socially structured belief systems. The concept of ideological hegemony also challenges mainstream assumptions about free thinking individuals and highlights **unequal power structures** in our society.

POWER

Power is a concept and a social reality. Perhaps because most contemporary societies depend on power inequalities—capitalist/communist, 'developed'/'developing', occidental/oriental—many people, including nurses, have difficulty in acknowledging this state of affairs and enquiring into these complexities. Power is a key issue which feminists as individuals and as groups of women have addressed in relation to practice and everyday life as well as theory and the exploration of ideas.

In our society, power commonly has negative connotations. This is not inevitable; power can be positive, negative or even both in the same instance. Power can be used positively for social justice purposes; or power can be used negatively for personal greed; it can also become negative when powerful emotions are not expressed in constructive ways. Feminists often describe examples of power used negatively as 'power over others', as opposed to the more positive possibilities of 'power with others' or 'power for others'.

Peter Bachrach and Morton Baratz propose the following definition of power.

> A power relationship exists when (a) there is a conflict over values or course of action between A and B; (b) B complies with A's wishes; and (c) B does so because he [sic] is fearful that A will deprive him of a value or values which he regards more highly than those which would have been achieved by noncompliance.
>
> *(Bachrach & Baratz 1970, p. 24)*

This definition shows that power is relational—that is, power is exercised and made manifest between people, rather than simply residing within one person no matter what he or she does. It is also an example of the negative use of power, or one person's use of power over or against another person.

When negative power is invoked it depends on the person wielding the power having access, or believed access, to sanctions. Sanctions may be positive or negative. Person B may force compliance by offering a reward, or removing an impediment, or by threatening a punishment or the removal of something positive. Presumably A's fear indicates that A believes that B has the capacity to offer the negative or positive sanction and that B is capable of doing so. Rewards or penalties may be specific or vague, and they may be available now or in the future. Negative power use may be underpinned by the potential for violence: from harassment to persecution, to psychological undermining, to emotional manipulation, to racist or sexist abuse, to unwanted sexual comments, propositions or actions, or from symbolic violence to overt physical aggression.

The main problem with this model of power, even though most people can recognise it as valid, is that power is only conceived of as being enacted between two individuals. Often, when this situation does occur, person B's capacity to wield power negatively derives from a structured power advantage. B may be a boss or supervisor and A an employee, or lower in the occupational hierarchy; B may have higher status than A; B may be an adult and A a child; B may be providing a necessary service to A; B may be wealthier and have greater access to significant people and resources in comparison to A.

A situation in which one person uses power negatively over another person may appear to be an interaction between two individuals. It may, in fact, be one actor embedded in structures of power advantage intimidating another actor who does not have equal access to power. In such a situation, power can be more fruitfully understood as the structured advantage of one group over another group. These actors do not commonly see themselves as part of a collective or group, but feel themselves to be two individuals in a 'power over' situation.

STRUCTURED INEQUALITIES

The structured inequalities that feminists focus on particularly are those relating to gender—that is, the power advantages which males in general have over females in general, in our society. This is a feminist interest which many men find disturbing, possibly because it might mean that women will gain a more incisive understanding of male behaviours, or resist the traditional forms of gendered power that men wield over women. Some women find the feminist interest in power disturbing, perhaps because they believe they are benefiting from male patronage or benevolence in the home or in the workplace.

To be of use as a conceptual analytical tool, structured power inequalities need to be understood as systematic and often invisible (Hartsock 1990, p. 168). Such systematic inequalities overlap in almost all the situations that could be analysed. Patriarchal powers may coincide with class, race, age, wealth, professional status, political influence, bureaucratic power and/or higher education. In certain circumstances, some of these structurally unequal systems of power work in concert with each other but in others some aspects of structured power will be working in different directions.

It is necessary to focus on structured inequality in order to try to explain the position and behaviours of women (and others) as subordinated groups of people. Subordinated means 'belonging to an inferior rank, grade, class, or order, and hence dependent upon the authority or power of another' (Shorter Oxford English Dictionary 1992). In order to explain structured power inequalities, Jean Baker Miller begins with 'permanent inequality' (1991, p. 6), which is ascribed or evident at birth. Such a position is a social given and precedes the birth of the person born into that category. The common criteria by which such statuses are determined are race and gender. In many societies, class, caste, religion and nationality are conditions into which one is born and from which one cannot readily extricate oneself.

Miller's use of the notion of 'permanent' inequality is virtually the same as my use of the term 'structured' inequality. From my perspective, the fact that such inequalities are structured, systematic or predetermined is essential to understanding the tenacity, irrationality and longevity of these processes. The term 'structured' also seems preferable, in relation to gender and ethnicity in particular, because it allows for the possibility of positive change and diminishes the sense of hopelessness that can be associated with the term 'permanent'.

Structured inequality has diverse and profound consequences for the social, political, economic, spiritual, practical, emotional and intellectual future of those born into the category designated as inferior. These **macro social factors** may even contribute to characteristics which mainstream individualistic psychology describes as 'personality', or which psychiatry may call 'personality disorders'.

CHARACTERISTICS COMMON IN MEMBERS OF SUBORDINATED GROUPS

The first and most significant point Miller makes about the lives of subordinated people is that they have to deal with basic personal or family survival issues (1991, p. 9) in an ongoing way in their daily lives. In our society, this means that some such people may have to expend energies to prevent their own homelessness. Others may be in financial jeopardy because of unemployment, part-time employment, very low rates of pay or because a pension or benefit is insufficient to cover their individual or family necessities.

The second characteristic of subordinated groups is their attendance to the needs of others. By virtue of living in circumstances that are structured by inequalities from childhood, subordinated groups study those who are dominant in order to accommodate to their demands, or even to anticipate them. Miller makes the following comment:

> Here . . . is where the long story of 'feminine intuition' and 'feminine wiles' begins. It seems clear that these 'mysterious' gifts are, in fact, skills, developed through long practice, in reading many small signals, both verbal and non-verbal.
>
> *(Miller 1991, p. 10)*

A third characteristic discussed by Miller is that some members of the subordinated group model their behaviours on those displayed by the dominating groups (p. 11). This results in layers of hierarchical domination and subordination in some social settings. Another consequence of this may be the conditional acceptance by the dominants of a specific individual member of the dominated group; and in this situation the individual may collude with the dominant group against other subordinated people. These processes are part of divide-and-conquer dynamics set up by the dominating groups. The conditionally accepted individual often gains, or is promised, personal privileges and breaks ranks with the rest of the subordinated group.

The fourth characteristic is that subordinates frequently absorb, believe and perpetuate the negative stereotypical myths about themselves that originate from within the dominant belief system (Miller 1991, p. 11). There are indigenous people who feel inferior to colonising peoples, and women who actually believe they are, by definition, less important than men. These negative stereotypes are often long-lived and include ideas such as women being incapable of administering large budgets, or being unable to make 'hard' decisions. When these myths are believed, they can even become truths in some instances, when subordinated people continue to support the known oppressive status quo because speaking out is risky and freedom is unknown and fearful (Hedin 1986, p. 54).

This commonly means that subordinated people cannot discern or name their own positive attributes, let alone recognise excellence. Consequently, oppressed people often undervalue themselves and their peers (in line with the dominants) and denigrate their skills or positive attributes. A more extreme example is hatred of self and others like oneself. Barbara Hedin says that these behaviours reveal that many members of subordinated groups 'house the oppressor within' (1986, p. 55) and abet their own oppression and that of others.

Resentments felt by subordinated people towards the dominating group are frequently expressed indirectly. Direct and honest responses may actually be dangerous, or believed to be dangerous, for subordinated people. Jokes, cautionary tales and personal anecdotes about bettering, or deceiving, a person from the dominant group often circulate in back rooms or other spaces where subordinated people can gather in safety without being seen or heard by any member of the dominant group.

IS THIS RELEVANT TO NURSING STUDENTS?

The account of feminist interests and principles, and the explorations of power relations between structurally unequal groups that I have set out in the first half of this chapter may, or may not, be meaningful to undergraduate nurse readers. As a nurse academic, I could hope that feminisms are unnecessary because all women and men are politically, economically and practically equal. I could hope that the disciplines we study are not androcentric, Eurocentric or ahistorical, and that theorists, teachers and practitioners are all aware of their assumptions about people and the world and have clarified their values, which are conducive to the well-being of readers, students and consumers. From my own perspective, we are still continuing to raise our awareness of these significant issues and only beginning to address them.

As preregistration students, you will assess these circumstances by virtue of the values acted out in your family, your particular life experiences of oppression and autonomy and the sophistication of the education in your high school, and by other conscious and unconscious criteria. Undergraduate nurses in the second half of the nursing program will have had opportunities to ascertain the level of sexism in academia, the commitment to medical or scientific values as opposed to nursing values in the curriculum, the level of supportiveness of clinical teachers and the hospital milieux.

Registered nurses studying in undergraduate or postgraduate programs bring extensive experience as nurses to their studies; they commonly recognise the unequal power dynamics and can relate to the descriptions and explications of oppressed group behaviours. Expert registered nurses often discuss clinical and personal constraints to the provision of caring nursing in their diverse workplaces at the present time. Recent nurse graduates may experience 'reality shock' with regard to patient care and interprofessional dynamics in hospitals; sometimes they perceive two nursing cultures, the older and the new, in the one clinical setting.

Inevitably, you must make up your own mind about the usefulness of these ideas and insights for yourself as a person and a nurse. From my own experience of listening to nursing students in the academic setting in the last decade, it seems that undergraduate students and registered nurses can experience undue professional difficulties in relation to client care and as nurses in the workplace. At least some of these problems and constraints are related to structural inequalities in hospitals and other health care settings.

Janice Thompson (1987) presents arguments in support of the relevance of feminism and critical theory, in the form of 'critical scholarship', for the discipline of nursing. She points out that nurses step into 'social structures and practices that are inherited as externally imposed sources of domination' (p. 31). This position indicates that structured inequalities precede the arrival of recent nurse graduates or new employees. Such a situation is like Miller's account of 'permanent inequality', where the individuals are born into pre-existing structures and have an inferior designation before their arrival. As hierarchies and dominating practices have tendencies to perpetuate themselves and the people they disadvantage, structural change requires collective action and perseverance by groups over a lengthy time frame.

CONSCIOUSNESS-RAISING

Feminist projects often involve the crucial processes of group consciousness-raising. If constructive changes are required, those involved need to name the problems and struggle to explain the mechanisms which cause or sustain the impediments to change. Julianne Cheek and Trudy Rudge (1994) argue for consciousness-raising processes that do not fall prey to the individualisation of nursing difficulties. Processes that seek answers within one person may further disempower the comparatively powerless by supporting the myth that if they understand the situation they should be able to change it by themselves.

It is at this juncture that the feminist drive for a unity of theory and practice becomes patently clear. Nurses may aim to improve patient care, or to create a workplace in which both nurses and consumers have their rights as people enshrined in practice. However, to achieve such practical aims, the nurses who endorse these ideals need first to look to their own experiences and their own feelings and think critically about strategies and barriers.

One of the first phases of critical thinking involves 'rupturing' or 'unraveling . . . layers of assumption and belief' (Thompson 1987, p. 36). This self-reflective process is likely to be circular, in that an awareness of our own assumptions is not self-evident in the first instance. Exploring assumptions and values precedes the capacity to declare our assumptions, and in some circumstances begins a mind-opening process that allows challenging material to be read, heard and understood.

Raphella Sohier (1992) states that the potential for change in nursing can be 'initiated by rejecting patriarchal definitions of life's purpose and meaning, as well as the social mythology that presents women with second-class roles' (p. 65). By making such a claim, she is indicating a belief that gender, and women's place in nursing and health care generally, is a key issue and that hegemonic ideologies permeate nursing. Androcentric ideals and orientations are not necessarily those most conducive to high quality nursing practice or consumer well-being.

A number of feminist writers have suggested that people go through phases in relation to embracing new knowledges and in the processes of consciousness-raising; these are highly likely to be interconnected. Katherine Heinrich and Barbara Witt (1993) observe that their students (most of the nurses taking their course on feminism and nursing are women) first identify 'the desire to understand, to connect' with new knowledges. Second, they strive to understand their experiences by reading about and discussing the lives of others. The third phase is that of judgement: after analysis and reflection, the course participants arrived at a conclusion or an 'expanded standpoint or perspective' (Heinrich & Witt 1993, p. 119).

Heinrich and Witt also note that group consciousness-raising is often understood as a process which develops through phases. They begin with acceptance of the status quo in relation to gender, followed by ambivalence about gendered roles. The new awareness often evokes anger in nurses who experience abuse of power by men (or by women in positions of authority) in their daily professional and/or personal lives; this stage is followed by nurses determining what their insights mean in relation to changes they can make, given their situation.

Consciousness-raising may be an essential ingredient in nurses' increased capacity to integrate 'tacit' and 'explicit' knowledges. Phyllis Schultz and Afaf Meleis (1988) consider that 'knowing the self, knowing that [explicit knowledge] and knowing how [tacit knowledge]—are the sum of what one knows. All three are brought to the caring situation' (p. 218). They suggest that nurses' ways of knowing may be similar to those revealed in Belenky et al.'s study of women's ways of knowing. Accordingly, the most complex form of knowing is evident when learners 'view all knowledge as contextual, experience themselves as creators of knowledge, and value both subjective and objective strategies . . . [and believe that] the knower is an intimate part of the known' (Schultz & Meleis 1988, p. 219).

Consciousness-raising involves a number of the feminist principles presented in the first sections of this chapter. Practice and theory are interrelated in nursing as in life in general. The processes of consciousness-raising involve feminist principles, in that personal values are explored and our own assumptions and those behind stereotypes are recognised and named. Nurses' experiences in private and professional life become starting points for the revaluing of intuitive knowledge and recognising the hegemonic devaluing of these ways of knowing in our society. Such processes implicitly challenge notions of objectivity, the separation of the private domain from the public, and the possibility that theories or ideas may have nothing to do with the practical realities of embodied people in their daily lives.

THE PERSONAL, THE POLITICAL, THE POSSIBLE

Cheek and Rudge (1994) argue for consciousness-raising to deal explicitly with structures of oppression, and Carolyn Emden (1995) notes that the discipline of nursing has been more interested in the 'cultural' aspects of feminism at the expense of 'structural' components (p. 30). These observations are correct from my perspective; however, I believe that the politicisation of nurses *en masse* in Australia remains at a tentative and early stage. For this reason I wish to support any constructive changes nurses are able to make at the personal or professional level, whether they be interpersonal or structural, ephemeral or long-term. Purposeful action is empowering.

Nurses—women and men—are embedded in complex interconnected structures of subtle and gross constraints. These factors and their longevity indicate that Miller's (1991) point about survival is relevant. Nurses by and large are dependent on the State for employment and are therefore not yet easily able to stand up for patients' rights or their own professional or personal rights when negative structural powers are brought to bear on a situation. Nurses also work closely, sometimes in an hour-by-hour proximity, with the medical profession who, as a group, have comparatively easy access to state policy-makers and the administrative and financial elite within hospitals. These realities make it difficult for nurses to initiate and sustain personal or professional change in the workplace. Our struggle for survival as individuals and as a group is essential for ourselves and our work and must not be rendered invisible or diminished by those of us who would target only major changes.

CLINICAL NURSING KNOWLEDGE AND FEMINISM

As feminisms have drawn on women's lived experience as the starting point for theory, Schultz and Meleis (1988) have located the self of the nurse as the foundation of knowing and caring. This indicates that consciousness-raising has much potential value for nurses as people and as professionals who work with patients. Personal knowledge requires understanding at the structural level and personal awareness is a prerequisite for the nurse's therapeutic use of self in client care. When the self of the nurse is a therapeutic facet of nursing practice, then taken-for-granted understandings of nursing clinical knowledges and the discipline of nursing may be questioned.

Expert clinical nursing knowledge is not supported by ideological hegemony, it is not merely an appendage of medical knowledge, it is not striving only for objectivity, it is not something that anybody (especially a woman) can do—even though some people may still make such claims in the 1990s. Nursing knowledges, like women's knowledges and the knowledges of colonised peoples, do not have mainstream claims to legitimacy in the way that biological knowledges, medical knowledges and economic knowledges do. Devalued or suppressed nursing knowledges benefit from the reclamation of clinical theory and practice in ways similar to those whereby feminist and post-colonial writings have benefited women's and indigenous people's knowledges.

The complexity of clinical nursing knowledges is partly addressed by Schultz and Meleis in the following account.

> Historically, clinical knowledge has been the product of a combination of personal knowing and empirics . . . Intuition and subjective knowledge are regaining their legitimacy as necessary components of humane care. The aesthetic and ethical patterns of knowing are also contributing to the development of clinical knowledge.
>
> *(Schultz & Meleis 1988, p. 219)*

They rightly point out that published accounts of clinical nursing knowledge often reflect 'received' or 'procedural' knowledges. Nurses have usually been too busy nursing even to document the subtleties of their practice. In other words, the experiential expertise of nurses resembles more the oral traditions of indigenous peoples, or the complex knowledges of women about birthing, child-raising and 'folk' medicine handed down through generations within our cultures until comparatively recent times.

'Clinical knowledge is manifested primarily in the acts of the practicing nurse; it is individual and personal' (Schultz & Meleis 1988, p. 219). Clinical nursing is personal from the perspective of the nurse and it is also personal from the perspective of the patient. This position questions prevailing beliefs about what nursing is, and displaces the discipline from one that hinges on techniques and technicalities to one that can be understood to be interactive in a multiplicity of ways. Such a reconceived discipline of nursing may allow nurses to apprehend patients and health as concepts and realities in ways that challenge traditional definitions.

CLINICAL NURSING, FEMINISM AND SELF

Feminist groups commonly aim to establish an egalitarian and caring framework and processes to benefit the group as a whole and support individuals with particular needs. Beverley Hall and Janet Allan (1994), by virtue of practising as nurses in a non-hierarchical and caring environment, have come to redefine clinical nursing. 'We have . . . identified the core of nursing practice as helping clients to fully use their sense of self as they cope with whatever changes they are finding in their physical, psychologic, spiritual, and social worlds' (Hall & Allan 1994, p. 111). This stunningly simple definition of clinical nursing, like many distilled ideas and practices, required a complex struggle on behalf of practitioners. They describe the processes as 'transformational' and note with irony that they had written about, and taught, nursing from a holistic perspective. However, actually relinquishing power over clients, along with the traditional focus on disease, required personal resources of an intellectual, emotional, reflective and political nature.

Hall and Allan (1994) state that, according to their philosophy of nursing care, 'there is a lack of separation between healer and client' (p. 111). This unity is similar to the unity of subject and object that I outlined as the second feminist principle earlier in the chapter. From my reading of Hall and Allan, they are not proposing a messy merging of two people in a romantic or sexual way but the sense of unity invokes emotionally mature nurses who can empathise with clients in distress, and who know what pain belongs to them and what emanates from the client.

Their definition of clinical nursing indicates that the health practices of the nurse are as important as those of the client. Such a unity of health and person for the nurse has not been endorsed by traditional nursing discourses, wherein the health of the nurse is invisible and considered to be irrelevant to client well-being. Their perception of health depends on the centrality of 'self in relation' to other people (Hall & Allan 1994, p. 110), and this is as pertinent for the nurse as it is for the consumer.

Hall and Allan 'conceptualise nursing practice as occurring within the client's worlds, not the professional world' (1994, p. 110). This perspective also surmounts the subject–object split by understanding nursing as truly patient-centred, rather than disease-centred, 'treatment'-centred, medical diagnosis-centred or nurse-centred. In this view, the clients are considered to be the ultimate source of healing possibilities, and experts on themselves and the difficulties being experienced (see Horsfall 1993). Feminist and client-centred therapies also begin from the premise that clients have the potential for growth and positive change, and that the therapist aims to facilitate these processes.

The nursing care and health of the client are not the only issues here. The understanding of ourselves as nurses is implicated. 'Patients facilitate the development of nursing expertise just as nurses assist the development of patient health and healing knowledges and skills' (Horsfall 1995, p. 6). Nurses become experts because clients teach us to be, if we take heed.

This demolition of the purported subject–object divisions in our society is furthered when the nurse 'forms a picture of self by shifting her or his energies back and forth between the self and the other' (Hall & Allan 1994, p. 114). In this instance, the person of the nurse evolves out of her or his interactivity and effectiveness in relation to clients. Inadequate nursing care has ramifications not only for patient well-being but for the well-being and sense of competence of the nurse.

To put this into a practical context, Hall and Allan (1994) point out that the social structuring of health care organisations does impede, and often prevents, the possibility of holistic nursing care. 'In these impoverished environments, the focus is not on caring so much as on establishing a relationship with the patient for the purpose of administering the medical treatment' (p. 115). From this perspective, nursing could be experienced by some patients as disempowering (Horsfall 1993) rather than therapeutic.

Instead of being agents of social control, nurses could re-view themselves as having interests in common with patients. Again, Hall and Allan put this into perspective.

> There is often a maze of power struggles between administrators and health professionals who hold different ideologies and engage in competitive behaviour that is gender based and discipline based and that is alienating to nurses and clients, who are often the ones with the least power.
>
> *(Hall & Allan 1994, p. 115)*

This indicates that the quality of clinical nursing care is often, ultimately, not dependent on the nurse and consumer but is contingent on hospital organisational structures. Feminist consciousness-raising encourages the growth of self on the one hand but never denies the actual social and political constraints to action and constructive change on the other. By accounting for both the microsocial and macrosocial factors, feminist processes aim to stop people from being blamed inappropriately for what is done to them. This means that individual nurses need to understand that their effectiveness and capacity to provide quality care can be impeded by structural forces beyond the realistic influence of the individual nurse alone.

Feminist interests, criticisms and principles can contribute to the theorising of nurses at the microsocial level of care and intersubjectivity. They can also enhance the ability of nurses to locate their practice in a complex but comprehensible macrosocial political, professional and organisational context. These awarenesses, when processed and internalised by nurses, are capable of having both a subtle and an overt impact on nursing care and patient well-being, as well as offering a less individualistic understanding of the limits to contemporary nursing practice.

In this section of the chapter I have argued that clinical nursing practice can benefit from the incorporation of feminist insights and the use of feminist principles. The clinical nurse begins with the lived experiences of the client and the nurse. The nurse and the client are both embodied people, not diseases or automatons. Nursing practice contains subjective and intuitive elements which are at least as valuable as objective and technical elements. Much healing emerges from the interactive and interpersonal realm and this implicates the value systems of both the patient and the nurse. This indicates a unity of subject and object and ultimately a unity of 'tacit' and 'explicit' knowledges, emotion and techniques.

FEMINISM IN THE CLASSROOM

Feminist principles are good educational principles. This is probably related to the fact that 1960s feminisms emerged out of women's political and practical struggles to face a world in which many felt that Western stereotypes of femininity were a more comprehensive version of the old Chinese custom of binding girls' feet. Endeavouring to understand the world in which we live, and to ascertain how to take steps to change devolves on group and individual empowerment and is educational, political and personal.

The feminist principles that I particularly endorse for educational benefits are those that engage the value systems of the learners–teachers. Values held by all parties ultimately impinge on classroom processes as much as bedside interactions. Similarly, clear communication is essential in both settings and this sometimes requires the use of basic strategies, such as appropriate language, multiple media (e.g. spoken, written, experiential, demonstration activities) and clarifying messages, and giving feedback to speaker and listener. Sometimes these processes lead back to the feminist principle of acknowledging assumptions and expectations in educational and therapeutic interactions. Both situations must be interactive if they are to be effective. As has been shown in earlier sections of this chapter, feminists have had a lengthy interest in, and commitment to, the centrality of interactivity to facilitate constructive change, whether it is related to health, learning or personal growth. This understanding of interactivity extends to the unity of teaching and learning, thinking and doing, and theory and practice, in both educational settings and those focused on health or sickness.

The positions I proposed in the section on feminist criticisms are also relevant to learning and teaching. The recognition that language is not neutral is an essential ingredient from both teaching and learning perspectives. If education is understood to be related to the development of skills for enquiry and the capacity to formulate a reasoned argument, then the refusal to accept information at face value is a central educational, and feminist, principle. By virtue of classroom discussions and reading different texts, the feminist position that there is no one truth becomes increasingly important for learning. (This does not deny the fact that in some clinical situations, once the nurse has verified certain danger signs, the emergency nursing response, at that juncture, is not debatable.)

The feminist principle that lived experiences are the starting point for theory could apply to nursing students as consumers of educational courses. If this were so, then courses should be student-centred and should begin where the group of students is— intellectually, emotionally and practically—at that specific point in time in the classroom. One step prior to this (which is not necessarily a facet of academic lore) is that the teacher must consider the students to be competent people with the capacity to learn, grow and become nurses (nurses being incredibly diverse). A shorthand expression of this is to work with students as adults (Horsfall 1990, pp. 7–14), as whole people and as active participants in their own learning by virtue of their lived experience. When educational processes are not open and respectful, then the 'hidden curriculum' conveys negative messages to students (Hedin 1987, p. 268) about what it means to be a nurse, an academic, a teacher, a person of influence, a professional in a position of authority.

Teaching and learning nursing in the classroom and clinical setting in a three-year degree program is not a simple matter for any participant. When writing an earlier paper, I aimed to find out what nurses said nurses do. Nurses may act as:

> caregivers; change agents; client advocates; comforters; communicators; consultants; decision-makers; ethical practitioners; family practitioners; financial administrators; health promoters; leaders; managers of client care; networkers; personnel managers; political lobbyists; primary prevention workers; quality assurance agents; rehabilitators; teachers.
>
> *(Horsfall 1990, p. 2)*

Such expectations, even when viewed as long-term goals, are awesome (Horsfall 1990, p. 4), from the perspective of both teachers and learners. However, my own position remains that, as teachers, we are still not especially successful in our endeavours to prepare students 'to the best of our collective capabilities, for the social, political and economic realities of nursing within the health industry' (Horsfall 1990, p. 6). If one of our imperatives is to relate ideas and models to practice, and vice versa, then these exigencies cannot be ignored.

When faced with such complex and changing futures, it is necessary to broach power issues—and these have certainly been of central interest to feminists. Nursing is crisscrossed by powered structures and interactions within organisational settings such as hospitals, universities and community or area health divisions. Power inequalities also permeate the classroom.

> As teachers we are [commonly] older than the students we teach, we have experiences as RNs, we have power in relation to passing and failing. We may be more educated, more intelligent and more self-confident. If we are not, some combination of those factors often results in the negative use of power over students—an abuse of our privileged positions.
>
> *(Horsfall 1992, p. 11)*

To deal with these realities, 'power differences between teacher and student should be owned, clarified and used constructively for student ends' (Horsfall 1992, p. 9). The positive future of the nursing profession requires empowered student nurses.

This, of course, does not mean that all recourse to power lies in the hands of academics. Like teachers, students have the capacity to wield positive or negative powers within the constraints of the particular rules, regulations and decision-making structures. Unfortunately, when students use power negatively it is often other students who are most affected, inside and outside the classroom, and students may need to develop skills collectively to manage these situations constructively.

FEMINIST CONTRIBUTIONS TO NURSING RESEARCH

As power permeates settings in which nurses practice and is implicated in the teaching of nursing, and even though its effects had been rendered invisible in research, it is now on the nursing research agenda, too. June Lowenberg (1993), in a discussion of methodologies, notes three major shifts in interpretive research directions. Highlighting life experiences and socially constructed realities is the first new direction; the second brings the interactivity of the researcher and the researched into focus and asks the researcher to reflect on his or her taken-for-granted assumptions (p. 63). The third change she discerns is 'the emphasis on the location of the researcher in relation to other participants in terms of power and status inequities' (Lowenberg 1993, p. 63). Lowenberg notes a fourth change whereby research is increasingly interdisciplinary (p. 64); sometimes in nursing this is not simply a team approach, but within the person of one nurse, several disciplinary knowledges are drawn on to extend the research insights. She considers that these influences partially derive from feminist critiques.

Dorothy Henderson (1995) begins with a similar concern: 'nursing practice and research that are grounded in emancipatory inquiry challenge the inequalities and injustices that affect health in this society' (p. 58). She articulates five distinguishing qualities of research (deriving from feminist and other critical theories) that are oriented towards effective social change (see King 1994, p. 21)—the participants are involved in the research from the planning stage until the end; experiential knowledge is valued; the research focuses on power relations and the empowerment of participants; consciousness-raising is the preferred method; and the goal is social action or change (Henderson 1995, pp. 61–2). In nursing practice this approach would require patients, potential clients, health educators and nurses to be research participants who would facilitate changes for the improvement of consumer health and well-being.

Judy Catalano (1994) focuses on factors that may contribute to increased nurse empowerment. If nurses collectively do not feel empowered in the clinical setting, it seems reasonable to begin with nurses. She takes up Gorman and Clark's 'empowerment framework', which outlines four categories of strategies fundamental to the development of nurse power in the practice setting:

1 using analytical nursing skills to promote 'organisational problem solving';

2 engaging nurses in change initiation;

3 strengthening collegiality; and

4 extending administrative 'sponsorship' or mentorship.

(Catalano 1994, p. 18)

In her research, Catalano then develops 10 teacher activities for each of the four categories. She found that, among the 104 nurse academics she surveyed, the majority of whom taught in clinical and classroom settings, there were two domains in which potentially empowering teaching activities were radically underused. These were the strategies that targeted nurse-initiated change, and the use of managerial mentorship and support (Catalano 1994, p. 185). This indicates that nurse students (undergraduate and postgraduate) are sometimes not being prepared with adequate skills and knowledge, nor an understanding of the necessary organisational supports that would enable them to manage change, rather than responding to imposed changes in the clinical setting.

Research studies such as those carried out by Catalano and Henderson (to give only two examples) have only emerged in the discipline of nursing during the last 10 years. Catalano's research into nurse academics' ability to use a range of teaching strategies to prepare graduates for the exigencies of power in the workplace is fruitful, in that educators may now explore these knowledge and practice domains and incorporate new approaches into teaching and curricula. Nurses in management positions can also reflect on their knowledge and strategies, and the circumstances in which certain approaches are likely, or unlikely, to be effective. As nurse clinicians' knowledge often resides within experiential and oral traditions, this could also be the case for nurse managers, who may then benefit from further research in these areas.

Henderson's research is powerful in different ways. She briefly documents some of the challenges that emerged when nine women—four residents in a drug treatment program, three staff women, the nurse researcher and a social work student—met to plan a women-only program. The small group was clearly a diverse mixture and crossed class, professional and ethnic divisions, as well as including both drug dependent and non-dependent experiences (Henderson 1995, p. 65). After meeting weekly for eight months, these women were able to work cohesively and respectfully and establish a woman-centred space in the treatment centre, and all participants gained from these feminist consciousness-raising processes. This research involved reflection and action with the aim of improving the health of drug-dependent women. The reflection revealed the social, political and economic factors implicated in their present health status; the actions were taken by individuals and the group to change these societal impediments (Henderson 1995, p. 67).

SUMMARY

In this chapter I have aimed to set out some key feminist principles. To be consistent with contemporary feminist viewpoints, I have chosen to speak of principles and knowledges rather than theories. My selection of feminist interests does not simply revolve around gender. Factors such as class, race and gender do not work in isolation but have intersecting effects on all people in our society. Consequently, a discussion of feminism in relation to nursing must take other structured power relations into account.

Even though 92 per cent of practising nurses are women, the impact of hierarchical structures in hospitals is likely to be similar for female and male nurses. Similarly, the ability of nurses to carry out effective nursing care often depends on the benevolence, or lack thereof, of the medical profession, which has the capacity to dominate and oppress nurses by virtue of ready access to formal and informal negative sanctions in the workplace and at the level of policy-making.

The feminist principles I have outlined are those which I believe are useful for nurses. As most feminisms begin with women's lived experience, so, too, the discipline of nursing should benefit from investigating the lived experiences of nurses and consumers, clarifying the assumptions and values that each party brings to the interactive processes of nursing care, health maintenance and healing. By articulating our 'tacit' and 'explicit' knowledges, we can continue to revalue our nursing knowledges for the benefit of the profession, patients and the well-being of society. An equally important issue for nurses is the fact that we need time to reflect on the structures that impede our practice, to put our individual frustrations into perspective, and to develop personal and group strategies via education or research to facilitate constructive changes.

GLOSSARY

Androcentric: this includes *andro*, a Greek root that means 'man' or 'male'. Androcentric therefore means male-centred.

Epistemology: comes from the Greek root for 'knowledge'. Epistemology relates to the grounds on which knowledge is based. At the present time many philosophers are questioning the foundations of ways of knowing and recognise that Western philosophy derives from European cultural assumptions. Feminist philosophers show that these cultural assumptions are not only Eurocentric but androcentric.

Ideological hegemony: ideology signifies a comparatively unified system of thought, beliefs and attitudes. Marxist use of the term indicates that ideologies support the vested political and economic interests of the ruling elite. Hegemony comes from the Greek word that means 'capable of command' and derives from the root meaning leader or chief. Consequently this word relates to the predominance of one State or leader. Ideological hegemony refers to predominant or mainstream belief systems.

Macrosocial factors: are those which derive from 'big' social forces in society. These are the subject matter of sociology. They include class, gender, ethnicity and institutionalised religion. Macrosocial factors affect microsocial groupings such as families, peers and neighbourhoods.

Transcendental reason: indicates a belief that some types of thinking are unrelated to the person who does the reasoning or thinking. Another term that has a similar meaning is 'absolute reason' which conveys the impression that there are some forms of thinking which are not affected by the social context in which they take place or are promoted.

Unequal power structures: refer to macrosocial structures, such as class or ethnicity, that create substantial differences in access to justice, health, autonomy or education—that is, to power—between specific groups in a given society.

QUESTIONS

1 The 'hidden curriculum' consists of the messages/perceptions you gain as students about nursing and nurses that are conveyed to you in classrooms, clinical settings and via the media, but are not part of the formal learning of nursing per se. What negative information have you taken up in this way? Attempt to explain why this occurs and how the processes may undermine future generations of nurses.

2 Which feminist principles do you consider to be most relevant to (a) teaching nursing students; (b) clinical nursing practice; and (c) nursing research?

3 What do you think are the personal/professional survival issues faced by registered nurses in hospital settings? Draw on Miller's explication of oppression and personal characteristics to explain some self-defeating nursing behaviours.

LEARNING ACTIVITY

Closely observe a registered nurse attending to a patient/s in a clinical setting for a short time, then interview the nurse about what she or he was doing, how and why. Explain the differences between what you thought occurred and what the nurse says she or he did, by applying the concepts of tacit and explicit knowledge.

FURTHER READING

Hall, B. & Allan, J. 1994, 'Self in relation: A prolegomenon for holistic nursing', *Nursing Outlook*, 15, pp. 110–16. This documentation of the authors' own holistic nursing work with HIV-infected clients in a consumer-based, health-oriented setting is inspiring.

Miller, J. Baker 1991, *Towards a New Psychology of Women*, Penguin, London. This is a very readable explanation of the connections between personal characteristics and the consequences of long-term experiences of oppressive social structures.

Reinharz, S. 1992, *Feminist Methods in Social Research*, Oxford University Press, New York. This is also easily understood, as well as being a comprehensive compilation of a diverse range of qualitative research approaches which the researcher considers to be feminist.

Schultz, P. & Meleis, A. 1988, 'Nursing epistemology: Traditions, insights, questions', *Image: Journal of Nursing Scholarship*, 20(4), pp. 217–21. This article is a good introduction to nurses' ways of knowing.

Sohier, R. 1992, 'Feminism and nursing knowledge: The power of the weak', *Nursing Outlook*, 40 (2), pp. 62–6. This article is an excellent introduction to concepts of social structure, feminism and holistic nursing.

16

NURSING THEORY
Whose Interests are Being Served?

SANDRA SPEEDY AND STEPHEN KERMODE

The authors wish to thank discourse participants Bev Taylor, Claire Brown, Nancy Emmanuel, Virginia King and Greg Gover for providing a nursing practitioner perspective.

LEARNING OBJECTIVES

When you have read this chapter you should be able to:

1 Discuss the nature and value of theory. *formal discussion*

2 Analyse some of the issues in the debate surrounding the relationship of theory to practice.

3 Identify a number of the political subtexts to the theory debate in nursing.

4 Describe the influence of paradigm debates on the theory discourse in nursing.

5 Explain the consequences *result importance.* of rejecting 'grand theory' in favour of a pluralist approach to theory discourse. *speak or write formally and at length*

most than one of this form.

Sandra Speedy, RN, BA (Hons), DipEd, MURP, EdD, is Professor and Dean of the Faculty of Health Sciences at Southern Cross University. Her research interests include women's health and the role of women in management.

Stephen Kermode, RN, BA, MHPEd, PhD, is Associate Professor of Nursing at Southern Cross University. His research interests include quality of life, quality of care and alternative health practices and professionalisation.

Bev Taylor, RN, RM, AssocDipNurseEd, BEd, GradDipEdAdmin, MEd, PhD, is Foundation Chair of Nursing at the Centre for Nursing and Health Care Practices, Faculty of Health Sciences, Southern Cross University. Her research interests lie in all areas of nursing, health and natural therapies.

Claire Brown, BA, MGenStud, is a lecturer in sociology in the Centre for Nursing and Health Care Practices, Southern Cross University. Her research interests focus on gender issues and, in particular, how these affect the shape of the health care system. Her research also focuses on the evaluation of programs offered by health service providers. She is currently engaged in research on men in nursing.

Nancy Emmanuel, RN, AssocDipNurseEd, BA, MEdAdmin, commenced her nursing studies at the Repatriation General Hospital, Concord, in the early 1960s. She has worked in a variety of acute settings and in aged care. She has been teaching since 1978 and returned to study in 1979. She is currently undertaking doctoral studies researching nursing assessment.

Virginia King, RN, RM, BA, MNA, spent 19 years in clinical nursing and midwifery positions before beginning an academic career in 1989. Her interest in theory and the theory of nursing stems from teaching is the foundation of nursing subjects which are offered in both pre- and post-registration nursing programs at Southern Cross University. She also teaches in health service management and midwifery units offered externally in Masters programs, where students are encouraged to uncover the theoretical bases of their professional practice. Her current research interests include NANDA nursing diagnoses and reflective practice paradigms.

Greg Gover, RN, BHSc (Nsg), Crit CareCert, works in the Intensive Care Unit at Lismore Base Hospital, and also holds a joint appointment in the Centre for Nursing and Health Care Practices, Southern Cross University. His research interests include pain management, emergency care protocol and sleep issues in intensive care units.

INTRODUCTION

This chapter provides you with the opportunity to observe a process of discursive critique which examined a particular issue related to nursing theory. The major question debated by six members of a group was: Whose interests are being served by nursing theory? The chapter begins with a description of the methodology and proceeds to examine the major themes arising from the debate. These included:

- defining what is meant by theory and nursing theory;
- examining the utility of nursing theory from the practitioners' and academics' viewpoint; and
- providing a pluralist view of nursing theory.

The chapter concludes with a summary and a postscript from participants, reflecting their views of the process and its outcome.

METHODOLOGY AND PROCESS

A small group of academics met for a total of six hours to consider and discuss the question, 'Nursing theory: Whose interests are being served?' The group comprised five nurse academics and a health sociologist. The combined total of nursing experience in academia was 79 years; combined clinical nursing experience was 103 years.

The process involved four stages.

1   The first stage comprised a taped dialogue between the participants on the topic, the focus of which was critical, scholarly and interesting. There were three two-hour sessions of debate. This dialogue was transcribed and edited.

2   The second stage consisted of examining the transcript to identify prominent themes and salient issues. These were then grouped and, drawing on the nursing and practice literature to demonstrate the validity of the claims made, were discussed in a narrative format, while supporting quotations from the dialogue were identified.

3   The third stage involved participants in critiquing the outcome and providing a brief personal transcript of their perception of this process.

4   The fourth stage involved a **critique** of the paper by a clinician who is a joint appointee—that is, a practising clinician who is also partly employed by the university to undertake clinical supervision of students, and who has an additional research role at the university.

There was an overall perspective which provided a framework for the task. The two major questions guiding debate were:

▨   *Whose interests are served by nursing theory?*

▨   *Who are the stakeholders in nursing theory?*

The question of 'whose interests are served by nursing theory?' is taken directly from the work of Habermas and subsequently Kemmis (1985). It seeks to identify who derives most benefit from the study and understanding of nursing theory. Reference to the stakeholders in nursing theory seeks to determine whether nurse academics, administrators, researchers, clinicians or patients derive most benefit from the study of nursing theory. The general consensus in this work is that patients (or clients) are the least likely to benefit from this thing called nursing theory. The next level of impact appears to be clinicians, as evidenced from the authors' experiences and from the literature.

In summary, this chapter is an attempt to understand the nature of the Nursing Theory **discourse** in terms of who might benefit from the development and continuance of the discourse. It attempts to identify the outcomes from the discourse in relationship to those who are involved in the discourse. More importantly, it was suggested that there is a tacit acceptance of this discourse in nursing literature without adequate criticisms in respect of the direction it may be taking us, or the extent to which it may represent little more than canonical dogma. Moreover, there is some evidence that nurses in clinical practice do not find the Nursing Theory discourse of particular relevance to them.

Broad questions which were used to focus the dialogue are listed below.

▨   Where did nursing theory come from, and why?

▨   What do nurses think theory is, and why?

▨   Does theory arise out of practice?

▨   Do practitioners/clinicians consciously use theory?

▨   Are theoretical concepts misapplied?

one of the things to be selected

- Are there <u>alternatives</u> to the biomedical model?

- What is the future of nursing theory?

- What evidence is there of nursing theory serving a purpose, from the point of view of nurses, patients, doctors, managers and any other relevant people involved in the health care delivery system?

The group agreed to a series of 'rules' for this process. These included:

- faithfulness to the method (outlined above);

- faithfulness to the question (whose <u>interests</u> are being <u>served</u>?);

    good manner

- basic <u>courtesies</u> of respect and listening;

- attempts to achieve equality of input opportunities; and

    name used instead of one's own

- the use of <u>pseudonyms</u> in-text.

Generally, these rules were adhered to, and participants will address the process and other issues in their <u>postscripts</u>.

The chapter proceeds to present <u>extracts</u> from the discourse which <u>exemplify</u> the major themes of the discourse. Each major theme is then discussed with <u>reference</u> to available literature in order to clarify and strengthen the theme. The major themes are:

1 positioning the discourse

2 the utility of theory

3 the <u>politics</u> of theory

4 a <u>pluralist</u> view of nursing theory.

more than one

POSITIONING THE DISCOURSE

Kim: There's been a lot written on what theory is and what theory isn't and I think part of the issue with nursing is that we are still trying to come to terms with what theory in nursing is. From my point of view, I don't see a lot of evidence that we are working towards resolution of that issue.

Jo: I think we haven't actually addressed the basic question, what is theory? What is it supposed to achieve? I'll just start up with what I believe theory is. I think theory attempts to make <u>universal</u> statements about certain things and if it can be shown that in one case it's not true, it's no longer a theory. So it has this sort of generalisability and universality that <u>transcends</u> every case and, because we've seen it like that, we've tended to go for a certain paradigm that would give us that sort of knowledge. Because we've made a shift from empirical, analytical knowledge into other forms of knowledge, it's really hard to say, well, is this still theory?

Kim: Nursing is having difficulty, in my view, in moving beyond describing or trying to describe into the <u>realm</u> of explanatory theory and I think that's part of the problem. I think where we're getting bogged down is we are preoccupied with the paradigm issues rather than the theory issues. I think paradigms are useful to provide the structure in which theory fits, but if it's not then going to help us deal with those issues of solving the problems that nursing is dealing with—and by problems I mean health problems—I think we are really wasting a lot of time and energy dealing with the paradigm issues, rather than the theoretical issues.

Rick: I think that this ties right back to one of the questions we posed. Is it related to the inability to define ourselves? Is the obsession with theory part of lack of identity and does it tie back into constantly looking for what is nursing?

Lyn: Why nursing theory at all? I think one view might be that there are a few scholars, in America basically, who really need to promote this mission, goal and vision of what they could do for nursing and so on, and theory is the way to go for them. But, it could be asked whether they are doing it to justify their existence or whether they really have this fantasy, or goal, vision, that nursing could only be developed with a theoretical basis because that's what developed disciplines do. I'm not sure they do—because, medicine, what theory has medicine?

Kim: Well, I think that's interesting, because what you are talking about then is a field of medicine and I think what you lapse into is the whole paradigm debate. Medicine has a wealth of theory, although predominantly set in one paradigm—a biomedical one. Take the example of cancer. There are two broad theories of cancer causation. One is the cellular transformation theory, the other one is the failed immuno-response theory. Both of these theories provide useful ways of explaining and predicting the phenomenon of cancer. Now, in my view, that is where the level of theoretical knowledge in nursing does not exist— the theoretical knowledge embedded in the question: How do we address this health problem and how do we explain, understand and deal with this health problem? To me, nursing is not far enough down this track. It is more preoccupied with defining itself.

Rick: And nursing is still trying to work out what nursing is, rather than what nursing can do.

Chris: I think that what we are saying is that it's necessary to have a theoretical base to what we do, but the scholarly body of literature that has come to be known as nursing theory isn't the way to go. And I agree with that.

Kim: That's exactly what I'm saying. The literature we associate with so-called 'Nursing Theory' is not, in my view, advancing the practice of nursing because it's not addressing the question: How do we best solve the problems that nurses deal with? And really I'm saying what Kuhn is saying and I know he said it in a sense of paradigms—its ability to solve the problem is what gives it power. Well, ask the question, 'Which theories are the most powerful theories?' In my view, the ones which best help us solve the most important problems are the most powerful theories. Nursing is preoccupied with dealing with paradigm issues, in my view, and has left data out of its deliberations. And I think that's where we've got to ask: What problems are we dealing with? How do we best deal with these problems? And what theoretical knowledge or understanding allows us to do that?

Almost none of the published material relating to Nursing Theory has done anything to advance the understanding of the vast majority of practising nurses about the activity they call 'nursing'. The **theory** discourse has probably had more to do with nurses trying to pursue their professional ambitions, and their ambitions as stakeholders in the world of science, than anything else. The quest for an identifiable body of knowledge which nursing can claim as its own has been as much a political exercise as it has been an academic exercise and the '. . . pursuit of nursing theory has been intertwined with the pursuit of professional status and the pursuit of control over work' (Kermode 1993, p. 105).

Nursing has struggled to understand the nature of its discipline because it has struggled to understand its place in the world. There are fundamental problems for nurses in how they see themselves as participants in the workplace and as members of a broader sociopolitical environment. Many of these issues derive from the politics of gender and many derive from nurses being primarily wage employees in large bureaucracies. Nursing literature is littered with pleas by nurses for other nurses to reconsider, reconceptualise, clarify and redefine what nursing is. This has not been as much a discourse on theory as it has been a discourse on power. While the language of the discourse resembles the language of theory, the agenda and **subtext** are essentially **political**. The literature on Nursing Theory provides many examples of the fundamentally political nature of the discourse.

Packard and Polifroni (1991), for instance, attribute the lack of a distinctive science of nursing to the fact that the reason for the science cannot be identified. They reject the notion of nursing as an applied science, because it implies application of 'some other discipline's knowledge' and is based on the misguided belief that improvement of nursing practice is the most important function of theory. They reject the American Nurses Association Social Policy Statement on nursing as inadequate because it constrains nurses to diagnosing and treating responses to health problems, while disqualifying nurses from considering the factors that contribute to health problems. They also decry the methodology debates in nursing as indicative of a deep philosophical dispute among nurses about the true essence of nursing. This discourse seems to be about imperialist claims for territory, the primacy of theory over practice and the preference for intellectual consensus over intellectual conflict.

The preoccupation of the Nursing Theory literature has been with **paradigm** issues, not with theory issues. Kuhn (1970) argued that a paradigm shift results from a group of practitioners seeking more successful ways of solving the problems that the group has come to recognise as acute. It would appear that the acute problem for nurses has been to position themselves in the world of work and in the world of science. The 'positioning' process inherent in paradigm debates is itself a political one. The process has to do with identifying the 'big ideas' which drive the ideology and which therefore characterise the paradigm. The process also involves identifying intellectual allies and intellectual foes for the purpose of validating the ideology.

Evidence of the persistence of the preoccupation with paradigms continues to be presented. Fawcett (1993), for instance, proposes the reconfiguring and rationalisation of previous paradigms in nursing literature into three general world views, which in her view simplifies the debate. Its purpose is to perpetuate the debate. She identifies four existing sets of paradigms in use in nursing (organismic/mechanistic; change/persistence; simultaneity/totality; and particulate–deterministic/interactive–integrative/unitary–transformative) and reconfigures and restates them as 'Reaction, Reciprocal Interaction and Simultaneous Action Worldviews'. Her attempt at paradigmatic parsimony is intended to simplify the debate but in fact she succeeds in perpetuating and complicating the debate through her invitation to proceed in further discourse. It is this discourse which Walker (1994, p. 164) argues is dominant in nursing and is distracting us from our other research efforts, most notably '. . . the things that we need to know in nursing'. He calls this the 'ontological imperative'.

Meleis (1991) argues that the preoccupation with paradigms is typical of the search for boundaries by groups who have no sense of identity. She argues that we ought to abandon this industrious futility in favour of developing theory in a multidisciplinary health care context, which will improve the impact of nursing services on health. Smith (1992), in criticising the position taken by Meleis, argues that in doing this the contribution of nursing in society will be marginalised or diluted. She stresses that Nursing Theory development is about 'nursing's struggle for emancipation' and that 'nurses have too much to lose not to contribute to the conceptual models that frame a perspective on the central focus that is distinctively nursing' (1992, p. 149). The essentially political nature of the Nursing Theory discourse remains evident in the literature that supports this view.

Packard and Polifroni (1991) echo the sentiments of many authors in the Nursing Theory literature, who entreat nurses to abandon the accumulated theoretical knowledge of other disciplines as a means of understanding the phenomena with which nurses are concerned, in favour of a unique 'nursing' understanding of these phenomena. This pursuit of 'truth' within a prescribed framework, while consciously rejecting accumulated wisdom, is akin to techniques employed by religious cults to indoctrinate and control their members. Intellectual control of any sort is anti-theoretical because it constrains individuals' ability to conceptualise their existence in ways that are meaningful to them. Rather than promoting the growth of knowledge, this approach constrains it and perpetuates the problems of theory development in nursing. Once again it is evidence of the politics embedded in the Nursing Theory discourse.

In a potted version of the history of Nursing Theory, King (1991) characterises problems in its development into three areas.

1 There was an early development of an anti-theoretical bias in nursing.

2 There has been poor development of concepts in nursing literature.

3 There is no specifically defined domain of nursing.

For these reasons, she argues, there has been continued confusion in the use of terminology in the Nursing Theory literature. Nursing Theory literature has been more preoccupied with the political question of the 'defined domain of nursing' than it has with the development of legitimate theory. Theory is, she maintains, '. . . a set of interrelated concepts with propositions that show relationships among the concepts, and lead to research questions or hypotheses that can be stated and tested in research' (King 1991).

The politics of ideas has been at the root of much of the Nursing Theory literature. The support for holism (and rejection of **reductionism** and **biomedicalism**), the support for concepts of health to drive health care provision (and rejection of concepts of illness), the support for naturalistic methods of enquiry (and rejection of **logical-positivism** and **empiricism**) are all evidence of the positioning process inherent in the paradigm debates with which nursing has been concerned. These processes have to a large extent been part of an attempt to carve out a legitimate and unique domain for nurses within health care. It has been noted, however, that what is missing from this literature is a strong sense of 'mutuality' between theory, practice and research in nursing (Kermode 1993). There is no sense of congruence between the academic interests associated with developing the discipline of nursing, the political interests associated with developing the profession of nursing, and the clinical interests associated with developing the practice of nursing. This is probably evidence that competing paradigms are in operation throughout the various nursing environments, and this competition is substituting for legitimate theoretical discourse that would advance the understanding of practising nurses about the activity they call 'nursing' and, more importantly, the experience of patients with nursing services.

Kim: If nurses are going to be faithful to a paradigm, and if what we mean is to take a social view of health, then let's become socially and politically active beings. We can do the jobs that society wants of us as doctors and nurses, but let's act as political agents to legitimately change the health of populations. Okay, that's one position. The other position is: look, we really like doing the work that nurses do, and that's what people want us to do. But we don't have a lot of strong theoretical knowledge in respect of what nurses do because we're preoccupied with the paradigm issues about what nurses ought to be.

Ngaire: To me a paradigm is, can be, all-encompassing and it's like if you put on a pair of spectacles . . . and when you put on that pair of spectacles, you see the world in a certain way and that prevents you from seeing the world, to some extent, in any other way. Now those spectacles can be really tight and block everything else around them, or if you become more flexible in your thinking, you can take those paradigm spectacles off and put another pair of paradigm spectacles on.

However, to me, there are some paradigms, that once you enter into them, it is very difficult to come out. I think the biomedical model is an extremely all-pervading paradigm that has practically become part of our culture and so, to step outside of that, for individuals, I find even for myself when I'm thinking about things, you slip back into it very easily . . . Once you have embraced the feminist paradigm, you can't stop being a feminist or not use that paradigm. It is, to me, a real ah-ha thing, and you look at it and that then to me explains so much of what you see in the world.

Jo: Yes, that's good, because if you are living it, it is because it's an ideology. It becomes so enculturated that you're no longer conscious of it.

Kim: I also think that moving from paradigm to **ontology** and being able to live and work within the paradigm, that will determine the sort of theoretical knowledge you develop. In other words, it will determine the way you explain the problems you are dealing with.

Jo: Because you have a degree of immersion in it.

Kim: And I think that's where you'll end up getting the link between the paradigm and the theory. And if you are immersed in the feminist paradigm, your ability to explain the problems you might be dealing with—health problems, whatever, will be derived out of that. The same as if you are immersed in the biomedical model, your first response to a health problem is 'There's got to be an organism causing this or there's got to be a genetic predisposition causing this'.

Rick: But the interesting thing there is what has now happened with the social model (which has been pointing out environmental factors for a number of years) is that the biomedical model has now incorporated it, reluctantly. Risk factors have become the new germs.

Kim: Yes, and I think possibly part of the problem where the paradigm issue is most contentious is what problems it successfully addresses, and I think what we are finding is that a lot of so-called problems are being introduced into paradigms which are not really problems, if you like, of health practice or whatever. They are political problems.

So when you say 'These factors are now the new organisms', I think you are exactly right, because how does the biomedical paradigm incorporate the political consequences of a whole bunch of new health professionals and, if you like, the new Public Health? How does it incorporate that and still survive? The paradigm is at fault because it perpetuates the individualisation of health.

Rick: Yes, the individualisation of responsibility for the planning of health.

Kim: It's an innately conservative status quo-maintaining view of health, designed to retain the existing power relationships.

Jo: . . . which serves their purposes as custodians of the human body, because while people are responsible for their own health and doctors are the custodians of the body, they get all the power related to the care of the body, or they get a large percentage of it. So how do we make a connection between paradigm and theory?

Kim: I think the connection, as I said before, is ontology. How you live a paradigm, and the extent to which it is possible for you to live a paradigm, will affect the way you will explain all the problems you deal with. What nursing now requires is to get beyond the politics of paradigms and develop a legitimate theory discourse.

THE UTILITY OF THEORY

There are two things that shape our theoretical understanding of the world. The first of these is the recurrence of phenomena which support our beliefs. The second of these is the absence of phenomena which challenge our beliefs. As consequences of our formal (research-based) and informal (experiential) encounters with phenomena, our understanding and ability to predict are shaped. This is what 'testing' of theoretical knowledge means. Theory which endures is that which is constantly supported by formal (research-based) and informal (experiential) data.

Popper (1968) insisted that if it was not possible to, at least, attempt to disprove a theory, then it should not be accepted as being true. His views presented the importance of 'falsification' as an approach to crystallising legitimate knowledge which can contribute to understanding and prediction of phenomena. The message in Popper's philosophy is that theory is only as strong as the methods by which it is produced, and that ideology without method produces little more than worthless dogma.

Phillips (1991) believes that nursing science itself is the most important phenomenon for nursing enquiry. He believes it to be characterised as a 'trinity' of education, practice and research. He rejects the notion that the client and nursing practice need to be studied in order to build nursing, and that 'nurses who come to see nursing science from the viewpoint of the trinity will acquire a new synthesis, a creative leap into the simultaneity paradigm of nursing' (1991). There is considerable evidence here of dogma but scant evidence of method.

A legitimate theoretical discourse, which moves beyond rhetoric about paradigms, is able to advance understanding beyond description and towards explanation and prediction. Meleis (1985) subscribes to the view that theory is first, about describing and labelling phenomena which are of concern to the practitioner. Second, it is about explaining the relationship between various phenomena. Third, it is about predicting the outcome effect of one phenomenon upon another. She goes on to describe the fourth level of theory as being the ability to prescribe as a result of the previous three levels.

Torres (1990) agrees that theory is about description, explanation and prediction but prefers 'control' as the final purpose of theory. Nursing Theory, if it remains at the descriptive level, is of little use to practitioners. Practitioners need to be able to predict the outcomes of their actions. This is an academic, professional and practice imperative. Real theoretical discourse will generate knowledge that helps clinicians make better judgements. The prime objective of theory discourse in nursing should be the provision of better nursing care. The most powerful value of any theory in a political, academic or clinical sense is that it produces better outcomes for those who use nursing services. In other words, theory needs to describe, explain and predict phenomena in ways that benefit patients. If society is better off because of theory, then the practitioners of this theory will be stronger, as will their discipline.

Marx (1976, p. 249) argued that '. . . if there is no way of testing a theory it is scientifically worthless, no matter how plausible, imaginative, or innovative it may be'. This is another shortcoming of the Nursing Theory discourse in nursing. The value of theoretical knowledge is that it stands up, not only to the rigours of research, but to the rigours of experience. We are born with the capacity to theorise about our existence. We learn to predict the outcomes of our actions in minute detail. We can predict, for instance, that if we walk across a busy road then we are likely to be hit by a car. Kelly (1969) argues that all human beings are scientists who constantly theorise and attempt to predict the consequences of their own existence. The same must be true of nurses and their understandings about nursing. Dale (1994) suggests that theory provides the basis for understanding reality, which in this case is the reality of nursing. She maintains that the so-called theory–practice gap in nursing is a myth and that what exists is a theory–theory gap, with practitioners operating on one theoretical level and academics operating on another. Congruence with experience is the key to theoretical integrity and only this will produce meaningful theoretical explanation, prediction and control of the phenomena with which nurses work.

Alexander (1982) argues that scientific theory exists in a two-dimensional continuum, ranging from general presuppositions on one end to data on the other end. Nursing Theory has been concerned with general presuppositions which are unsupported by data. So-called 'grand theory' has produced dogma for its devotees, but is essentially data-free. The willingness to let data inform theory is a novelty in nursing. There is a need to escape from preoccupation with the political issue of what nursing 'is' and focus on explaining the things that nurses can 'do', in order to advance theoretical discourse in nursing. Ironically, a strong body of explanatory/predictive theory related to the effectiveness of nurses in what they 'do' is likely also to have far more significant political impact than all our collective musings about what nursing 'is'.

THE POLITICS OF THEORY

As indicated in earlier sections of this chapter, nursing has chosen to develop its profession and discipline for a variety of reasons, not the least of which can be linked with its history, with social movements in health care and with the women's movement in particular. Nursing reforms in the 1950s and 1960s have promoted examination of the purpose of nursing and the roles of participants within it. Nursing theory has been used to assist in this process.

Although the term 'nursing theory' was not used extensively in the 1970s, several concepts were promoted to nurses. These concepts, which had their origins in World Health Organization reports, included:

- nursing care as distinct from medical care;

- the focus in nursing to be on the whole person—physical, psychological, emotional and spiritual;

- the extension of nursing care from the individual to the family and community; and

- the shift in focus from acute hospital to primary health care.

Although not regarded as a theory, the nursing process was an influential import which provided impetus to nursing to start thinking about the nature of nursing work.

Kim: . . . theory . . . this is something that is politically driven. It was a way of building nursing into something radical which it currently wasn't. It was a way of making nursing work more satisfactory to nurses. So it was a patently political agenda.

Jo: I think in all those cases, the early theories anyway, jumped on the bandwagon of the so-called science and used the language and assumptions of science to validate us as political people for maybe a movement towards so-called professional status and all the benefits that gives. That seduction to science and scientific approaches stayed with us a very long time. I don't think we moved away from it before the 1970s. . . .

I think there was an unquestioning acceptance initially but I think that's being questioned now. I suppose we have to look at the extent to which nursing theory is talked about in hospital schools in the 1970s.

Clearly, nursing theory in hospitals at that time was a non-issue, but began to be promoted in the college and, eventually, the university system. But it could be claimed that nurse academics accepted and adopted, often unquestioningly, the importation of nursing theory, particularly from North America. While many innovations have been important and useful to nursing in Australia, it is imperative, as pointed out by Beunza et al. (1994), that these ideas be 'critically appraised for contextual relevance within and between countries' (p. 48). We must be aware of the dangers of adopting 'inappropriate modes of nursing practice', and strive to adapt innovations to suit the particular cultural context.

It was not until the 1980s that formal published critiques of nursing theory began to appear, although some candid statements about the usefulness of nursing theory prior to that time can be found in the literature. For example, Jolley and Brykczynska (1993) quote King (1971) as stating that: 'If theory is not useful it really is not worth the effort to develop it.' As a member of the discourse group noted: nursing theory is unhelpful if it does not assist in problem solving. Nevertheless, the patently political agenda in using nursing theory to promote the discipline of nursing has been championed and promoted by academic nurses in the higher education system. A survey of Australian nursing schools indicated that 88 per cent of respondents reported that their undergraduate curricula were based on, or guided by, nursing theory. This contrasted with 63 per cent for graduate nursing programs (Speedy 1990). It is clear that nursing theory has been adopted by Australian nurse academics; the degree to which this has occurred uncritically is unknown, as is the transference of nursing theory to the practising arena by students, both undergraduate and postgraduate. This is also the conclusion of Abu-Saad (1993), while also noting that '[N]ursing theories and nursing paradigms have replaced the medical model in most nursing school curricula at all levels of nursing education' (p. 292).

It is assumed that nursing theory development will facilitate the scholarly development of the discipline of nursing, which in turn will enhance the professionalisation for which nursing continues to strive (Gruending 1985). It has also been suggested that nurses' professional identity problems are linked to their obsession with theory and knowledge development, as evidenced in the previous section. The efficacy of these strategies has been questioned, as can be seen in the discourse, and the supporting literature that follows.

Kim: I think you can't disentangle the whole theory discourse from the professionalisation discourse. They become one and the same and, in fact, what we are really talking about in nursing now is the politics of ideas. It's not so much the utility of ideas at the workplace but the political advantage that we get from pursuing certain ideology . . . I really think the theory discourse now is a political one, more than anything else, and I think more so in Australia than anywhere else.

Lyn: Who is making mileage out of the theory–practice debate?

Kim: I think academics are. I think academics are making huge mileage out of it because we are getting papers and improve our CVs which improve our credentials and get us promoted and get us jobs. I think we are keeping it alive in a way . . . If you look at the pursuit of the theory discourse and the professionalisation of nursing, they are both tied closely to the pursuit of the capitalist ideal . . . It has happened to secure greater market power for practising nurses.

And so has questioning of the questioning, which is perceived as heretical at worst, and ignorant at best. For example, Whall (1993), in a paper entitled 'Let's get rid of all nursing theory', abhors this 'brash and uninformed opinion' that questions the relevance and utility of nursing theory. She makes a number of salient points, suggesting that nursing models have helped nursing to become a fully developed discipline, and that to 'get rid of all nursing theory' would 'lead to a repetition within nursing of several great mistakes of the past', mistakes which created much confusion and wasted time and effort, thus reducing 'nursing to a trade-like status, not to that of a scientific discipline'.

Smith (1993, p. 165) articulates the value of nursing theory to administrative practice, primarily to provide leadership for the introduction of theory-based practice models, as well as to guide the practice of nursing administration. The arguments are based on political imperatives, rather than scientific imperatives.

As suggested in the previous section, it is essential that nursing is fully aware of the dangers inherent in dogmatism, the major one being its effect in retarding future development (Rodgers 1991). She provides a number of examples of dogmatism in nursing, including the 'nursing is an art and a science' statement, and the rigidification of nursing practice, procedures and 'pre-printed plans', which all indicate the 'right way' to provide nursing care. Rodgers advocates critical analysis of extant authority and tradition, which in turn provides the potential for consideration of alternative perspectives that may be more appropriate. The discourse group also made the comment below, while recognising the historical and structural factors militating against serious critique.

Ngaire: The thing about nursing theory is that it is not debated. It is either being sold to us as religion, almost as religion, and in the journals there are very few critical articles. If you pick up a sociology journal, you've got postmodernism with everybody tearing it to shreds. Nursing has never generated that debate.

Jo: I think it's connected to the fact that a lot of them have come out of America where the scholars are treated as icons; there's not a lot of critique of their work and some of the scholars themselves don't really change. It's about never being subject to critique and debate which is an open spirit of enquiry and reformation and so therefore one stays with our old ideas, or is stuck in the paradigm.

Ngaire: Maybe the way for nursing to go ahead is to generate this position of question and debate.

Jo: I think Australian scholarship's doing that . . . when I hit the university system . . . I started to realise that there could be an alternate view. But here again, it's the unquestioning acceptance of something that's stated as truth.

Kim: I believe that was probably part of an intellectual and cultural cringe that Australia was suffering from at the time. I actually think about it and groan. And I think that what we are starting to see in Australia is the real influence of Australian culture on theory development in nursing . . . Australians are innately sceptical. This can be a very healthy intellectual quality.

Not surprisingly, the value of nursing theories is supported by a wide range of theorists, including Kim (1994) and Barrett (1993), who asserts that nursing actions must be based in 'substantive knowledge of nursing and that nursing science frameworks known variously as nursing models, nursing theories, or nursing science conceptual systems constitute this substantive nursing knowledge'. She suggests that Nursing Centers will provide for nursing's unique contribution to 21st-century health care, and that they should be guided by a particular nursing theory, which would attract nursing practitioners and clients. Barrett recommends that these centres use nursing frameworks and that these be 'reflected in legislation similar to Canadian standards that strongly recommend that nursing theory provide the scientific basis for nursing education and practice' (p. 117). The issue of 'theory by legislation' creates another potential minefield, since this would be a very potent example of dogma suppressing data that did not accord with the specific theory being proposed.

Parse (1990) supports the views of Kim (1994) and Barrett (1993), noting that the use of theory-based practice in hospitals is becoming more common as an alternative mode of practice in settings that value nursing frameworks. This, accordingly, 'makes an important difference to nurses and the people they serve'; it results in greater satisfaction with work, and has a role in stabilising the workplace.

Notwithstanding these theorists' preferences, there is increasing evidence that nurses in North America are also questioning the value of nursing theory. One only has to hook into the NURSENET Global Forum for Nursing Issues to observe the debate, particularly but not exclusively in relation to the continuing education arena, where it is clear that the curriculum is market-driven, given that these programs are voluntary and must be paid for by the participant. One communication indicates that continuing education programs must be clinical in nature and very practical. The communicant says: 'since all of our programs must be self-supporting it would be a risk to plan one on nursing theory that would have to be cancelled with about $1000 sunk costs' (Perry 1994). The ongoing discourse makes very clear that clinical nurses have major difficulties in seeing the relevance and value of nursing theories and models for practice.

For example, Romeo (1994) despairs about having completed university studies after 17 years of experience in paediatric nursing, and wonders why she completed her studies. Her observations are that nurses spend a great deal of time defining their role, striving for recognition and value, and 'making sense' of their work. For her, the 'division between clinical practice and academia seems just as wide as it was when I began nursing'. Similar criticism of nursing theories occurs in Europe (see, for example, Lundh, Soder & Waerness 1988).

This debate is alluded to by Smith (1991) who acknowledges that many practising nurses were educated without nursing theory and 'some feel disenfranchised and devalued by the definition of professional nursing practice as grounded in nursing theory. Their identities are threatened as they are confronted by a definition of practice that is foreign to them' (p. 147), so that when it is suggested that nursing theory is discovered through practice, they are affirmed. The gap therefore between nursing theory and practice occurs as a result of viewing practitioners as atheoretical and technical, and scientists/scholars as artificial and pedantic. [Or 'elite class–working class' in Maeve's (1994) terms (see below)]. She does conclude, however, that we can only uncover what nurses do by 'identifying the disciplinary perspective and theoretical basis of nursing that distinguishes it from all other professional disciplines (p. 147)'. So nursing theory, it is argued, is an essential component of the professional discipline that is nursing; to be atheoretical is to reduce nursing to the status of a technology or craft. Once again, issues of status and prestige permeate the discourse.

Kim: What do nurse clinicians think theory is? We all talk to nurses, what do they think nursing theory is?

Jo: Well, they think it's beyond them. They think that what we do here is not relevant to their practice. That we're these ivory tower dwellers and we make these grand statements that have got no relevance to what they do every day.

They don't really understand unless they've got to do tertiary study and then they swallow it like a bitter pill. . . .

Kim: And are they right? Yes, I think they're right. I think they're 100 per cent right. . . . there's a difference between what nurses see in published theory and what theory really is. So theory is the stuff that they are carrying around with them that they don't know they've got, and the ways that they explain and predict and act out, rather than this published stuff that they call capital N capital T, Nursing Theory.

Jo: If we think that nurses think that theory is this thing and they don't actually live that, what is it to them in their existence?

Ngaire: Could we say that if you did take a theory that nurses have in practice, they might then have a theory about being powerless, a theory that encompasses the biomedical model, a theory that nurses' role was only bedside care and not looking at other things.

In assessing the value of nursing theory and its debates to clinical nurses, it has been reported to us on many occasions that nursing theories are 'beyond' them, that they are 'not smart enough to understand them', that theories are unnecessary, and that the debate devalues their role in patient care. This validates the views of Smith (1991) (above) and others. This view is also reinforced by practising nurses who have difficulty in articulating their knowledge and who are therefore subsequently silenced (Josefson 1988), or who choose to remain silent rather than criticise or oppose nursing theory advocates. Hence, theory becomes a political tool in the hands of professionalisers.

Turner (1986) provides a compelling analysis of the complaint system in nursing that derives from the 'vocabulary of complaint' concept proposed by Hughes (1951). This is demonstrated in nursing by 'whingeing in the pan room' and is a means of rebelling against structures and authority, while allowing nurses to remain silent and be silenced. Jolley and Brykczynska (1993) suggest that, on the nursing theory issue, nurses 'prefer to vote with their feet (or minds) and simply side-step the entire issue, while enduring linguistic agonies in muted silence' (p. 153). Silence, then, becomes a substitute for complaint.

Such views are reinforced by the fact that, historically, clinical nurses were not valued for what they were and did. Part of this was located in the attitudes of nurses themselves, who failed to view clinical practice as an end in itself, and not just a means to an end. Many nurses, legitimately, move from clinical practice to management and education. But the view that clinical practice was somehow of lesser importance has had the effect of devaluing direct nursing care and encouraging defection of the nurse as clinical practitioner (Wiles 1994).

Maeve (1994) develops the 'carrier bag theory of nursing practice', which reinterprets how nursing is known and practised, explicitly to acknowledge and value nursing's oral and experiential traditions. This is based on the assumption that 'nursing has been effectively divided into two worlds—academia and the world of practice' (Maeve 1994, p. 9). Consequently, there is what she labels an 'elite class–working class gap, as well as a gap between **epistemes**, or "knowing that" versus "knowing how"' (p. 9). Maeve asserts that the carrier bag theory is about scholarship embedded in practice and about the clinicians who create that scholarship—bedside scholars. She continues the argument, suggesting that the actual practice of nursing is different from theories of practice, since each reality is generated by different people living in different worlds, and that the gap is between the 'intelligentsia of the high hard ground [who] have claimed and assumed for themselves the guiding role for the profession of nursing' (p. 10) and bedside nurses.

Bedside nurses, on the other hand, are only expert if they meet quantifiable standards 'set forth by the intelligentsia or at the behest of the intelligentsia who compete with each other for awards such as those promoted by schools of nursing for excellence in practice' (p. 11), which increasingly alienates practising nurses. With relatively few exceptions, they are not encouraged to consider themselves experts, since the 'intelligentsia of the high hard ground have claimed this distinction for themselves' (p. 14). Clinical nurses, too, collude with these beliefs; their contribution is 'always invisible partly because she is "woman", partly because she is (and, sadly, often of her own admission) "just a nurse"' (Walker 1994). Until nursing conceptualises nursing practice as scholarly, and nurses engage in the process of deconstructing and reconstructing practice, there will continue to exist the elite class–working class gap, with retarded development of the discipline of nursing.

There is a view from the clinical domain that nursing theory is being used to justify the existence of academic nurses within the university setting. Some justification may be found in the fact that perusal of biographical data preceding the publications of various theorists indicates that many of them generated their theories as a requirement of their postgraduate studies. This raises the question as to why these works were created: was it purely for academic requirements, or was it based in nursing practice, for the practical benefit of practitioners? Two texts that support the former assertion are authored by George (1990) and Chinn and Kramer (1991).

Nursing academics (and nurse practitioners for that matter) might like to think that they 'are building a bridge, each from their own bank of the river, and that, although we may not live to see the day, the spans will meet' (O'Gorman 1994, p. 182). He proceeds to point out that there is increasing nervousness about achieving this union, because the two parties are building on different rivers. This is an issue that needs to be addressed by academic nursing and practising clinicians. Are they building on different rivers?

The issues raised by Sheehan (1994), pertinent to the psychology discipline, might be raised for nursing. These include the features of professionalism, training and structure of the profession, and the validity of the scientist–practitioner model of training. Nurse academics have, until the more recent past, operated on the assumptions of a traditional model of science informing practice. Many are now recognising the limitations that such a model imposes (Watson 1985; Meleis 1987, 1991; Holmes 1990), and are exploring the potential of alternative ways of conceptualising 'nursing science', particularly if it can establish further independence from medicine and the limiting medical model. Hoshmond and Polkinghorne (1992) suggest that alternative conceptions of the science–practice relationship must be based on the commendable goal of science and practice mutually informing each other (Sheehan 1994). There has been much useful debate in the nursing literature addressing the issue of the theory–practice nexus, but there may be other questions that need addressing—such as the one above: Are we building on different rivers?

A similar question has been posed by Holter (1988) and explored further by Dale (1994). As Dale asserts, the value of theory is purported to be purposive action, evidenced in planning, direction and outcomes. Non-theory-based activity is therefore random. On this logic, nursing activity must be based on theory. However, as was noted in the previous section, rather than accepting a gap between theory and practice, Dale suggests that the gap is a 'theory–theory gap'—that is, the theory taught in the classroom by academics is different from the theory on which practice is based. The gap here is between the theoretical perspectives held by practitioners and academics, and exists because there is a lack of development of experiential knowledge. The solution, according to Dale (1994), lies in the development of the clinical nurse teacher's role and greater emphasis on clinical teaching. There are Australian nurse theorists attempting to close this gap, most notably Lawler (1991) and Taylor (1994).

In reality, in their teaching and promotion of nursing theory, nurse theorists and nurse academics often succeed in mystifying nursing, making theory and practice abstract, complex and, in some cases, less accessible, particularly by the use of jargon (Lundh et al. 1988; Meleis 1991; Randell 1992; Jolley & Brykczynska 1993; McCoppin & Gardner 1994). Nursing theories do run the risk of complicating the obvious, and sometimes appear trivial or largely a matter of common sense.

This process creates and further potentiates divisiveness in nursing, specifically between educators and clinicians. McCoppin and Gardner (1994) quote an Australian nurse who, while accepting the need for nursing theory in practice, also criticised the obscure and patronising way theorists expressed themselves. She added that she was 'left with the feeling that the nurse theorist was 'an apologist for a vocation which will never gain professional acceptance unless The Theory is "discovered" . . . ' (James 1976 cited in McCoppin & Gardner 1994, p. 40). This instance can be interpreted as a clash of cultures, with the importation into one culture of the product of another. American theories were designed by American nurses and, as previously suggested, must be contextually examined for their relevance and capacity for transfer to other cultures.

A further potential problem is that of confusing the patient, since it is nurses who have the knowledge and techniques essential for nursing care. Nurses who need to wield power and control can use intellectualisation and abstractions of theory to retain superiority over their patients. Nursing theory in this situation then becomes a weapon.

One of the problems of the theory–practice, or theory–theory debate is that, although there is a strong commitment to theory arising out of practice, nursing practice, at present, occurs within a paradigm, the biomedical model, that does not acknowledge the value of nursing work.

The inherently practical nature of nursing is such that clinical nurses who do see some relevance of theory to their practice do so because of that theory's capacity to describe, explain, predict and assist in problem solving at the work-face level.

The process of theorising is, however, an intellectual activity. Our experience of the world is what creates the parameters within which we produce theory. To say that practice informs theory is a truism. Equally, however, our understandings of the world shape the way we perceive and interact with the world. To say that theory informs practice is likewise a truism. The extent to which formal, published theoretical discourse helps to inform practice is the contentious issue. Our theoretical understandings are invariably trapped in the paradigm(s) that are sourced in the social, political and cultural forces underscoring our experience. Having uncovered the paradigm(s) that are propping up our theory, it is then possible to look again at the phenomena of concern to nurses with a fresher and less filtered gaze.

To safeguard the practice of nursing, there is a need to focus on a better understanding of the phenomena with which nurses deal. Succumbing to the compulsion to present grand theory as a substitute for this will do nothing to secure the future of nursing work. This is not meant to downplay the importance of discourse on matters concerning paradigms but rather to refocus theoretical endeavour on the work that nurses do.

Kim: . . . what I'm arguing for is development of theory that solves the problems that nurses find important . . . if theory is not defined as something that helps us solve the problems we deal with, whether that's purely by describing and explaining them to help us understand them; if it's not defined in that way, then in my view, theory is useless . . . the predictive thing is something that may or may not happen down the track. I still think there is value in purely going as far as explanatory theory.

Jo: Because of the contextual nature of the nursing relationship . . . we need theories about this sort of nursing and that sort of nursing. So when it's centred in a context, it'll have explanatory power within that context only . . . if you can't explain anything, what's the point? What's the point of asking about the nature of existence if there's not a point?

Ngaire: Maybe it was nursing's efforts to come to terms with dealing with the complexities of the human being. You have the complexity of the human being, the complexity of their problems and the complexity of their context.

A PLURALIST VIEW OF NURSING THEORY

In a debate which examined nursing theory in the 21st century with a number of nursing theorists, including Johnson, Neuman, Orem, Parse, Rogers and Roy, the question was raised regarding multiple models versus unified theory (Randell 1992). Roy suggested that pluralism would diminish and that polarisation around a few selective conceptualisations would occur. Johnson, Neuman, Rogers and Parse all disagreed. Johnson advocated searching questions about the usefulness of models in practice, education and research, as well as its significance on actions and decisions regarding the patients. Neuman opted for a diversity of models, greater creativity and newer thinking. Rogers believed that if there was no commitment to nursing as a science, then we did not need higher education. She also opted for more than one paradigm, which Parse concurred with, in addition to indicating that diversity is enriching in all our endeavours.

Munhall (1992) argues for the adoption of 'various modes of thinking that create meaning and provide direction for one's own pedagogy' (p. 371). She suggests that debate is not necessary but that dialect is essential. Using the metaphor of a pendulum, she demonstrates that some approaches to nursing provide useful knowledge and skills but that others enable nursing care to be contextualised so that we can 'hear our different voices'. So, for example, the 1960s and 1970s were characterised by a technical–rational model of knowledge in which there was certainty of outcomes, while the late 1980s were characterised by 'open-ended **humanism**', including **phenomenology**, **hermeneutics**, and **feminist** and **critical theory**. The general tenor of Munhall's argument is that, whatever approach is used, be it constrained by positivist and 'objective' methods, or more subjective, person-oriented and meaningfully defined, the aim is to provide as many avenues of development for nursing as are valuable and useful. Therefore, rather than have polarisation of the pendulum, Munhall advocates a swinging pendulum approach to the development of the discipline of nursing that will capitalise on any approach that will ultimately enhance it. She, too, makes a plea for pluralism. Failure to do so will, as indicated earlier, result in doctrinaire and prejudiced thinking.

The uncritical acceptance of nursing theory will, in the longer term, retard the development of nursing as a discipline and profession. So will dogmatism and territoriality.

Kim: . . . if we look at the theory discourse in nursing, where it's going, where it ought to go, in my opinion, the things we should guard against most are bigotry and the pursuit of political correctness . . . the pluralistic approach to the theory debate in nursing is what we mean . . . . We have to allow the duplicity of ideas and arguments. If we achieve that alone, we will have safeguarded the intellectual inheritance of future nurses, because we run the risk of creating an intellectual desert or theoretical desert in nursing if we allow bigotry and political correctness to dictate what is published.

Jo: But are we ever inflexible and unwilling to change our minds because it shakes our foundations and it makes us step outside ourselves? I think that, in fairness to nurses who have been struggling out there in the bunkers for years, their lives are so unpredictable . . . if they can just keep something steady from day to day by the rigidity of their own thought and work patterns, then there's one thing that doesn't change . . . to have an open area of critique is about trusting one another, to hear what we've got to say and know it's not a personal attack on our person. I don't think that nurses have actually felt good about themselves and one another to be able to develop those critiques.

But it's important not to de-mark knowledge and say, 'This is my property and you can't have it', but to offer it to other people and say 'This is something that's been generated from my experience, here you are, work with it. Tell me what you think about it.' Because I think there is a demarcation mentality about who owns knowledge. Everything and everyone owns knowledge but we've tended to mark off disciplines and say 'This is my turf' and the motive in that was, I think, about fee for service and all the professionalisation things that have occurred. But it's a far freer and more mature thing to say, 'I've found this, what do you think about it? From the experience of my being something, like a nurse, I've found this.' Because we've tended to take parts of philosophy, say, and assume it as our own and philosophy hasn't fought back, it's encouraged questioning. So, you know, that's a mature discipline that can do that.

Chris: So we may in fact have come full circle now. The early nursing theorists looked to territorialise their health practice and define what nursing is, and now we are not going to have anything to do with that?

Jo: Well, yes and no, I think. Yes and no in the sense that all those things can coexist. There may be some need to safeguard, say, the future role of registered nurses. We can't just throw the baby out with the bath water.

For Rodgers (1991), '[C]ontinuing progress in nursing . . . warrants an examination of, and release from, the dogma that may impede future development' (p. 177). Vigilance regarding the existence of dogma must be exercised in nursing practice, and in the professional discipline. For example, with respect to the structure of the nursing discipline, dogmatism was apparent in avoiding the dangers 'inherent in a reliance upon theories "borrowed" from other disciplines and developing nursing theory as a legitimate science and profession' (Rodgers 1991, p. 178). Although the intensity of debate regarding 'borrowed' versus 'unique' theories and knowledge has diminished, it is clear that nursing theory still endeavours to identify concepts and phenomena important to nursing.

A well-known example of dogmatic thinking was the promotion of a 'grand theory of nursing'. Much early theory development was directed towards the development of a grand theory that would explain the work of nurses in practice, while enhancing the development of the discipline. This notion is, however, incompatible with many basic assumptions in nursing, including the contextual and inclusive approach taken by nurses in response to their clients. As was discussed in the group, everyone has a theory whether it is valid or not. This position argues for the value of reflective theory and practice, which has been promoted by Australian nurses in the last decade. It was the view of the group members that reflective theory and practice provided greatest value because it is situated in nursing practice and considers the person in context. This is not to deny the contributions of theoretical constructs, but emphasises that these must be developed with a focus on the specific context.

Jo: [this] required a lot of living in the practice and working with people and developing a maturity that went beyond the knowledge and skills to a freedom. When you develop a sort of spontaneity in the moment, you develop a freedom that goes beyond the rule of the knowledge and skills. You're . . . on a tightrope without the net because you're that confident. And those conditions were like that, and so rather than say this was a grand theory that should be applied uniformly to make nursing practice over the world top notch, it was to say that in the experience of these people, these qualities came out and in the experience of the patients, they responded to that . . .

Rick: And the theory is of use to nursing practice?

Jo: Yes, it's of use, and I would call it a reflective theory and it is of use if it resonates for someone else who sees its usefulness for them . . . it's a rational process, but I also say it's intuitive and that brings the whole philosophical argument of what is intuition? So, I think that what we have done . . . is make statements that automatically exclude other possibilities, and what I would like to see is an inclusive set of possibility-generating theories that will allow other realities to coexist at multiple levels and in multiple dimensions so that I don't have this grand theory that knocks everything else on the head, but it allows it to stay parallel or be intertwined with other possibilities.

The value of reflection is based on the assumption (and largely accepted view) that there are different types of knowing. There is no question that we can acquire all the knowledge we need for living and working independently, and that we must depend on 'knowledge acquired by, reflected on and communicated to us by others' (John 1994, p. 161). Several writers in this area have elaborated levels of knowing, including Schön (1987), Shotter (1990) and Kitchener (1983). In broad terms, this equates to knowing in action, reflection in action, reflection on reflection in action (in order to produce an explicit verbal account) and reflection on that account (John 1994).

Clinicians need to operate at the 'reflection on reflection in action' level to take account of the uniqueness of each situation, and thus are frequently impatient with the perceived lack of relevance of nursing theories. Hence their need for 'applicable knowledge which, of necessity, is likely to be situated, local and context limited and may be expressed in narrative, rather than in paradigmatic propositional form' (John 1994, p. 162). This operates against fitting practice into predetermined categories, since it is essential to allow theory to emerge from the clinicians' accounts of reflections on their practice. Many extant nursing theories have not been derived from practice, although there have been exceptions (e.g. Paterson & Zderad 1976; Roper, Logan & Tierney, 1980).

These views accord with those espoused by Maeve (1994), who believes that clinical knowledge cannot be taught, but only demonstrated. She continues: 'Knowledge and scholarship, then, are inherently embedded in the practice of nursing in a unique, non-reproducible way' (p. 11). As previously noted, Maeve proposes the 'carrier bag theory of nursing practice' which is concerned 'directly with improvements in practice that occur at the micro level when one nurse shares what she has learned with another' (p. 14). These improvements in practice are necessarily and always related to the patient's perception and experience of that success, that is, the patient in context. Such an approach will allow the practice nurse to find the moral good embedded in practice, as well as the scholarship in that practice. Nursing has not conceptualised nursing practice as scholarly and so, for nursing to have a future, scholarship should be redefined 'in a way that allows the bedside nurse the stature and status of a scholar' (p. 15). The meanings and values inherent in practice then become the focus of nursing's development.

SUMMARY

This chapter has advocated that theory discourse must become more focused on the things nurses do that affect the health of their patients, rather than on the rhetoric of self-justification. This perspective will assist nurses in presenting to their various communities an understanding of their work that is not simply descriptive but explains and predicts the outcomes of their work. It has also been noted that the irony of this development is that it will be more politically effective than any deliberate attempts to promote nursing's professionalisation agenda by other means.

We have also emphasised the importance of recognising the paradigms that source and support our theoretical understandings about the things we do as nurses. It is imperative, however, that our theoretical gaze is focused on the phenomena with which our practice is concerned. In a statement that attempts to predict the future of nursing theory, Meleis (1991) suggests that nursing theories will become theories for health care, developed by a range of health professionals, including nurses. She believes that nursing will be a driving and unique force in theory development, but that theorists' names will not be attached to the theory proposed. The focus will move from theories to phenomena, a change that will be instrumental in bringing different communities of scholars together. Only then will it be possible to have a truly pluralist perspective.

POSTSCRIPT FROM PARTICIPANTS

Kim: Often you don't know what you know or even what you feel till you start to engage in a discourse on the topic. Too often, theory discourse in nursing is one-sided; more like diatribe than discourse. Talking with your colleagues can ground it in a way that cuts through the rhetoric and the dogma and exposes the ideas. Theorising is thinking. If this chapter says anything, I hope it says that we are all theoreticians, struggling to understand our world. Our experience shapes our understanding from the day we are born. For the activity we call 'nursing', we need to understand why we do what we do and what happens when we do it. This is nursing theory.

Rick: It was an enjoyable experience to be involved in this debate. While the topic of theory is often one which many people perceive as dry, the discussions we had proved this to be an incorrect perception. Obviously, the issue of theory is one we should all approach more passionately if nursing is going to have a major say in the delivery of health care.

Ngaire: Nurses in practice do have theories about what they do; it is just that they are largely unarticulated. Perhaps this is what the task is—to try to tease out what theories/ideas underpin nursing practice in Australia. Lawler (1991) has already started to do this and has articulated some of the unwritten rules of nursing—Taylor (1994) likewise. Perhaps we need to focus on these as heralding new thinking for Australian nursing. Another way forward for nursing is exploration of the phenomena that create nursing's context—the Australian health care system. I think nursing ought to be more critical of the present system of health care, and generate and work with others on alternative models to the dominant medical model. The idea of one encompassing theory for nursing, I think, is dead or, if not, should be killed. I think we have to recognise that there is also an anti-intellectual bias of Australians and Australian nursing which has tended to marginalise nurse teachers in the past and nurse academics in the present.

Jo: The process of sharing information and opinions about theory allowed me to use other people's ideas as triggers for my own. I enjoyed the sense of being part of a process that generated enthusiasm and excitement around what might be considered a 'dry subject'. At the end of the project I felt as though I had been able to clarify and further my own ideas about theory.

Chris: I came to these round-table discussions on nursing theory, hoping to find some answers to my growing disenchantment with the whole notion of nursing theory and the theory/practice debate. Having for several years coordinated an external unit of study, written largely around the theses produced by American nurse theorists, a situation which necessitated my reading hundreds of essays on nursing theory, I was increasingly frustrated by the unquestioning acceptance of this writing by my students. However, the fact emerged from our group discussion that the body of literature that has come to be known as nursing theory had virtually developed into a sacred cow for many nurse academics. If academics were reluctant to challenge it, why should students?

It was thus a heartening experience to join with my colleagues in systematically debunking the myths that have crept into the Australian nursing lexicon from the American nurse scholars, many of whom developed their own 'theory' of nursing. In an effort to understand what theory is, members of the group attempted to explain the theories they espoused in their personal lives. By the end of our meetings, there was general consensus that this was the preferred approach to theory: the study of nursing theory ought to be replaced by reflecting on what it is that we do in nursing and health care practices, thereby uncovering the theory that is embedded in clinical practices.

We resolved that theory has a definite place in nursing, and that it can serve the interests of practitioners. The group process itself provoked some stimulating discussion and was a convenient method of obtaining different views on a contentious subject. However, I did find it difficult at times to contribute to the dialogue and felt that the group at six members was too large.

Lyn: As one member of the group unable to be present at all the discussions, and charged with the task of using supporting literature to elaborate the emergent themes, the exercise proved to be quite fascinating. It was as if I was one small step removed. To discover in the transcript the views of my colleagues, able to intuitively agree with many of these views (and disagree with others), then to weave in the appropriate literature, was an exciting and challenging venture. The exercise clearly provided an opportunity for colleagues to legitimise scholarly debate at the informal level, where one most expects it to occur, yet finds environmental constraints militating against these opportunities. Exposing these ideas to clinical practitioners was intended; in the event, only one practitioner responded to the request to examine the paper and provide critical comments. These were valuable and useful: they provided a grounded perspective that accorded with that generated by the academic group. I would recommend this exercise to enquiring academics, but would also include clinicians within the discussion group.

GLOSSARY

Biomedicalism: explanations of health and ill-health which are based entirely on measurable biological variations such as microorganisms and genetic abnormalities.

Critical theory: an approach to understanding social and political reality which is critical in the sense that the intention of analysis is to lead to human emancipation. It posits a critical approach as a way of exposing to those most affected the nature of the historical and contemporary forces that control, shape and manipulate their lives.

Critique: the art of criticism.

Discourse/Discursive: words, talk, conversation and formal discussion.

Empiricism: the belief that all knowledge is based on experience, observation and/ or experiment.

Episteme: a way of knowing or understanding.

Feminist theory: that which advocates the rights and equality of women in social, political and economic spheres, and has a commitment to the fundamental alteration of women's role in society.

Hermeneutics: the science of interpretation aimed to produce understanding. Often used in relation to interpretation of texts, but has wider implications.

Humanism: any system or mode of thought or action in which human interests and questions predominate.

Logical–positivism: a scientific paradigm which is based on the belief that something is meaningful only if it can be verified by one's physical senses; it forms the basis of the classical 'scientific method'; it is a form of empiricism.

Ontology: the study of the nature of 'being'; study of the 'lived experience'.

Paradigm: a 'world-view' or way of interpreting the world; creationism and evolutionism are examples of paradigms.

Phenomenology: a form of interpretation aimed at full and objective description of phenomena related to understanding the meaning of the phenomena described.

Pluralist: a system which recognises more than one ultimate truth or principle.

Political subtexts: ideas related to power and influence which may be implicit in a discourse but which are not explicit or obvious.

Postmodernism: relating to the critique of modern, capitalist, industrialised bourgeois society; new political and social strategies which embrace pluralism and diversity of cultures and values.

Reductionism: attempts to explain phenomena by reducing them to their smallest parts; in health care, molecular biology is a good example of reductionist science.

Theory: in its simplest form a theory is a way of describing or explaining something; a set of concepts linked by propositions; the theory of gravity, for instance, explains why things that go up tend to come down again.

QUESTIONS

1 What do you understand 'nursing theory' to be? Is your understanding consistent with what you read about 'nursing theory'?

2 Think of a nursing activity you engage in. How do you explain what you do and why you do it? Are you able to predict the likely consequences of this activity?

3 In some of the nursing activities you engage in, are there different views about what should be done and why it should be done? What makes you choose the approach that you take?

4 What sort of literature helps you most in understanding and carrying out your nursing practice? Are you happy with the quality of this literature? Why or why not?

LEARNING ACTIVITY

Can you find three recent nursing publications which provide you with a better understanding and rationale for engaging in any nursing activities? What is it about these publications that is helpful to you?

FURTHER READING

Gray, G. & Pratt, R. (eds) 1991, *Towards a Discipline of Nursing*, Churchill-Livingstone, Melbourne.

McCoppin, B. & Gardner, H. 1994, *Tradition and Reality: Nursing and Politics in Australia*, Churchill-Livingstone, Melbourne, particularly Chapter 2.

REFERENCES

Abu-Saad, H.H. 1993, 'Nursing: the science and the practice', *International Journal of Nursing Studies,* 30(3), pp. 287–94.

Advisory Committee to the Multicultural Nursing Workforce Project 1991, *Responding to a Multicultural Society: Issues and Strategies for Nurse Education,* Office of Ethnic Affairs and Ethnic Health Unit, Melbourne.

Agan, R. 1987, 'Intuitive knowing as a dimension of nursing', *Advances in Nursing Science,* 10 (1), pp. 63–70.

Aggleton, P. & Chalmers, H. 1987, 'Models of nursing, nursing practice and nursing education', *Journal of Advanced Nursing,* 12, pp. 573–81.

Alexander, J. 1982, *Theoretical Logic in Sociology,* vol. 1, University of California Press, Berkeley.

Alfano, G.J. 1988, 'A different kind of nursing', *Nursing Outlook,* 36:1, Jan/Feb, pp. 34–7, 39.

Alfaro, R. 1990, *Applying Nursing Diagnosis and Nursing Process: A Step-by-Step Guide,* 2nd edn, J.B. Lippincott, Philadelphia.

Alfaro-LeFevre, R. 1994, *Applying Nursing Diagnosis and Nursing Process: A Step-by-Step Guide,* 3rd edn, J.B. Lippincott, Philadelphia.

Allan, H. 1993, 'Feminism: A concept analysis', *Journal of Advanced Nursing,* 18, pp. 1547–53.

Allen, D. 1985, 'Nursing research and social control: Alternative models of science that emphasise understanding and emancipation', *Image* XVII(2), pp. 58–64.

Allen, D. 1988, 'The challenges of gender for the development of nursing sciences', in *Proceedings of the 5th Nursing Science Colloquium: Strategies for Theory Development,* eds C. Bridges & N. Wells, Boston University School of Nursing, Boston.

Allen, D., Benner, P. & Diekelmann, L. 1986, 'Three paradigms for nursing research: Methodological implications', in *Nursing Research Methodology: Issues and Implementation,* ed. P. Chinn, Aspen, Maryland.

Allison, S.E., McLaughlin, K. & Walker, D. 1991, 'Nursing theory: A tool to put nursing back into administration', *Nursing Administration Quarterly,* 15(3), pp. 72–8.

Andersen, B. 1991, 'Mapping the terrain of the discipline', in *Towards a Discipline of Nursing,* eds G. Gray & R. Pratt, Churchill Livingstone, Melbourne.

ANF 1989, *Nursing in Australia: A National Statement,* prepared on behalf of Australian Nursing Federation, College of Nursing Australia, NSW College of Nursing, Florence Nightingale Committee, Australia.

Angeles, P.A. 1992, *The HarperCollins Dictionary of Philosophy,* 2nd edn, HarperCollins, New York.

ANRAC 1990, Oct., Nursing Competencies Assessment Project: *Report to the Australasian Nurse Registering Authorities Conference Vol. 1—The Project Report.* Assessment and Evaluation Research Unit, Education Department, University of Queensland.

Argyris, C. & Schön, D. 1974, *Theory in Practice,* Jossey-Bass, San Francisco.

Aristotle 1976, *Ethics,* Penguin Books, London.

Aristotle 1988, *De Anima* (On the soul), Penguin Books, London.

Arnold, E. & Boggs, K. 1989, *Interpersonal Relationships. Professional Communication Skills for Nurses*, Saunders, Philadelphia.

Aspinall, M.J. 1976, 'Nursing diagnosis—the weak link', *Nursing Outlook*, 24 (7), pp. 433–7.

Australasian Nurse Registering Authorities Conference 1990, *ANRAC National Competencies for the Registration and Enrolment of Nurses in Australia*, Nurses Board of South Australia, Adelaide.

Australian Concise Oxford Dictionary 1987, Oxford University Press, Melbourne.

Australian Diabetes Educators Association (ADEA) Newsletter 1989, 'Role of the diabetes educator', Newsletter No. 27, October, Diabetes Australia, Canberra, pp. 11–13.

Australian Nursing Council Inc. 1993, *National Competencies for the Registered and Enrolled Nurse in Recommended Domains*.

Australian Nursing Council Inc. 1994, *Registration and Enrolment of Nurses and the ANCI Competencies*, Canberra.

Australian Nursing Federation 1983, *Standards for Nursing Practice*, North Fitzroy, Melbourne.

Australian Nursing Federation 1989, *Standards for Nursing Care*, Victoria.

Bachrach, P. 1967, *The Theory of Democratic Elitism: A Critique*, Little, Brown, Boston.

Bachrach, P. & Baratz, M. 1970, *Power and Poverty*, Oxford University Press, New York.

Bandman, E.L. & Bandman, B. 1990, *Nursing Ethics through the Life Span*, 2nd edn, Appleton & Lange, Norwalk, Connecticut.

Bandura, A. 1977, *Social Learning Theory*, Prentice-Hall, Englewoods Cliffs, New Jersey.

Barnum, B.J. 1987, 'Holistic nursing and nursing process', *Holistic Nursing Practice*, 1 (3), pp. 27–35.

Barnum, B.J.S. 1990, *Nursing Theory: Analysis, Application, Evaluation*. 3rd edn, Scott, Foresman/Little, Brown, Glenview, Illinois.

Barrett, E.A.M. 1993, 'Nursing Centers without nursing frameworks: What's wrong with this picture?' *Nursing Science Quarterly*, 6(3): pp. 115–17.

Bates, E. & Linder-Pelz, S. 1990, *Health Care Issues*, 2nd edn, Allen & Unwin, Sydney.

Belenky, M., Clinchy, B., Goldberg, N. & Tarule, J. 1986, *Women's Ways of Knowing: The Development of Self, Voice, and Mind*, Basic Books, New York.

Benhabib, S. 1990, 'Epistemologies of postmodernism: A rejoinder to Jean-Francois Lyotard', in *Feminism/Postmodernism*, ed. L. Nicholson, Routledge, New York.

Benner, P. 1984, *From Novice to Expert: Excellence and Power in Clinical Nursing Practice*, Addison-Wesley, Menlo Park, California.

Benner, P. 1989, 'The moral dimensions of caring', published proceedings of The Wingspread Invitational Conference on Knowledge about Care and Caring, State of the Art and Future Development, American Academy of Nursing, Kansas, Missouri.

Benner, P. & Wrubel, J. 1989, *The Primacy of Caring: Stress and Coping in Health and Illness*, Addison-Wesley, Sydney.

Bennett, M. 1986, 'Nursing diagnosis in the beginning', *Australian Journal of Advanced Nursing*, 4 (1), pp. 41–6.

Beunza, I., Boulton, N., Ferguson, C. & Serrano, R. 1994, 'Diversity and commonality in international nursing', *International Nursing Review*, 41(2), pp. 47–56.

Bevis, E.O. 1972, *Curriculum Building in Nursing: A Process*, C.V. Mosby, St Louis.

Bevis, E.O. 1988, 'New directions for a new age', in *Curriculum Revolution: Mandate for Change*, National League for Nursing, Pub. No.15–2224, New York.

Bevis, E.O. & Watson, J. 1989, *Toward a Caring Curriculum: A New Pedagogy for Nursing*, National League for Nursing, Pub. No. 15–2278, New York.

Birx, E.C. 1993, 'Critical thinking and theory-based practice', *Holistic Nurse Practitioner*, 7(3), pp. 21–7.

Bottorff, J.L. 1993, 'The use and meaning of touch in caring for patients with cancer', *Oncology Nursing Forum*, 20(10), pp. 1531–8.

Bottorff, J.L. & Morse, J.M. 1994, 'Identifying types of attending: Patterns of nurses' work', *Image: The Journal of Nursing Scholarship*, 26(1), pp. 53–60.

Bowers, B. 1994, 'Critical path, caremap and case management systems', paper presented at the Eleventh Biennial Conference on the Classification of Nursing Diagnosis, Tennessee, US.

Bowman, G.S., Thompson, D.R. & Sutton, T.W. 1983, 'Nurses' attitudes towards the nursing process', *Journal of Advanced Nursing*, 8, pp. 125–9.

Brookfield, S.D. 1987, *Developing Critical Thinkers*, Open University Press, Milton Keynes.

Brown, L. 1986, 'The experience of care: Patient perspectives', *Topics in Clinical Nursing*, 8(2), pp. 56–62.

Bruni, N. 1991, 'Nursing knowledge: Processes of production', in *Towards a Discipline of Nursing*, eds G. Gray & R. Pratt, Churchill Livingstone, Melbourne.

Buber, M. 1965 *Between Man and Man*, Macmillan, New York.

Buber, M. 1970, *I and Thou*, Charles Scribner, New York.

Buchanan, B.F. 1987, 'Conceptual models: An assessment framework', *Journal of Nursing Administration*, 7(10), pp. 22–6.

Buckenham, J.E. & McGrath, G. 1983, *The Social Reality of Nursing*, Adis Health Science Press, Sydney.

Burns, N. & Grove, S. 1993, *The Practice of Nursing Research: Conduct Critique & Utiliation*, W.B. Saunders, Sydney.

Byrne, A. 1995, 'Migrants' new life often jobless', *The Sydney Morning Herald*, 23 February, p. 8.

Cameron, B.L. 1993, 'The nature of comfort to hospitalized medical surgical patients', *Journal of Advanced Nursing*, 18, pp. 424–36.

Campbell, I. 1990, 'Diabetic autonomic neuropathy', in *Diabetes Clinical Management*, eds R.B. Tattersall & A.M. Gale, Churchill Livingstone, Edinburgh.

Carlson, J.H., Craft, C.A., McGuire, A.D. & Popkess-Vawter, S. 1991, *Nursing Diagnosis: A Case Study Approach*, W.B. Saunders, Sydney.

Carnevali, D. 1983, *Nursing Care Planning: Diagnosis and Management*, 3rd edn, J.B. Lippincott, Philadelphia.

Carpenito, L.J. 1992, *Nursing Diagnosis: Application to Clinical Practice*, 4th edn, J.B. Lippincott, Philadelphia.

Carpenito, L.J. 1994, personal communication, Perth, November.

Carper, B.A. 1978, 'Fundamental patterns of knowing in nursing', *Advances in Nursing Science*, 1(1), pp. 13–23.

Carr, D. 1981, 'Knowledge in practice', *American Philosophical Quarterly*, 18(1), pp. 53–71.

Carr, W. & Kemmis, S. 1986, *Becoming Critical: Knowing through Action Research*, rev. edn, Deakin University Press, Geelong.

Carroll-Johnson, R.M. (ed.) 1991, *Classification of Nursing Diagnoses: Proceedings of the Ninth Conference*, J.B. Lippincott, Philadelphia.

Carstens, J. 1984, 'The effects of an in-service program on nurses' ability to identify valid nursing diagnosis', in *Classification of Nursing Diagnoses: Proceedings of the Third and Fourth National Conferences*, eds M.J. Kim & D.A. Moritz, McGraw-Hill, New York.

Cassmeyer, V.L. 1987, 'Interventions for persons with diabetes mellitus and hypoglycemia', in *Medical-Surgical Nursing Concepts and Clinical Practice*, eds W.J. Phipps, B.C. Long & N.F. Woods, C.V. Mosby, St Louis.

Castles, M.R. 1984, 'Interrater agreement in the use of nursing diagnoses', in *Classification of Nursing Diagnoses: Proceedings of the Third and Fourth National Conferences*, eds M.J. Kim & D.A. Moritz, McGraw-Hill, New York.

Catalano, J. 1994, 'A survey of educators' activities to empower nurses for practice', *Nursing Outlook*, 42, pp. 182–87.

Caudill, W. & Weinstein, H. 1969, 'Maternal care and infant behaviour in Japan and America', *Psychiatry*, 32, pp. 12–43.

Cauthen, K. 1985, 'Imaging the future: New visions and new responsibilities', *Zygon*, 20(3), pp. 321–39.

Chalmers, H. 1990, 'Nursing models: Enhancing or inhibiting practice', *Nursing Standard*, 5(11), pp. 34–40.

Charlesworth, Max 1982, *Science, Non-science and Pseudo-science*, Deakin University Press, Geelong, Victoria.

Cheek, J. & Rudge, T. 1994, 'Been there, done that? Consciousness raising, critical theory and nurses', *Contemporary Nurse*, 3, pp. 58–63.

Chenitz, C. & Swanson, C. 1986, *From Practice to Grounded Theory: Qualitative Research in Nursing*, Addison-Wesley, Menlo Park, California.

Chinn, P. & Jacobs, M. 1987, 'The evaluation of theory', in *Theory and Nursing: A Systematic Approach*, C.V. Mosby, St Louis.

Chinn, P. & Kramer, M. 1991, *Theory and Nursing: A Systematic Approach*, 3rd edn, Mosby-Year Book Inc., St Louis.

Chinn P., Wheeler C. & Roy A. 1988, Theoretical framework—exploratory study of friendship among women nurses, unpublished manuscript.

Chinn, P.L. & Jacobs, M.K. 1983, *Theory and Nursing: A Systematic Approach*, 2nd edn, C.V. Mosby , St Louis.

Chinn, P.L. & Kramer, M.K. 1995, *Theory and Nursing: A Systematic Approach*, 4th edn, Mosby, St Louis, Chapters 4 and 5.

Chittock, R. 1968, Assignment report, April to June 1968, WHO, Manila, in P. Wood (1990), *Nursing: Progress through Partnership 1921–1991*, AGPS, Canberra.

Chopoorian, T. 1986 'Reconceptualizing the environment', in *New Approaches to Theory Development*, ed. P. Moccia, National League for Nursing, New York.

Clarke, J. 1982, 'Development of models and theories on the concept of nursing', *Journal of Advanced Nursing*, 7, pp. 129–34.

Clay, T. 1987, *Nurses: Power and Politics*, Heinemann Nursing Books, London.

Cody, W.K. & Mitchell, G.J. 1992, 'Parse's theory as a model for practice: The cutting edge', *Advances in Nursing Science*, 15(2), pp. 52–65.

Commission on Catholic Health Care 1988, *A New Vision for a New Century*, Catholic Health Ministry, Farmington Mills, Michigan.

Commonwealth Department of Community Services and Health 1989, *National Women's Health Policy: Advancing Women's Health in Australia*, AGPS, Canberra.

Comstock, D. 1982, 'A method for critical research', in *Knowledge and Values in Social and Educational Research*, eds E. Bredo & W. Feinberg, Temple University Press, Philadelphia.

Connelly, A.M., Keele, B.S., Kleinbeck, S.V.M., Schneider, A.K. & Cobb, A.K. 1993, 'A place to be yourself: From the client's perspective', *Image: Journal of Nursing Scholarship*, 25(4), pp. 297–303.

Connelly, C.E. 1993, 'An empirical study of a model of self-care in chronic illness', *Clinical Nurse Specialist*, 7(5), pp. 247–53.

Considine, M. 1988, 'The corporate management framework as administrative science: A critique', *Journal of Public Administration*, 47(1), pp. 4–18.

Cook, E. 1942, *The Life of Florence Nightingale*, Macmillan, New York, in J. Fitzpatrick and A. Whall (1983) *Conceptual Models of Nursing: Analysis and Application*, Robert J. Brady Co., Bowie, Maryland.

Cooney, C. & Watts, R. 1992, 'Nursing diagnosis: Implications for health, with particular concerns for community nursing', *Contemporary Nurse*, 1(2), pp. 101–3.

Coultan, M. & Mellor, B. 1995, 'Chasing the Asian vote', *The Sydney Morning Herald*, 8 February, p. 16.

Cowling, R.W. 1989, 'Parse's theory of nursing', in *Conceptual Models of Nursing: Analysis and Application*, eds J.J. Fitzpatrick & L.L. Whall, Appleton & Lange, Norwalk.

Cox, H., Hickson, P. & Taylor, B. 1992, 'Exploring reflection: Knowing and constructing practice', in *Towards a Discipline of Nursing*, eds G. Gray & R. Pratt, Churchill Livingstone, Melbourne.

Cox, K., Lumby, J. & White, J. 1995, Practice as a discipline, unit of study in Master of Clinical Education, School of Medical Education, University of New South Wales.

Crane, Sue 1989, 'Joint appointments: The Deakin experience', *Australian Journal of Advanced Nursing*, 6:3, March–June, pp. 21–25.

Cunning, B. & Pflederer, D. 1986, 'Taking the nursing process gamely', *Nursing Management*, 17 (5), pp. 49–50.

Dale, A.E. 1994, 'The theory–theory gap: The challenge for nurse teachers', *Journal of Advanced Nursing*, 20, pp. 521–24.

Daly, J., Cody, W.K. & Romanini, J. 1994, 'Nursing theory and critical care nursing', in *Critical Care Nursing: Australian Perspectives*, eds J. Romanini & J. Daly, Harcourt Brace, Sydney.

Davis, A. & George, J. 1993, *States of Health: Health and Illness in Australia*, 2nd edn, HarperEducational, Pymble.

de Certeau, M. 1984, *The Practice of Everyday Life*, translated by S. Pendall, University of California Press, Berkley.

Deatrick, J.A. & Fischer, D.K. 1994, 'The atypical becomes typical: The work of oncology nurses', *Oncology Nursing Forum*, 21(8) (Suppl.), pp. 35–40.

Department of Human Services and Health 1995, *Nursing Education in Australian Universities: Report of the National Review of Nurse Education in the Higher Education Sector, 1994 and Beyond*, AGPS, Canberra.

Derrida, J. 1983, 'The time of a thesis: Punctuations', in *Philosophy in France Today*, ed. A. Montefiore, Cambridge University Press, Cambridge.

Dewey, J. 1958, *Experience and Nature*, Dover, New York.

Diabetes Control and Complications Trial Research Group 1993, 'The effect of intensive treatment of diabetes on the development and progression of long-term complications in insulin-dependent diabetes mellitus', *New England Journal of Medicine*, Sept., 239, pp. 977–86.

Dickoff, J. & James, P. 1968, 'Theory in a practice discipline, Part 1', *Nursing Research*, 17(5), pp. 415–35.

Dickoff, J., James, P. & Wiedenbach, E. 1968, 'Theory in a practice discipline: Part 1. Practice oriented theory', *Nursing Research*, 5, pp. 415–35.

Dickoff, J., James, P. & Wiedenbach, E. 1968b, 'Theory in a practice discipline: Part II, Practice oriented research', *Nursing Research* 17(6), pp. 545–54.

Diekelmann, N., Allen, D. & Tanner, C. 1989, *The NLN Criteria for Appraisal of Baccalaureate Programs: A Critical Hermeneutic Analysis,* National League for Nursing, New York.

Diers, D. 1986, 'To profess . . . to be a professional', *Journal of Nursing Administration,* 16(3), pp. 25–30.

Dilthey, W. 1988, *Introduction to the Human Sciences* (trans. R. Betanzos), Wayne State University Press, Detroit.

Dobson, S. & Penman, A. 1994, *Clinical Health Goals and Targets for Western Australia,* vol. 1, Health Department of Western Australia, Perth.

Doheny, M., Cook, C. & Stopper, C. 1987, *The Discipline of Nursing,* 2nd edn, Appleton & Lange, Norwalk, Connecticut.

Doherty, M.K., Sirl, M.B. & Ring, O.L. 1963, *Modern Practical Nursing Procedures,* 10th edn (revised by W.B. Smith, Y.L. Lew and M.L. Tomlinson), Dymocks, Sydney.

Donaghue, S. (1975), *Goals in Nursing Education, Part 1: Changing Patterns of Nursing Education in Australia,* College of Nursing, Melbourne, Australia.

Donahue, M.P. 1985, *Nursing: The Finest Art. An Illustrated History,* C.V. Mosby, St Louis.

Donaldson, S. K. & Crowley, D. M. 1978, 'The discipline of nursing', *Nursing Outlook,* 26, pp. 113–20.

Donnelly, P., Johnson, D., Maloney, S. & O'Brien, B.B. 1990, 'Establishing a professorial nursing unit', *Australian Nurses Journal,* 20:2, Sept., pp. 13–14.

Donnolly, G.F. 1987, 'The promise of nursing process: An evaluation', *Holistic Nursing Practice,* 1(3), pp. 1–6.

Dowd, T.M., Grabau, A.M., Kolbe, M.R., Munn, D.K., McCabe, B.W. & Smith, D.R. 1987, 'A replication study evaluating the use of a focused data collection tool for the generation of nursing diagnoses', in *Classification of Nursing Diagnoses: Proceedings of the Seventh Conference,* ed. R.M. McLane, C.V. Mosby, St Louis.

Draper, P. 1990, 'The development of theory in British nursing: Current position and future prospect', *Journal of Advanced Nursing,* 15, pp. 12–15.

Drew, P. 1995, 'Made in Japan', *The Sydney Morning Herald, Good Weekend,* 25 February, pp. 25–30.

Duffy, M. & Muhlenkamp, A.F. 1974, 'A framework for theory analysis', *Nursing Outlook,* 22(9), pp. 570–75.

Duldt, B. & Giffin, K. 1985, 'Assumptions', in *Theoretical Perspectives for Nursing,* eds B. Duldt & K. Giffin, Little, Brown, Boston, US.

Dunlop, M. 1992, *Shaping Nursing Knowledge: An Interpretive Analysis of Curriculum Documents from NSW, Australia,* Royal College of Nursing Australia, Melbourne.

Dunlop, M.J. 1986, 'Is a science of caring possible?' *Journal of Advanced Nursing,* 11:6, pp. 661–70.

Dunn, W., Brown, C. & McGuigan, A. 1994, 'The ecology of human performance: A framework for considering the effect of context', *American Journal of Occupational Therapy,* 48(7), pp. 595–607.

Durdin, J. 1991, *They Became Nurses: A History of Nursing in South Australia 1836–1980,* Allen & Unwin, North Sydney.

Eben, J.D., Gashti, N.N., Hayes, S.E., Marriner-Tomey, A., Nation, M.J. & Nordmeyer, S.B. 1994, 'Dorothea E. Orem', in *Nursing Theorists and their Work,* 3rd edn, ed. A. Marriner-Tomey, Mosby-Year Book Inc., St Louis.

Echartsberg, R. van 1981, 'Maps of the mind', in *The Metaphors of Consciousness,* eds R.S. Valle & R. van Echartsberg, Plenum, New York.

Edelson, M. 1970, *Sociotherapy and Psychotherapy,* University of Chicago Press, Chicago.

Ellis, R. 1968, 'Characteristics of significant theories', *Nursing Research,* 17(3), pp. 217–22.

Ellis, R. 1985, Foreword to 1st edn, in L. Nicoll 1992, *Perspectives on Nursing Theory,* 2nd edn, J.B. Lippincott, Philadelphia.

Emden, C. 1991, 'Becoming a reflective practitioner', in *Towards a Discipline of Nursing,* eds G. Gray & R. Pratt, Churchill Livingstone, Melbourne, pp. 335–55.

Emden, C. 1991, 'Ways of knowing in nursing', in *Towards a Discipline of Nursing,* eds G. Gray and R. Pratt, Churchill Livingstone, Melbourne, pp. 11–31.

Emden, C. 1995, 'A magnificent chaos: Feminist (nursing) comments on Western philosophy', *Nursing Inquiry,* 2, pp. 29–35.

English, J. & Morse, J.M. 1988, 'The "difficult" elderly patient: Adjustment or maladjustment?', *International Journal of Nursing Studies,* 25(1), pp. 23–39.

Estabrooks, C.A. & Morse, J.M. 1992, 'Toward a theory of touch: The touching process and acquiring a touching style', *Journal of Advanced Nursing,* 17, pp. 448–56.

Estes, S.D. & Hart, M. 1993, 'A model for the development of the CNS role in adolescent health promotion self-care', *Clinical Nurse Specialist,* 7(3), pp. 111–15.

Evans, M. 1991, 'Professional ethics and reflective practice: A moral analysis' in *Towards a Discipline of Nursing,* eds G. Gray & R. Pratt, Churchill Livingstone, Melbourne.

Ewan, C., Bryant, E. & Calvert, D. (eds) 1991, *Health Implications of Long Term Climatic Change,* National Health and Medical Research Council, AGPS, Canberra.

Ewan, C., Young, A., Bryant, E. & Calvert, D. 1994, *National Framework for Environmental and Health Impact Assessment,* National Health and Medical Research Council, AGPS, Canberra.

Eysenck, M. & Keane, M.T. 1990, *Cognitive Psychology: A Student's Handbook,* Lawrence Erlbaum, Hove, England.

Eysenck, M.W. 1993, *Principles of Cognitive Psychology,* Lawrence Erlbaum, Hove, England.

Fawcett, J. 1980, 'A framework for analysis and evaluation of conceptual models of nursing', *Nurse Educator,* 5(6), pp. 10–14.

Fawcett, J. 1984, 'The metaparadigm in nursing: Present status and future refinements', *Image,* 3, pp. 84–7.

Fawcett, J. 1984, *Analysis and Evaluation of Conceptual Models of Nursing,* F.A. Davis, Philadelphia.

Fawcett, J. 1988, *Analysis and Evaluation of Conceptual Models on Nursing,* 2nd edn, F.A. Davis, Philadelphia.

Fawcett, J. 1993, 'From a plethora of paradigms to parsimony in worldviews', *Nursing Science Quarterly,* 6(2), pp. 56–8.

Fawcett, J. 1993b, *Analysis and Evaluation of Nursing Theories*, F.A. Davis, Philadelphia.

Fawcett, J. & Carino, C. 1987, 'Hallmarks of success in nursing practice', *Advances in Nursing Science*, 11(4), pp. 1–8.

Fay, B. 1975, *Social Theory and Political Practice*, Unwin Hyman Books, Sydney.

Fernandez, R. Brennan, M.L., Alvarez, A.R. & Duffy, M.R. 1990, 'Theory-based practice: A model for nurse retention', *Nursing Administration Quarterly*, 14(4), pp. 47–53.

Field, L. & Winslow, E.H. 1985, 'Moving to a nursing model', *American Journal of Nursing*, October, pp. 1100–1.

Field, P.A. & Morse, J.M. 1985, *Nursing Research. The Application of Qualitative Approaches*, Chapman & Hall, London.

Fine, G. A. & Rosnow, R. L. 1978, 'Gossip, gossipes, gossiping', *Personality and Social Psychology Bulletin*, 4, pp. 161–68.

Fitch, M., Rogers, M., Ross, E., Shea, H., Smith, I. & Tucker, D. 1991, 'Developing a plan to evaluate the use of nursing conceptual frameworks', *Canadian Journal of Nursing Administration*, March/April, pp. 22–28.

Fitts, P.M. & Posner, M.I. 1967, *Human Performance*, Brooks/Cole Publishing Co., Belmont, California.

Fitzpatrick, J. & Whall, A. 1983, *Conceptual Models of Nursing: Analysis and Application*, Robert J. Brady, Bowie, Maryland.

Fitzpatrick, J., Kerr, M., Saba, V., Hoskins, L., Hurley, M., Mills, W., Rottkamp, B., Warren, J., & Carpenito, L. 1989, 'Nursing diagnosis: Translating nursing diagnosis into ICD code', *American Journal of Nursing*, April, pp. 493–95.

Fitzpatrick, J.J. & Whall, A.L. (eds) 1989, *Conceptual Models of Nursing: Analysis and Application*, 2nd edn, Appleton & Lange, Norwalk, Connecticut.

Flaskerud, J.H. & Halloran, E.J. 1980, 'Areas of agreement in nursing theory development', *Advances in Nursing Science*, 3(1), pp. 1–7.

Flax, J. 1992, 'The end of innocence', in *Feminists Theorize the Political*, eds J. Butler & J. Scott, Routledge, New York.

Fortin, J.D. & Rabinow, J. 1979, 'Legal implications of nursing diagnosis', *Nursing Clinics of North America*, 14(3), pp. 553–61.

Foster, P.C. & Janssens, N.P. 1990, 'Dorothea Orem', in *Nursing Theories: The Base for Professional Nursing Practice*, 3rd edn, ed. J.B. George, Appleton & Lange, Connecticut.

Foucault, M. 1972, *The Archeology of Knowledge*, Tavistock, London.

Foucault, M. 1984, *The History of Sexuality, Vol. 1: An Introduction*, Vintage Books, New York.

Fox, D.J. 1982, *Fundamentals of Research in Nursing*, 4th edn, Appleton-Century-Crofts, Norwalk, Connecticut.

Fredette, S.L. & O'Neil, E.S. 1987, 'Can theory improve diagnoses? An examination of the relationship between didactic content and the ability to diagnose in clinical practice', in *Classification of Nursing Diagnoses: Proceedings of the Seventh Conference*, ed. A.M. McLane, C.V. Mosby, St Louis.

Freire, P. 1972, *Pedagogy of the Oppressed*, Penguin, Harmondsowrth.

Freire, P. 1994, *Education for Critical Consciousness*, Continuum, New York.

French, P. 1992, 'The quality of nurse education in the 1980s', *Journal of Advanced Nursing*, 17, pp. 619–31.

Frey, M.A. & Denyes, M.J. 1989, 'Health and illness self-care in adolescents with IDDM: A test of Orem's theory', *Advances in Nursing Science*, 12(1), pp. 67–75.

Friedson, E. 1983, 'The theory of professions: State of the art', in *The Sociology of the Professions*, eds R. Dingwall & P. Lewis, Macmillan, London.

Fry, S.T. 1994, *Ethics in Nursing Practice*, International Council of Nurses, Geneva.

Funnell, M.M., Anderson, R.M., Arnold, M.S., Barr, P.A., Donnelly, M., Taylor-Moon, D. & White, N.H. 1991, 'Empowerment: An idea whose time has come in diabetes education', *The Diabetes Educator*, 17(1) Jan./Feb., pp. 37–41.

Gadow, S. 1980, 'Existential advocacy: Philosophical foundation of nursing', in *Nursing: Images and Ideals*, eds S. Spicker & S. Gadow, Springer, New York.

Gardner, D.L., Kelly, K., Johnson, M., McCloskey, J.C. & Mass, M. 1991, 'Nursing administration model for administrative practice', *Journal of Nursing Administration*, 21(3), pp. 37–41.

Gardner, H. (ed.) 1989, *The Politics of Health: The Australian Experience,* Churchill Livingstone, Melbourne.

Gardner, K.G. & Wheeler, E.C. 1987, 'Patients' perceptions of support', *Western Journal of Nursing Research,* 9(1), pp. 115–31.

Gebbie, K., & Lavin, H. 1974, 'Classifying nursing diagnoses', *American Journal of Nursing,* 74 (2), pp. 250–53.

Gendron, D. 1994, 'The tapestry of care', *Advances in Nursing Science,* 17(1), pp. 25–30.

George, J.B. 1990, *Nursing Theories: The Base of Professional Practice*, 3rd edn, Prentice-Hall, New Jersey.

Gibb, H., O'Brien, B.B., Bradford, J. & Curtis, P. 1993, Action research into the nursing management of continence, unpublished research report, Julia Farr Foundation, Adelaide, South Australia.

Giddens, Anthony 1989, *Sociology*, Polity Press, Cambridge.

Gilkey, H.H. 1953, 'Does higher education have an obligation for nursing education?' *School and Society,* 77, pp. 101–103, in J.A. Thibodeau, 1983, *Nursing Models: Analysis and Evaluation*, Monterey, California.

Gilligan, C. 1982, *In a Different Voice: Psychological Theory and Women's Development*, Harvard University Press, Harvard.

Giorgi, A. 1970, *Psychology as a Human Science: A Phenomenologically Based Approach*, Harper & Row, New York.

Giorgi, A. 1985, 'Sketch of a phenomenological method', in *Phenomenology and Psychological Research*, ed. A. Giorgi, Duquesne University Press, Pittsburgh.

Glaser, B. & Strauss, A. 1967, *The Discovery of Grounded Theory*, Aldine, Chicago.

Glaser, B.G. 1978, *Theoretical Sensitivity*, Sociology Press, Mill Valley, California.

Glaser, B.G. 1992, *Basics of Grounded Theory Analysis: Emergence vs Forcing*, Sociology Press, Mill Valley, California.

Gordon, M. 1976, 'Nursing diagnosis and the diagnostic process', *American Journal of Nursing,* 76(8), pp. 1298–1300.

Gordon, M. 1987, *Nursing Diagnosis: Process and Application*, 2nd edn, McGraw-Hill, New York.

Gordon, M. 1989, 'Strategies for teaching diagnostic reasonings', in *Classification of Nursing Diagnoses: Proceedings of the Eighth Conference*, ed. R.M. Carroll-Johnson, J.B. Lippincott, Philadelphia.

Gortner, S.R. 1983, 'The history and philosophy of nursing science and research', *Advances in Nursing Science,* 5(2), pp. 1–8.

Gott, M. 1984, *Learning Nursing*, Royal College of Nursing, London.

Gray, G. & Pratt, R. (eds) 1991, *Towards a Discipline of Nursing*, Churchill Livingstone, Melbourne.

Gray, G. & Pratt, R. (eds) 1992a, *Issues in Australian Nursing 3*, Churchill Livingstone, Melbourne.

Gray, G. & Pratt, R. (eds) 1992b, *Towards a Discipline of Nursing*, Churchill Livingstone, Melbourne.

Gray, G. & Pratt, R. (eds) 1995a, *Issues in Australian Nursing 4*, Churchill Livingstone, Melbourne.

Gray, G. & Pratt, R. (eds) 1995b, *Issues in Australian Nursing 5,* Churchill Livingstone, Melbourne.

Gray, G. & Pratt, R. (eds) 1995c, *Scholarship in the Discipline of Nursing*, Churchill Livingstone, Melbourne.

Greenwood, J. 1984, 'Nursing research: A position paper', *Journal of Advanced Nursing*, 9, pp. 77–82.

Greenwood, J. 1988, 'More considerations concerning the application of nursing models to curricula: A reply to Lorraine Smith', *Nurse Education Today*, 8, pp. 187–90.

Greenwood, J. 1990, Learning to care: Thought and action in the education of nurses, unpublished PhD thesis, Leeds University, England.

Greenwood, J. 1993, 'The apparent desensitization of student nurses during their professional socialisation: A cognitive perspective', *Journal of Advanced Nursing*, 18, pp. 1471–9.

Greenwood, J. & King, M. 1995, 'Nursing orthopaedic patients: Profoundly absorbing work', in *Issues in Nursing 5,* eds G. Gray & R. Pratt, Churchill Livingstone, Melbourne.

Griffin, A.P. 1980, 'Philosophy and nursing', *Journal of Advanced Nursing*, 5:2, pp. 261–72.

Griffin, A.P. 1983, 'A philosophical analysis of caring in nursing', *Journal of Advanced Nursing*, 8:4, pp. 289–95.

Gross, E. 1986, 'What is feminist theory?' in *Feminist Challenges*, eds C. Pateman & E. Gross, Allen & Unwin, Sydney.

Gruending, D.L. 1985, 'Nursing theory: A vehicle of professionalism?', *Journal of Advanced Nursing*, 10(6), pp. 553–8.

Grundy, S. 1987, *Curriculum: Product or Praxis?* The Falmer Press, Bascombe, Lowes.

Grundy, S. & Kemmis, S. 1988, 'Educational action research in Australia: The state of the art', in *The Action Research Reader*, 3rd edn, eds S. Kemmis & R. McTaggart, Deakin University, Geelong, Victoria, pp. 321–35.

Guzzetta, C. 1990, 'Holistic nursing: Unravelling the mysteries and weaving the tapestry', *Conference proceedings: Fourth National Nursing Education Conference*, Melbourne.

Guzzetta, C.E. & Dossey, B. 1983, 'Nursing diagnosis: Framework, process and problems', *Heart and Lung,* 12(3), pp. 281–91.

Guzzetta, C.E., Bunton, S.D., Prinkey, L.A., Sherer, A.P. & Seifert, P.C. 1989, *Clinical Assessment Tools for Use with Nursing Diagnoses*, C.V. Mosby, St Louis.

Habermas, J. 1965, *Knowledge and Human Interests* (trans. 1986 Jeremy Shapiro), Polity Press, Cambridge.

Hagell, E.I. 1989, 'Nursing knowledge: Women's knowledge. A sociological perspective', *Journal of Advanced Nursing*, 14, pp. 226–33.

Haire-Joshu, D. 1992, *Management of Diabetes Mellitus: Perspectives of Care across the Life Span*, Mosby-Year Book Inc., St Louis.

Hall, B. & Allan, J. 1994, 'Self in relation: A prolegomenon for holistic nursing', *Nursing Outlook*, 15, pp. 110–16.

Hall, L.E. 1964, 'Nursing—what is it?', *Canadian Nurse*, 60:2, pp. 150–54.

Hardy, L.K. 1986, 'Identifying the place of theoretical frameworks in an evolving discipline', *Journal of Advanced Nursing*, 11, pp. 103–7.

Hardy, M.E. 1974, 'Theories: Components, development, evaluation', *Journal of Nursing Research*, 23(2), pp. 101–8.

Hargreaves, I. 1981, 'The nursing process', in *Nursing Science in Nursing Practice*, ed. James P. Smith, Butterworths, London.

Harmer, B. & Henderson, V. 1955, *Textbook of the Principles and Practice of Nursing*, 5th edn, Macmillan, New York.

Hart, G. 1991, 'Research for action: Promoting excellence in clinical teaching', National Conference on the Discipline of Nursing: New Horizons in Nursing Theory, Education, Practice and Research, University of Sydney, June.

Hartsock, N. 1990, 'Foucault on power: A theory for women?' in *Feminism/Postmodernism*, ed. L. Nicholson, Routledge, New York.

Hedin, B. 1986, 'A case study of oppressed group behaviour in nurses', *Image: Journal of Nursing Scholarship*, 18:2, pp. 53–57.

Hedin, B. 1987, 'Nursing education and social constraints: An indepth analysis', *International Journal of Nursing Studies*, 24:3, pp. 261–70.

Heidegger, M. 1962, *Being and Time*, Harper & Row, New York.

Heinrich, K. & Witt, B. 1993, 'The passionate connection: Feminism invigorates the teaching of nursing', *Nursing Outlook*, 41:3, pp. 117–24.

Henderson, D. 1995, 'Consciousness raising in participatory research: Method and methodology for emancipatory nursing inquiry', *Advances in Nursing Science*, 17:3, pp. 58–69.

Henderson, V. 1966, *The Nature of Nursing: A Definition and its Implication for Practice, Research, and Education*, Macmillan, New York.

Henderson, V. 1977, *Basic Principles of Nursing Care*, International Council of Nurses, Geneva.

Henderson, V. 1982, 'The nursing process—is the title right?', *Journal of Advanced Nursing*, 7, pp. 108–9.

Henderson, V. 1987, 'Nursing process—a critique', *Holistic Nursing Practice*, 1(3), pp. 7–18.

Henderson, V. & Nite, G. 1978, *Principles and Practices of Nursing*, 6th edn, Macmillan, New York.

Henning, M. 1991, 'Comparison of nursing diagnostic statements using a functional health pattern and a health/history/body systems format', in *Classification of Nursing Diagnoses: Proceedings of the Ninth Conference*, ed. R.M. Carroll-Johnson, J.B. Lippincott, Philadelphia.

Heydebrand, W. 1983, 'Organization and praxis', in *Beyond Method*, ed. G. Morgan, Sage, Beverley Hills.

Hillson, R. 1992, *Diabetes: A Beyond Basics Guide*, Optima, Little Brown, London.

Hillson, R. 1994, *Diabetes: A New Guide*, Optima, Little Brown, London.

Hinds, P.S. & Chaves, D.E. 1992, 'Context as a source of meaning and understanding', *Qualitative Health Research*, 2(1), pp. 61–74.

Hinshaw, A. 1989, 'Nursing diagnosis forging the link between theory and practice', in

Classification of Nursing Diagnoses: Proceedings of the Eighth Conference, ed. R.M. Carroll-Johnson, J.B. Lippincott, Philadelphia.

Hockey, L. 1981, *Recent Advances in Nursing: Current Issues in Nursing*, Churchill Livingstone, Melbourne.

Hohnson, D.E. 1974, 'Development of theory: A requisite for nursing as a primary health profession', *Nursing Research*, 23(5), pp. 372–77.

Holden, R.J. 1991, 'An analysis of caring: Attributions, contributions and resolutions', *Journal of Advanced Nursing*, 16, pp. 893–8.

Holmes, C.A. 1990, 'Alternatives to natural science foundations for nursing', *International Journal of Nursing Studies*, 27, pp. 187–98.

Holter, I.M. 1988, 'Critical theory: A foundation for the development of nursing theories', *Scholarly Inquiry for Nursing Practice*, 2(3), pp. 223–32.

Horsfall, J. 1990, 'An education for professional autonomy, or a pedagogy for oppressed nurses', paper presented to National Nurse Education Conference, Melbourne, Nov., 1994.

Horsfall, J. 1992, 'Humanism, feminism and problem-based learning', in *Proceedings National Nursing Conference*, Problem-based Learning in Nursing Education and Practice, Melbourne.

Horsfall, J. 1993, 'Ask and adequately inform: RPN Responsibilities working with the long-term mentally ill', *Proceedings Psychiatric Nursing Conference*, RMIT, Melbourne.

Horsfall, J. 1995, 'Madness in our methods: Nursing research, scientific epistemology', *Nursing Inquiry*, 2:1, pp. 2–9.

Hoshmond, L.T. & Polkinghorne, D.E. 1992, 'Redefining the science-practice relationship and professional training', *American Psychologist*, 47, pp. 55–66.

Hoskins, K.W. & Macve, R.H. 1993, 'Accounting as discipline: The overlooked supplement', in *Knowledges: Historical and Critical Studies in Disciplinarity*, eds E. Messer-Davidow, D.R. Shumway & D.J. Sylvan, University Press of Virginia, Charlottesville.

Hovenga, E. 1991, 'An Australian nursing data dictionary', *Proceedings of the National Nursing Diagnosis Conference*, Gold Coast, Queensland.

Howard, R.W. 1987, *Concepts and Schemata: An Introduction*, Cassell Education, London.

Hughes, E.C. 1951, 'Studying the nurses' work', *The American Journal of Nursing*, 51, pp. 294–95.

Hughes, J. 1990, *The Philosophy of Social Research*, Longman, London.

Husserl, E. 1976, *Ideas*, Humanities Press, New York.

Hutchinson, S.A. 1986, 'Creating meaning: Grounded theory of NICU nurses', in *From Practice to Grounded Theory*, eds W.C. Chenitz & J.M. Swanson, Addison-Wesley, Menlo Park, California, pp. 191–204.

Hutchinson, S.A. & Webb, R.B. 1989, 'Teaching qualitative research: Perennial problems and possible solutions', in *Qualitative Nursing Research—A Contemporary Dialogue*, ed. J.M. Morse, Aspen, Rockville, Maryland, pp. 285–302.

Ingram, R. 1991, 'Why does nursing need theory?' *Journal of Advanced Nursing*, 16, pp. 350–53.

Irurita, V. 1993, 'From person to patient: nursing care from the patient's perspective', occasional paper, School of Nursing, Curtin University of Technology, Perth, WA.

Irurita, V., Williams, A. & Reeves, G. 1994, A study comparing nurses' and patients' perceptions of the quality of nursing care, unpublished report, Department of Nursing Research, Sir Charles Gairdner Hospital, Perth, WA.

Iyer, P.W., Taptich, B.J. & Bernocchi-Losey, D. 1991, *Nursing Process and Nursing Diagnosis*, 2nd edn, W.B. Saunders, Philadelphia.

Jackson, T., Mitchell, S. & Wright, M. 1989, 'Community development continuum', *Community Health Studies*, 13(1), pp. 66–73.

Jacobs-Kramer, M. & Chinn, P. 1988, 'Perspectives on knowing: A model of nursing knowledge', *Scholarly Inquiry for Nursing Practice*, 2(2), pp. 129–39.

Jacox, A.K. 1974, 'Theory construction in nursing: An overview', in L. Nicoll 1992, *Perspectives on Nursing Theory*, 2nd edn, J.B. Lippincott, Philadelphia.

Jacox, A.K. & Webster, G. 1986, 'Competing theories of science', in L. Nicoll 1992, *Perspectives on Nursing Theory*, 2nd edn, J.B. Lippincott, Philadelphia.

James, J. 1976, 'Activating Theory', *The Lamp*, May, pp. 23–25.

Jennings, B.M. 1987, 'Nursing theory development: Successes and challenges', *Journal of Advanced Nursing*, 2(1), pp. 63–69.

Jenny, J. & Logan, J. 1992, 'Knowing the patient: One aspect of clinical knowledge', *Image: Journal of Nursing Scholarship*, 24(4), pp. 254–58.

John, I.D. 1994, 'Constructing knowledge of psychological knowledge: towards an epistemology of psychological practice', *Australian Psychologist*, 29(3), pp. 158–63.

Johns, Christopher 1991, 'The Burford Nursing Development Unit holistic model of nursing practice', *Journal of Advanced Nursing*, 16:4, pp. 1090–98.

Johns, Christopher (ed.) 1994, *The Burford NDU Model: Caring in Practice*, Blackwell Science, Oxford.

Johnson, C. & Hales, L. 1989, 'Nursing diagnosis anyone? Do staff nurses use nursing diagnosis effectively?', *Journal of Continuing Education in Nursing*, 20(1), pp. 30–5.

Johnson, J. 1994, 'A dialectical examination of nursing art', *Advances in Nursing Sciences*, 17(1), pp. 1–14.

Johnson, N. & Baumann, A. 1992, 'Selecting a nursing model for psychiatric nursing', *Journal of Psychosocial Nursing*, 30(4), pp. 7–12.

Jolley, M. & Brykczynska, G. 1993, *Nursing: Its Hidden Agendas*, Edward Arnold, London.

Jonas, C. 1995, 'Evaluation of the human becoming theory in family practice', in Parse, R.R. (ed.), *Illuminations: The Human Becoming Theory in Practice and Research*, National League for Nursing Press, Pub. No. 15–2670, New York.

Jonas, C.M. 1987, 'Kings' goal attainment theory: Use in gerontological nursing practice', *Perspectives*, 11(4), pp. 9–12.

Jonas, C.M., Pilkington, B., Lyon, P. & McDonald, G.E. 1992, *Parse's Theory of Human Becoming Learning Modules*, St Michael's Hospital, Toronto.

Jones, D. & Smith, L. 1981, 'Introduction', in *Deprivation, Participation and Community Action*, eds L. Smith & D. Jones, Routledge & Kegan Paul, London.

Jones, W. T. 1975, *A History of Western Philosophy: Kant and the Nineteenth Century*, 2nd edn, Harcourt Brace Jovanovich, New York.

Josefson, I. 1988, 'The nurse as engineer—the theory of knowledge in research in the care sector', in *Knowledge, Skill and Artificial Intelligence*, eds B. Goranzon & I. Josefson, Springer-Verlag, London.

Kamsler, A. 1990, 'Her-story in the making. Therapy with women who were sexually abused in childhood', in *Ideas for Therapy with Sexual Abuse*, eds M. Durrant & C.White, pp. 9–37.

Kanitsaki, O. 1988, 'Transcultural nursing: Challenge to change', *Australian Journal of Advanced Nursing*, 5(3), pp. 4–11.

Kearney, J. 1993, *Healthy Participation: Achieving Greater Public Participation and Accountability in the Australian Health Care System*, Background Paper No. 12, National Health Strategy, Canberra.

Keck, J.F. 1989, 'Terminology of theory development', in *Nursing Theorists and their Work*, 2nd edn, ed. A. Marriner-Toomey, C.V. Mosby, St Louis.

Keen, P. 1991, 'Caring for ourselves', in *Caring and Nursing: Explorations in Feminist Perspectives*, eds R. Neil & R. Watts, National League of Nursing, New York.

Kellerman, D.F. (ed.) 1973, *The International Webster New Encyclopedic Dictionary*, Tabor House, New York.

Kelly, B. 1991, 'The professional values of English undergraduates', *Journal of Advanced Nursing*, 16, pp. 867–72.

Kelly, G. 1969, *Clinical Psychology and Personality: The Selected Papers of George Kelly*, George Wiley & Sons, New York.

Kemmis, S. 1985, 'Action research and the politics of reflection', in *Reflection: Turning Experience into Learning*, eds D. Boud, R. Keogh & D. Walker, Kogan Page, London.

Kennedy, M. M. 1983, 'Working knowledge', *Creation, Diffusion, Utilisation*, 5(2), pp. 193–211.

Keohane, N.S. & Lacey, L.A. 1991, 'Preparing the woman with gestational diabetes for self-care: Use of a structured teaching plan by nursing staff', *Journal of Obstetric Gynecologic and Neonatal Nursing*, 20(3), pp. 189–93.

Kermode, S. 1993, 'The power to be different: Is professionalization the answer?', *Contemporary Nurse*, 2(3), pp. 102–9.

Kermode, S. & Brown C. 1995, 'Where have all the flowers gone? Nursing's escape from the radical critique', *Contemporary Nurse*, 4:1, March, pp. 8–15.

Kidd, P. & Morrison, E. 1988, 'The progression of knowledge in nursing: A search for meaning', *Image*, 20 (4), pp. 222–24.

Kierkegaard, S. 1958, *Philosophical Fragments*, Princeton University Press, Princeton.

Kierkegaard, S. 1959, *Either/Or*, Anchor Books, New York.

Kim, H.S. 1989, 'Theoretical thinking in nursing: Problems and prospects', in *Recent Advances in Nursing: Theories and Models*, ed. J.A. Akinsanya, Churchill Livingstone, Edinburgh.

Kim, H.S. 1994, 'Practice theories in nursing and a science of nursing practice', *Scholarly Inquiry for Nursing Practice*, 8(2), pp. 145–58.

Kim, M.J., Suhayda, R., Waters, L. & Yocum, C. 1984, 'The effect of using nursing diagnosis in nursing care planning', in *Classification of Nursing Diagnoses: Proceedings of the Third and Fourth National Conferences*, eds M.J. Kim & D.A. Moritz, McGraw-Hill, New York.

King, I. 1991, 'Nursing theory 25 years later', *Nursing Science Quarterly*, 4(3), pp. 94–95.

King, I.M. 1971, *Toward a Theory for Nursing: General Concepts of Human Behaviour*, Wiley, New York.

King, K. 1994, 'Method and methodology in feminist research: What is the difference?', *Journal of Advanced Nursing*, 20, pp. 19–22.

Kitchener, K.S. 1983, 'Cognition, metacognition, and epistemic cognition', *Human Development*, 26, pp. 222–32.

Klein, J.T. 1993, 'Blurring, cracking, and crossing: Permeation and the fracturing of disciplines', in *Knowledges: Historical and Critical Studies in Disciplinarity*, eds E. Messer-

Davidow, D.R. Shumway & D.J. Sylvan, University Press of Virginia, Charlottesville.

Kockelmans, J.J. 1978, *Edmund Husserl's Phenomenological Psychology: A Historico-critical Study*, Humanities Press, Atlantic Highlands.

Komter, A. 1991, 'Gender, power and feminist theory', in *The Gender of Power*, eds K. Davis, M. Leijenaar & J. Oldersma, Sage, London.

Kozier, B., Erb, G. & Blais, K. 1992, *Concepts and Issues in Nursing Practice*, 2nd edn, Addison-Wesley, Redwood City, California.

Kuhn, T.S. 1970, *The Structure of Scientific Revolutions*, University of Chicago Press, Chicago.

Labonte, R. 1989. 'Commentary: Community empowerment: Reflections on the Australian situation', Community Health Studies, 13(3), pp. 347–49.

Lacey, A.R., 'Theory of knowledge', in *A Dictionary of Philosophy*, 2nd edn, Routledge & Kegan Paul, London.

Lague, D. 1995, 'Trading with the tigers', *The Sydney Morning Herald*, 7 February, p. 12.

Lampe, S. & Hitchcock, A. 1987, 'Documenting nursing diagnosis using focus charting', in *Classification of Nursing Diagnoses: Proceedings of the Seventh Conference*, ed. A.M. McLane, C.V. Mosby, St Louis.

Larson, P.J. 1984, 'Important nurse caring behaviours perceived by patients with cancer', *Oncology Nursing Forum*, 11(6), pp. 46–50.

Larson, P.J. 1987, 'Comparison of cancer patients' and professional nurses' perceptions of important nurse caring behaviours', *Heart and Lung*, 16(2), pp. 187–93.

Lather, P. 1986, 'Research as praxis', *Harvard Educational Review*, 56(3), pp. 257–77.

Lawler, J. 1991, 'In search of an Australian identity', in *Towards a Discipline of Nursing*, eds G. Gray & R. Pratt, Churchill Livingstone, Melbourne.

Lawler, J. 1991, *Behind the Screens: Nursing, Somology and the Problem of the Body*, Churchill Livingstone, Melbourne.

Lawler, J. 1991, What you see is not always what you get: Seeing, feeling and researching nursing. Keynote address given to First International Conference of the Centre for Nursing Research Inc., Adelaide, July 15–17.

Leedy, S. & Pepper, J. 1989, *Conceptual Bases of Professional Nursing*, J.B. Lippincott, Philadelphia.

Leininger, M. 1994, 'Evaluation criteria and critique of qualitative research studies', in *Critical Issues in Qualitative Research Methods*, ed. J. Morse, Sage Publications, London.

Leininger, M.M. (ed.) 1991, *Culture Care Diversity and Universality: A Theory of Nursing*, National League for Nursing, New York.

Lenoir, T. 1993, 'The discipline of nature and the nature of disciplines', in *Knowledges: Historical and Critical Studies in Disciplinarity*, eds E. Messer-Davidow, D.R. Shumway & D.J. Sylvan, University Press of Virginia, Charlottesville.

Levine, M. 1969, *Introduction to Clinical Nursing*, Davis, Philadelphia.

Levine, M. 1973, *Introduction to Clinical Nursing*, 2nd edn, Davis, Philadelphia.

Levine, M.E. 1988, Book review—Parse, R.R., *Nursing Science Quarterly*, 1, pp. 184–85.

Lewis, T. 1988, 'Leaping the chasm between nursing theory and practice', *Journal of Advanced Nursing*, 13, pp. 345–51.

Limrandi, B.J. 1982, Book reviews—Parse, R.R., *Western Journal of Nursing Research*, 4(1), pp. 105–6.

Lister, P. 1991, 'Approaching models of nursing from a postmodern perspective', *Journal of Advanced Nursing*, 16, pp. 206–12.

Livingstone, P.G. (Chair), Committee to advise on Desirable Developments in Nurse Education Report, Board of Advanced Education, Queensland, August 1976, in R.L. Russell (1990), *From Nightingale to Now: Nurse Education in Australia*, W.B. Saunders, Sydney.

Lloyd, G. 1984, *The Man of Reason: 'Male' and 'Female' in Western Philosophy*, Methuen, London.

Lowenberg, J. 1993, 'Interpretive research methodology: Broadening the dialogue', *Advances in Nursing Science*, 16:2, pp. 57–69.

Lowry, L. 1988, 'Operationalizing the Neuman Systems Model: a course in concepts and process', *Nurse Education*, 13(3) pp. 19–22.

Ludwig-Beymer, P., Ryan, C.J., Johnson, N.J., Hennessy, K.A., Gattuso, M.C., Epsom. R. & Czurylo, K.T. 1993, 'Using patient perceptions to improve quality care', *Journal of Nursing Care Quality*, 7(2), pp. 42–51.

Lumby, J. 1991, 'Threads of an emerging discipline: Praxis, reflection, rhetoric and research', in *Towards a Discipline of Nursing*, eds G. Gray & R. Pratt, Churchill Livingstone, Melbourne.

Lundh, U., Soder, M. & Waerness, K. 1988, 'Nursing theories: A critical view', *Image: Journal of Nursing Scholarship*, 20(1), pp. 36–40.

Maeve, M.K. 1994, 'The carrier bag theory of nursing practice', *Advances in Nursing Science*, 16(4), pp. 9–22.

Mager, R. 1962, *Preparing Instructional Objectives*, Feron Publishers, Belmont, CA.

Mahan, W. 14/10/1994, *Nursenet: A Global Forum for Nursing Issues*, Email.

Mahler, H. 1977, 'The meaning of primary health care', *Australian Nurses' Journal*, 7(6), pp. 22–25.

Mallick, M.J. 1981, 'Patient assessment-based on data not intuition', *Nursing Outlook*, October, pp. 600–605.

Manning, J., Broughton, V. & McConnell, E. A. 1995, 'Reality based scenarios facilitate knowledge network development', *Contemporary Nurse*, 4, pp. 16–21.

Manock, H. 1973, 'How can nursing in Australia grow?', *Australian Nurses' Journal*, 2(1), pp. 30–31.

Marriner, A. 1979, *The Nursing Process*, 2nd edn, C.V. Mosby, St Louis.

Marriner, A. 1986, *Nursing Theorists and their Work*, C.V. Mosby, St Louis.

Marriner-Tomey, A. (ed.) 1989, *Nursing Theorists and their Work*, 2nd edn, C.V. Mosby, St Louis.

Marriner-Tomey, A. 1994, *Nursing Theorists and their Work*, 3rd edn, C.V. Mosby, Sydney.

Marx, M. 1976, 'Formal Theory', in *Theories in Contemporary Psychology*, 2nd edn, eds M. Marx & F. Goodson, Macmillan, New York.

Maslen, G. 1995, 'The last gasp', *The Sydney Morning Herald, Good Weekend*, 25 February, pp. 18–23.

Masso, M. 1990, 'Nursing process: Help or hindrance?', *Journal of Advanced Nursing*, 7(3), pp. 12–16.

Mayberry, A. 1991, 'Merging nursing theories, models, and nursing practice: More than an administrative challenge', *Nursing Administration Quarterly*, 15(3), pp. 44–53.

Mayer, D.K. 1986, 'Cancer patients' and families' perceptions of nurse caring behaviours', *Topics in Clinical Nursing*, 8(2), pp. 63–69.

Mayer, D.K. 1987, 'Oncology nurses' versus cancer patients' perceptions of nurse caring behaviours: A replication study', *Oncology Nursing Forum*, 14(3), pp. 48–53.

McCaugherty, D. 1991, 'The theory–practice gap in nurse education: Its causes and possible solutions. Findings from an action research study', *Journal of Advanced Nursing*, 17, pp. 1055–61.

McClosky, J. & Bulechek, G. 1993, 'The NIC taxonomy structure', *Image*, 25(3), pp. 187–92.

McCoppin, B. & Gardner, H. 1994, *Tradition and Reality: Nursing and Politics in Australia*, Churchill Livingstone, Melbourne.

McCourt, A. 1986, 'Nursing diagnoses: Key to quality assurance', in *Classification of Nursing Diagnoses: Proceedings of the Sixth Conference*, ed. M.E. Hurley, C.V. Mosby, St Louis.

McCulloch, S.J. 1995, 'Utilisation of the Neuman Systems Model: University of South Australia', in *The Neuman Systems Model*, 3rd edn, ed. B. Neuman, Appleton-Lange, Connecticut.

McFarlane, J. 1976, 'A charter for caring', *Journal of Advanced Nursing*, 1, pp. 187–96.

McGlone, M. 1990, 'Healing the spirit', *Holistic Nursing Practice*, 4(4), pp. 77–84.

McHugh, M.K. 1991, 'Does the nursing process reflect quality care?', *Holistic Nursing Practice*, 5(3), pp. 22–28.

McKnight, J. 1987, 'Regenerating community', *Social Policy*, 17(3), pp. 54–61.

McLane, A.M., Lancour, J. & Gotch, P. 1986, 'Nursing diagnoses in nursing practice', in *Classification of Nursing Diagnoses: Proceedings of the Sixth Conference*, ed. M.E. Hurley, C.V. Mosby, St Louis.

McLaughlin, A.M. & Carey, J.L. 1993, 'The adversarial alliance: Developing therapeutic relationships between families and the team in brain injury rehabilitation', *Brain Injury*, 7:1, pp. 45–59.

McMahon, R. & Pearson, A. (eds) 1991, *Nursing as Therapy*, Chapman Hall, London.

McMurray, A. 1995, Personal communication, Edith Cowan University, WA.

McTaggart, R. & Garbutcheon-Singh, M. 1988, 'A fourth generation of action research', in *The Action Research Reader*, 3rd edn, eds S. Kemmis & R. McTaggart, Deakin University, Geelong, Victoria, pp. 409–28.

McWhinney, I.R. 1966, 'General practice as an academic discipline', *The Lancet*, 19 February, pp. 419–23.

McWilliams, B., Murphy, F. & Sobiski, A. 1988, 'Why self-care theory works for us', *Canadian Nurse*, October, pp. 38–40.

Meade, C. & Kim, M.J. 1984, 'The effect of teaching on documentation of nursing diagnosis', in *Classification of Nursing Diagnoses: Proceedings of the Third and Fourth National Conferences*, eds M.J. Kim & D.A. Moritz, McGraw-Hill, New York.

Meleis, A.I. 1985, *Theoretical Nursing: Development and Profession*, J.B. Lippincott, Philadelphia.

Meleis, A.I. 1987, 'Revisions in knowledge development: A passion for substance', *Scholarly Inquiry for Nursing Practice*, 1(1), pp. 5–19.

Meleis, A.I. 1991, 'Directions for nursing theory development in the 21st century', *Nursing Science Quarterly*, 5(3), pp. 112–17.

Meleis, A.I. 1991, *Theoretical Nursing Development & Progress*, 2nd edn, J.B. Lippincott, Philadelphia.

Melia, K.M. 1981, Student nurses' accounts of their work and training: A qualitative analysis, unpublished PhD thesis, Edinburgh University.

Melia, K.M. 1987, *Learning and Working: The Occupational Socialisation of Nurses*, Tavistock, London.

Mellor, B. 1995a, 'Orient Express', *The Sydney Morning Herald*, 4 February, pp. 1A, 4A.

Mellor, B. 1995b, 'Pacific city', *The Sydney Morning Herald*, 6 February, pp. 8–9.

Mellor, B. & Mills, S. 1995, 'Now it's Sydney, New South Asia', *The Sydney Morning Herald*, 4 February, pp. 1, 10.

Mercer, R.T. 1994, 'Maternal role attainment', *Nursing Theorists and their Work*, 3rd edn, ed. A. Marriner-Tomey, Mosby-Year Book Inc., St Louis.

Merleau-Ponty, M. 1962, *The Phenomenology of Perception*, Routledge & Kegan Paul, London.

Merleau-Ponty, M. 1963, *The Structure of Behaviour*, Beacon Press, Boston.

Merleau-Ponty, M. 1974, *The Phenomenology of Perception*, (trans. C. Smith) Humanities Press, New York.

Metcalf, E. 1991, 'The orthopaedic critical path', *Orthopaedic Nursing*, 10, pp. 25–31.

Miller, G.A. 1956, 'The magical number seven plus or minus two: Some limits on our capacity for processing information', *Psychological Review*, 63, pp. 81–97.

Miller, J. Baker 1991, *Towards a New Psychology of Women*, Penguin, London.

Millett, M. 1995, 'Migrants rush Sydney, now the pressure is on services', *The Sydney Morning Herald*, 23 February, pp. 1, 8.

Mitchell, G. 1991, 'Nursing diagnosis: an ethical analysis', *Image*, 23(2), pp. 99–101.

Mitchell, G.J. 1990, 'Struggling in change: From the traditional approach to Parse's theory based practice', *Nursing Science Quarterly*, 3(4), pp. 170–76.

Mitchell, G.J. 1991, 'Nursing diagnosis: An ethical analysis', *Image Journal of Nursing Scholarship*, 23(3), pp. 99–103.

Mitchell, G.J. 1995, 'Evaluation of the human becoming theory in practice in an acute care setting', in *Illuminations: The Human Becoming Theory in Practice and Research*, ed. R.R. Parse, National League for Nursing Press, Pub. No. 15–2670, New York.

Mitchell, G.J. & Cody, W.K. 1992, 'Nursing knowledge and human science: Ontological and epistemological considerations', *Nursing Science Quarterly*, 5(2), pp. 54–61.

Moch, S. 1990, 'Personal knowing: Evolving research and practice', *Scholarly Inquiry for Nursing Practice*, 4 (2), pp. 155–65.

Moorhouse, C. 1992, *Registered Nurse: The First Years of a Professional Nurse*, La Trobe University Press, Bundoora, Melbourne.

Morse, J. 1994, 'Qualitative research: Fact or fantasy', in *Critical Issues in Qualitative Research Methods*, ed. J. Morse, Sage Publications, London.

Morse, J.M. 1983, 'An ethnoscience analysis of comfort: A preliminary investigation', *Nursing Papers*, 15 (1), pp. 6–19.

Morse, J.M. (ed.) 1988, *Recent Advances in Nursing. Issues in Cross-cultural Nursing*, Churchill Livingstone, Edinburgh.

Morse, J.M. (ed.) 1989, *Qualitative Nursing Research: A Contemporary Dialogue*, Aspen, Rockville, Maryland.

Morse, J.M. 1991, 'Negotiating commitment and involvement in the nurse–patient relationship', *Journal of Advanced Nursing*, 16, pp. 455–68.

Morse, J.M. 1992, 'Comfort: The refocusing of nursing care', *Clinical Nursing Research*, 1(1), pp. 91–106.

Morse, J.M., Solberg, S.M., Neander, W.L., Bottorff, J.L. & Johnson, J.L. 1990, 'Concepts of caring and caring as a concept', *Advances in Nursing Science*, 13(1), pp. 1–14.

Mulkeen, H. 1989, 'Diabetes: Teaching the teaching of self-care', *Nursing Times*, 18–25 January, 85(3), pp. 63–65.

Munhall, P. 1992, 'A new age ism. Beyond a toxic apple', *Nursing and Health Care*, 13(7), pp. 370–75.

Munhall, P. 1993, '"Unknowing": Toward another pattern of knowing in nursing', *Nursing Outlook*, 41(93), pp. 125–28

Murray, M. 1976, *Fundamentals of Nursing*, Prentice-Hall, New Jersey.

Myers, J.L. & Spiers, M.A. 1987, 'Nursing diagnostic skills: A content analysis of spontaneously generated nursing diagnoses', in *Classification of Nursing Diagnoses: Proceedings of the Seventh Conference*, ed. A.M. McLane, C.V. Mosby, St Louis.

Nagle, L.M. & Mitchell, G.J. 1991, 'Theoretic diversity: Evolving paradigmatic issues in research and practice', *Advances in Nursing Science*, 14(1), pp. 17–25.

National Aboriginal Health Strategy Working Party 1989, *A National Aboriginal Health Strategy*, Aboriginal and Torres Strait Islander Commission, Canberra.

National Health and Medical Research Council 1974, *The Role of the Nurse in Australia*, adapted from the Report of the 76th Session of the Council, May 1973, AGPS, Canberra.

National Health and Medical Research Council 1984, *The Role of the Nurse in Australia*, Report to the 96th Session of the Council, Oct. 1983, AGPS, Canberra.

National Health and Medical Research Council 1991, *The Role of the Nurse in Australia*, prepared for the NHMRC Health Care Committee by M.A. Robinson, AGPS, Canberra.

Nelson, M. 1993, 'Critical pathways in the emergency department', *Journal of Emergency Nursing*, 19 (2), pp. 110–14.

Neuman, B. (ed.) 1982, *The Neuman Systems Model: Application to Nursing Education and Practice*, Appleton-Century-Crofts, Connecticut.

Neuman, B. (ed.) 1989, *The Neuman Systems Model*, 2nd edn, Appleton-Lange, Connecticut.

Neuman, B. (ed.) 1995, *The Neuman Systems Model*, 3rd edn, Appleton-Lange, Connecticut.

Newell, R. 1993, 'Anxiety, accuracy and reflection: The limits of professional development', *Journal of Advanced Nursing*, 17:4, pp. 1326–33.

Newman, M. 1986, *Health as Expanding Consciousness*, C.V. Mosby, St Louis.

Newman, M.A., Sime, A.M. & Corcoran-Perry, S.A. 1991, 'The focus of the discipline of nursing', *Advances in Nursing Science*, 14(1), pp. 1–6.

Nicoll, L.H. (ed.) 1986, *Perspectives on Nursing Theory*, Scott, Foresman & Co., Glenview, Illinois.

Nightingale, F. 1859/1970, *Notes on Nursing*, Duckworth, London.

Noble, J. (Chair) 1974, Report of the Nurses' Education Board on the Future Development of Nurse Education in NSW, in R.L. Russell (1990) *From Nightingale to Now: Nurse Education in Australia*, W.B. Saunders, Sydney.

Nutbeam, D., Wise, M., Bauman, A., Harris, E. & Leeder, S. 1993, *Goals and Targets for Australia's Health in the Year 2000 and Beyond*, AGPS, Canberra.

O'Brien, B. & Pearson, A. 1993, 'Unwritten knowledge in nursing: Consider the spoken as well as the written word', *Scholarly Inquiry for Nursing Practice*, 7 (2), pp. 111–27.

O'Brien, B.B. 1992, Nursing praxis: An exploration of changing nursing practice in the evolution of an embryonic nursing unit, unpublished PhD thesis, Faculty of Nursing, Deakin University, Geelong, Victoria.

O'Brien, B.B. 1993, Structure, process and outcomes: Action research study of four wards at Julia Farr Centre, unpublished research report funded by the Centre for Nursing Research and the South Australian Health Commission, Adelaide.

O'Brien, B.B. & Marshall, K. 1987, A survey of nurses' attitudes to nursing assessment, unpublished research report, Julia Farr Centre and Royal Adelaide Hospital, Adelaide.

O'Brien, B.B. & Pope, J. 1994, 'Julia Farr Centre Nursing Development Unit: A model for practice', in *The Burford NDU Model: Caring in Practice*, ed. C. Johns, Blackwell Science, Oxford.

O'Connell, B. 1992, *A Comparative Study Evaluating the Effectiveness of Nursing Assessment Formats*, Nursing Research Unit, Curtin University of Technology, Perth, Western Australia.

O'Connell, B. 1995, 'Diagnostic reliability: A study of the process', *Nursing Diagnosis*, 6(3), pp. 99–107.

O'Gorman, J.G. 1994, 'A commentary on the observations of Nixon, of Sheehan, and of Gillam on the practices and needs in psychological training', *Australian Psychologist*, 29(3), pp. 181–83.

Orem, D.E. 1971, *Nursing: Concepts of Practice*, McGraw-Hill, New York.

Orem, D.E. 1980, *Nursing: Concepts of Practice*, 2nd edn, McGraw-Hill, New York.

Orem, D.E. 1985, *Nursing: Concepts of Practice*, 3rd edn, McGraw-Hill, New York.

Orem, D.E. 1991, *Nursing: Concepts of Practice*, 4th edn, Mosby-Year Book, St Louis.

Packard, S.A. & Polifroni, E.C. 1991, 'The dilemma of nursing science: Current quandaries and lack of direction', *Nursing Science Quarterly*, 4 (1), pp. 7–13.

Padrick, K.P., Tanner, C.A., Putzier, D.J. & Westfall, U.E. 1987, 'Hypothesis evaluation: A component of diagnostic reasoning', in *Classification of Nursing Diagnoses: Proceedings of the Seventh Conference*, ed. A.M. McLane, C.V. Mosby, St Louis.

Palmer, G.R. & Short, S.D. 1994, *Health Care and Public Policy: An Australian Analysis*, 2nd edn, Macmillan Education Australia, South Melbourne.

Parker, J. 1991, 'An interpretation of person and environment', in *Towards a Discipline of Nursing*, Churchill-Livingstone, Melbourne.

Parse, R. 1987, *Nursing Science: Major Paradigms, Theories, and Critiques*, W.B. Saunders, Sydney.

Parse, R.R. 1974, *Nursing Fundamentals*, Medical Examination Publishing, New York.

Parse, R.R. 1981, *Man-Living-Health: A Theory of Nursing*, Wiley, New York.

Parse, R.R. 1987, *Nursing Science: Major Paradigms, Theories and Critiques*, Saunders, Philadelphia.

Parse, R.R. 1989, 'Parse's man-living-health model and administration of nursing service', in *Dimensions of Nursing Administration: Theory, Research, Education, Practice*, eds B. Henry, C. Arndt, M. Di Vincenti & A. Marriner-Tomey, Blackwell Scientific Publications, Cambridge.

Parse, R.R. 1990, 'Health: A personal commitment', *Nursing Science Quarterly*, 3(3), pp. 136–40.

Parse, R.R. 1990, 'Nursing theory-based practice: A challenge for the 90s', *Nursing Science Quarterly*, 3(2), p. 53.

Parse, R.R. 1992, 'Human becoming: Parse's theory of nursing', *Nursing Science Quarterly*, 5, pp. 35–42.

Parse, R.R. (ed.) 1995, *Illuminations: The Human Becoming Theory in Practice and Research*, National League for Nursing Press, Pub. No. 15–2670, New York.

Parse, R.R., Coyne, B.A. & Smith, M.J. 1985, *Nursing Research: Qualitative Methods*, Robert J. Brady Co., Bowie, Maryland.

Pateman, C. 1970, *Participation and Democratic Theory*, Cambridge University Press, Cambridge.

Paterson, J. & Zderad, L. 1976, *Humanistic Nursing*, Wiley, New York.

Patton, M.Q. 1990, *Qualitative Evaluation and Research Methods*, 2nd edn, Sage, Newbury Park, California.

Pearson, A. 1983, *The Clinical Nursing Unit*, Heinemann Medical Books, London.

Pearson, A. 1984a, 'A centre for nursing', *Nursing Times*, 18 July, pp. 53–54.

Pearson, A. 1984b, 'The essence of advanced nursing is being there', *Nursing Mirror*, 159:8, 5 September, p. 16.

Pearson, A. 1984c, 'The Burford experience', *Nursing Mirror*, 159:22, 12 December, pp. 32–35.

Pearson, A. 1985, Introducing new norms in a nursing unit and an analysis of the process of change, unpublished PhD thesis, Dept of Social Science and Administration, University of London, Goldsmiths College.

Pearson, A. 1988, 'Theorising nursing: The need for multiple horizons' in *Expanding Horizons in Nursing Education*. Proceedings of the National Nursing Education Conference, Perth, Western Australia, Dec. 1988.

Pearson, A. 1988, Interview on nursing diagnosis, (videotape), Curtin University of Technology, Perth.

Pearson, A. (ed.) 1988, *Primary Nursing: Nursing in the Burford and Oxford Nursing Development Units*, Croom Helm, London.

Pearson, A. 1992, 'Knowing nursing: Emerging paradigms in nursing', in *Knowledge for Nursing Practice*, eds K. Robinson & B. Vaughan, Butterworth-Heinemann, Oxford.

Pearson, A. & Vaughan, B. 1986, *Nursing Models for Practice*, Heinemann Nursing, London.

Pearson, A., Punton, S. & Durant, I. 1992, *Nursing Beds: An Evaluation of the Effects of Therapeutic Nursing*, Scutari Press, Harrow, Middlesex.

Perry, S.H. 1994, NURSENET—A Global Forum for Nursing Issues.

Perspectives on Nursing Theory, Study Guide for the Distance Education topic in the Master of Nursing, Flinders University of South Australia. (The material on role statements in Australia was first developed in a different form for the topic, *Perspectives on Nursing Theory*, at Flinders University by this author.)

Phelan, A. 1995, 'Our great ethnic mix', *The Northern Herald* (courtesy *The Sydney Morning Herald*), 2 March, p. 4.

Phillips, J. 1991, 'Phenomena for nursing science inquiry and the trinity of nursing', *Nursing Science Quarterly*, 4(1), pp. 3–4.

Phillips, J.R. 1987, 'A critique of Parse's man-living-health theory', in *Nursing Science: Major Paradigms, Theories and Critiques*, ed. R.R. Parse, Saunders, Philadelphia.

Pincombe, J., O'Brien, B.B., Cheek, J. & Ballantyne, A. 1995, Being there: Critical aspects of nursing for aged and extended care, unpublished research report funded by the University of South Australia, Adelaide.

Plato 1987, *The Republic*, Penguin, Harmondsworth.

Polanyi, M. 1967, *The Tacit Dimension*, Doubleday, New York.

Polanyi, M. 1975, *Personal Knowledge: Towards a Post-critical Philosphy*, Routledge and Kegan Paul, London.

Pollock, S.E. 1993, 'Adaptation to chronic illness: A program of research for testing nursing theory', *Nursing Science Quarterly*, 6(2), pp. 86–92.

Pope, Judith 1993, Locked in syndrome: Nursing in the Julia Farr Centre Nursing Development Units, poster presentation at 'Research in Nursing: Turning Points' National Conference facilitated by the Centre for Nursing Research, Glenelg, South Australia, 21–23 October.

Popper, K. 1968, *The Logic of Scientific Discovery*, Hutchinson, London.

Pratt, R. 1992, 'The health of Planet Earth: The greening of nurses', in *Issues in Australian Nursing 3*, eds G. Gray & R. Pratt, Churchill Livingstone, Melbourne.

Price, P.J. 1993, 'Parents' perceptions of the meaning of quality nursing care', *Advances in Nursing Science*, 16(1), pp. 33–41.

Prideaux, G. 1991, 'Working with the nursing process: A question of attitude', *Proceedings of the National Nursing Diagnosis Conference*, Gold Coast, Queensland.

Procter, N. & Cheek, J. 1995, 'Nurses' role in world catastrophic events: War dislocation effects on Serbian Australians', in *The Neuman Systems Model*, 3rd edn, ed. B. Neuman, Appleton-Lange, Connecticut.

Proctor, S. 1989, 'The functioning of nursing routines in the management of a transient workforce', *Journal of Advanced Nursing*, 14, pp. 180–89.

Pugliese, L. 1989, 'The theory of man-living-health: An analysis', in *Conceptual Models for Nursing Practice*, ed. J.P. Riehl-Sisca, Appleton & Lange, Norwalk.

Randell, B.P. 1992, 'Nursing theory: The 21st century', *Nursing Science Quarterly*, 5(4): pp. 176–84.

RANF 1982, 'Quality assurance program: Definition, conceptual framework, implementation guidelines', *Australian Nurses' Journal*, 11(6), pp. 12–14.

RANF 1983, *Standards for Nursing Practice*, RANF National Professional Development Committee, Melbourne.

RANF 1984, *Nursing: A Statement*, RANF, Melbourne.

RANF, College of Nursing Australia, National Florence Nightingale Committee of Australia, 1982 'Goals in nursing', position paper, in *Nursing Targets: Education 1989–2000: Proceedings of the Nursing Education Targets Projects*, April 1988 to March 1990.

Rapley, P., O'Connell, B. & Tibbett, P. 1995, 'The diagnostic conundrum: Does the assessment make the difference?', *Proceedings of the Second National Nursing Diagnosis Conference*, Perth, Western Australia.

Rappaport, J. 1987, 'Terms of empowerment/exemplars of prevention: Toward a theory for community psychology', *American Journal of Community Psychology*, 15, pp. 121–47.

Rappoport, R.N. 1970, 'Three dilemmas in action research', *Human Relations*, 23:6, pp. 499–513.

Reason, P. & Hawkins, P. 1988, 'Storytelling as inquiry', in *Human Inquiry in Action: Developments in New Paradigm Research*, ed. P. Reason, Sage, London, pp. 79–102.

Reed, P.G. 1986, 'A model for constructing a conceptual framework in the clinical specialty', *Journal of Nursing Education*, 25(7), pp. 295–99.

Reid, J. & Trompf, P. 1991, *The Health of Aboriginal Australia*, Harcourt Brace Jovanovich, Sydney.

Reid, J.C. (Chair, Steering Committee) 1994, *Nursing Education in Australian Universities*. Report of the National Review of Nurse Education in the Higher Education Sector— 1994 and beyond, AGPS, Canberra.

Reinharz, S. 1992, *Feminist Methods in Social Research*, Oxford University Press, New York.

Report of a Working Party of Nominees (1975), *Goals in Nursing Education, Part II*. Melbourne, Royal Australian Nursing Federation, College of Nursing Australia, The National Florence Nightingale Committee of Australia, The NSW College of Nursing.

Reynolds, B. 1993, 'Criteria to evaluate nursing theories and models', *Journal of Psychological Nursing*, 31(12), pp. 5–6.

Reynolds, B. & Cormack, D.F.S. 1990, 'An evaluation of the Johnson Behavioural System Model of Nursing', *Journal of Psychological Nursing*, 16(9), pp. 1122–30.

Riehl-Sisca, J. 1989, *Conceptual Models for Nursing Practice*, 3rd edn, Appleton & Lange, California.

Riemen, D.J. 1986, 'Noncaring and caring in the clinical setting: patients' descriptions', *Topics in Clinical Nursing*, 8(2), pp. 30–36.

Rifkin, S. 1981, 'The role of the public in the planning, management and evaluation of health activities and programmes, including self-care', *Social Science*, 15A, pp. 377–86.

Robinson, Mardi 1988, 'The theory–practice gap in nursing', in *Bridging the Gap!*, published proceedings of a conference held at Deakin University, Geelong, 7–8 November, pp. 6–11.

Rodgers, B.L. 1989, 'Concepts, analysis and development of nursing knowledge: The evolutionary cycle', *Journal of Advanced Nursing*, 14, pp. 330–35.

Rodgers, B.L. 1991, 'Deconstructing the dogma in nursing knowledge and practice', *Image: Journal of Nursing Scholarship*, 23(3), pp. 177–81.

Rogers, M.E. 1970, *An Introduction to the Theoretical Basis of Nursing*, F.A. Davis, Philadelphia.

Rogers, M.E. 1980, 'Nursing: A science of unitary man', in *Conceptual Models for Nursing Practice*, 2nd edn, eds J.P. Riehl & C. Roy, Appleton-Century-Crofts, Norwalk.

Rogers, M.E. 1987, 'Rogers' science of unitary human beings', in *Nursing Science: Major Paradigms, Theories and Critiques*, ed. R.R. Parse, Saunders, Philadelphia.

Rogers, M.E. 1990, 'Nursing: Science of unitary, irreducible, human beings: update 1990, in *Visions of Rogers' Science-Based Nursing*, ed. E.A.M. Barrett, National League for Nursing, Pub. No. 15–2285, New York.

Romeo, S. 1994, NURSENET—A Global Forum for Nursing Issues.

Roper, N., Logan, W. & Tierney, A. 1980, *The Elements of Nursing*, Churchill Livingstone, Edinburgh.

Roper, N., Logan, W.W. & Tierney, A.J. 1985, *The Elements of Nursing*, 2nd edn, Churchill Livingstone, Edinburgh.

Roy, C. 1984, *Introduction to Nursing. An Adaptation Model*, Prentice-Hall, New Jersey.

Roy, C. & Andrews, H.A. 1991, *The Roy Adaptation Model: The Definitive Statement*, Appleton & Lange, Norwalk, Connecticut.

Russell, R.L. 1990, *From Nightingale to Now: Nurse Education in Australia*, W.B. Saunders/Balliere Tindall, Sydney.

Rysman, A. R. 1977, 'How the gossip become a woman', *Journal of Communication*, 26, pp. 176–80.

Saba, V. 1991, 'The international classification of diseases (ICD): Classification of nursing diagnosis', in *Classification of Nursing Diagnoses: Proceedings of the Ninth Conference*, ed. R.M. Carroll-Johnson, J.B. Lippincott, Philadelphia.

Saggers, S. & Gray, D. 1991, *Aboriginal Health and Society. The Traditional and Contemporary Aboriginal Struggle for Better Health*, Allen & Unwin, Sydney.

Salvage, J. 1988, Partners in care? An exploration of the theory and practice of the New Nursing in the UK, unpublished thesis, part of an MSc in Sociology with special reference to medicine, Royal Holloway & Bedford New College.

Salvage, J. 1989, 'Building centres of excellence', *Nursing Standard*, 48:3, 26 August, pp. 53–56.

Salvage, J. 1990, 'The theory and practice of the "New Nursing"', *Nursing Times* , 86:4, 24 January, pp. 42–45.

Salvage, J. & Kershaw, B. (eds) 1986, *Models for Nursing,* John Wiley & Sons, Chichester.

Samarell, N. & Fawcett, J. 1992, 'Enhancing adaptation to breast cancer: The addition of coaching to support groups', *Oncology Nursing Forum*, May 19(4), pp. 591–6.

Sanford, A.J. 1984, *Cognition and Cognitive Psychology*, Lawrence Erlbaum, New Jersey.

Santopinto, M.D.A. & Smith, M.C. 1995, 'Evaluation of the human becoming theory in practice with adults and children', in *Illuminations: The Human Becoming Theory in Practice and Research,* ed. R.R. Parse, National League for Nursing Press, New York.

Sarantakos, S. 1993, *Social Research*, Macmillan, Melbourne.

Sarter, B. 1988, 'Philosophical sources of nursing theory', *Nursing Science Quarterly*, 1(2), pp. 52–59.

Sartre, J.P. 1966, *Being and Nothingness*, Washington Square Press, New York.

Sauber, S. R. 1983, *The Human Service Delivery System,* Columbia University Press, New York.

Sax, S. (Chair) Aug. 1978, *Nurse Education and Training,* Report of the Committee of Inquiry into Nurse Education and Training to the Tertiary Education Commission, Canberra, in R.L. Russell (1990), *From Nightingale to Now: Nurse Education in Australia,* W.B. Saunders, Sydney.

Sax, S. 1990, *Health Care Choices and the Public Purse,* Allen & Unwin, Sydney.

Schaefer, K.M. & Pond, J.B. 1994, 'Levine's conservation model as a guide to nursing practice', *Nursing Science Quarterly*, 7(2), pp. 53–54.

Schön, D.A. 1983, *The Reflective Practitioner: How Professionals think in Action,* Basic Books, New York.

Schön, D.A. 1987, *Educating the Reflective Practitioner: Towards a New Design for Teaching and Learning in the Professions,* Jossey-Bass, San Francisco.

Schultz, P. & Meleis, A. 1988, 'Nursing epistemology: Traditions, insights, questions', *Image*, 20 (4), pp. 217–21.

Schultz, P. & Schultz, R. 1987, Nodding's caring and public policy: A linkage and its nursing implications, unpublished paper.

Scott, M. 1995, 'New schools of thought', *The Sydney Morning Herald,* 9 February, pp. 10–11.

Seed, A. 1991, Becoming a registered nurse: The students' perspective. A longitudinal, qualitative analysis of emergent views of a cohort of student nurses during their three-year training for general registration, unpublished PhD thesis, Leeds Polytechnic, CNAA.

Seidel, J.V. 1988, *The Ethnograph,* Version 3.0 [computer program], Qualis Research Associates, Corvallis, OR.

Serrell, M. 1990, Clinical nurses' ability to structure diagnostic statements, unpublished Master's thesis, Curtin University of Technology, Perth, Western Australia.

Sheehan, P.W. 1994, 'Psychology as a science and a profession: An Australian perspective', *Australian Psychologist*, 29(3), pp. 174–77.

Shelley, S.I. 1984, *Research Methods in Nursing and Health,* Little, Brown, Boston.

Shoemaker, J. 1984, 'Essential features of nursing diagnoses', in *Classification of Nursing Diagnoses: Proceedings of the Fifth Conference*, eds M.J. Kim, G. McFarland & A. McLane, C.V. Mosby, St Louis

Short, S. Sharman, E. & Speedy, S. 1993, *Sociology for Nurses: An Australian Introduction*, Macmillan Education, Melbourne.

Shotter, J. 1990, *Knowing of the Third Kind*, ISOR, Utrecht.

Silver, M. 1988, Nursing units: Report of a visit to Deakin University, unpublished report to the South Australian Health Commission, Adelaide.

Silver, M. 1989, 'Career structure for nurses: The South Australian experience', in *Issues in Australian Nursing 2*, eds G. Gray & R. Pratt, Churchill Livingstone, Melbourne.

Sims, S.E.R. 1991, 'The nature and relevance of theory for practice', *Towards a Discipline of Nursing*, eds G. Gray and R. Pratt, Churchill Livingstone, Melbourne, pp. 51–72.

Sipple, J. 1989, A model for curriculum change based on retrospective analysis, unpublished ED. D. Dissertation, University of South Carolina.

Sloboda, J. 1986, 'Acquiring skill', in *The Skilful Mind: An Introduction to Cognitive Psychology*, ed. A. Gelately, Open University Press, Milton Keynes, UK.

Smeltzer, C. & McCreary Juhasz, A. 1990, 'Relationships of nurses' education and experience to implementing the nursing process', *Journal of Nursing Quality Assurance*, 4(4), pp. 7–16.

Smith, D. & Hatton, N. 1993, 'Critical reflection on action in professional education', paper presented at the 5th National Practicum Conference, Macquarie University, Sydney, Feb. 1993.

Smith, L. 1994, 'An analysis and reflections on the quality of nursing research in 1992', *Journal of Advanced Nursing*, 19, pp. 385–93.

Smith, M. 1992, 'Enhancing esthetic knowledge: A teaching strategy', *Advances in Nursing Science*, 14(3), pp. 52–9.

Smith, M.C. 1991, 'Nursing practice: Guided by or generating theory?', *Nursing Science Quarterly*, 3(4), pp. 147–8.

Smith, M.C. 1992, 'The distinctiveness of nursing knowledge', *Nursing Science Quarterly*, 5(4), pp. 148–9.

Smith, M.C. 1993, 'The contribution of nursing theory to nursing administration practice', *Image: Journal of Nursing Scholarship*, 25(1), pp. 63–7.

Smith, M.C. & Hudepohl, J.H. 1988, 'Analysis and evaluation of Parse's theory of man-living-health', *Canadian Journal of Nursing Research*, 20(4), pp. 43–58.

Smith, P. & Redfern, S. 1988, 'The quality of care and students' educational experience in hospital wards', in *Changing Perspectives in Nursing Research*, eds J. Wilson-Barnett & S. Robinson, John Wiley, Chichester.

Smits, M.W. & Kee, C.C. 1992, 'Correlates of self-care among the independent elderly: Self-concept affects well-being', *Journal of Gerontological Nursing*, 18(9), pp. 13–18.

Soares-O'Hearn, C.A. 1987, 'The relationship between a structural-functional health/illness pattern (SHIP) tool and the generating of nursing diagnoses: A qualitative and quantitative study', in *Classification of Nursing Diagnoses: Proceedings of the Seventh Conference*, ed. A.M. McLane, C.V. Mosby, St Louis.

Sohier, R. 1992, 'Feminism and nursing knowledge: The power of the weak', *Nursing Outlook*, 40:2, pp. 62–6.

Sohn, K.S. 1991, 'One method for comparing different nursing models', *Nursing and Health Care*, 12(8), pp. 410–12.

Solomon, R.C. 1988, *Continental Philosophy since 1750: The Rise and Fall of the Self*, Oxford University Press, Oxford,

Sorrentino, E.A. 1991, 'Making theories work for you', *Nursing Administration Quarterly*, 15, pp. 54–59.

South Australian Health Commission 1990, *A Social Health Atlas of South Australia*.

Spacks, P.M. 1982, 'In praise of gossip', *Hudson Review*, 35, pp. 19–38.

Speedy, S. 1990, 'Nursing theory and nursing education: Ships that pass in the night?', Fourth National Nursing Education Conference, Nov., Melbourne.

Speedy, S.C. 1989, 'Theory-practice debate: setting the scene', *Australian Journal of Advanced Nursing*, 6(3), pp.12–20.

Spry, J.M. & O'Brien, B.B. 1993, 'Farrway: A clinical nursing information system', read by J. Spry (theme 14), International Congress of Nurses Quadrennial Congress, Madrid, Spain, 24 June 1993.

Stanhope, M. & Lancaster, J. 1984, *Community Health Nursing: Process and Practice for Promoting Health*, C.V. Mosby, St Louis.

Stanley, F. (Chair) 1994, *Australia's Health 1994*, Australian Institute of Health and Welfare, AGPS, Canberra.

Staunton, P. 1991, 'Report writing', in *Law for Nurses* (video), Camperdown, NSW Nurses Association.

Stepanas, T.V. 1991, 'Types of diabetes', in *Diabetes and You: An Owner's Manual*, eds P. Moffitt, P. Phillips & B. Ayers, Diabetes Australia.

Stevens Barnum, B. 1990, *Nursing Theory: Analysis, Application and Evaluation*, 3rd edn, Little, Brown, Boston.

Stevens Barnum, B. 1994, *Nursing Theory: Analysis, Application and Evaluation*, 4th edn, J.B. Lippincott, Philadelphia.

Storch, J.L. 1986, 'In defence of nursing theory', *Canadian Nurse*, Jan., pp. 16–20.

Strauss, A. 1987, *Qualitative Analysis for Social Scientists*, Cambridge University Press, New York.

Strauss, A. & Corbin, J. 1990, *Basics of Qualitative Research. Grounded Theory Procedures and Techniques*, Sage, California.

Street, A. 1991, *From Image to Action: Reflection in Nursing Practice*, Deakin University Press, Geelong, Victoria.

Street, A.F. 1991, *Inside Nursing: A Critical Ethnography of Clinical Nursing Practice*, SUNY, Albany, New York.

Streubert, H.J. & Carpenter, D.R. 1995, *Qualitative Research in Nursing: Advancing the Humanistic Imperative*, J.B. Lippincott, Philadelphia.

Sullivan, G.C. 1989, 'Evaluating Antonovsky's Salutogenic model for its adaptability to nursing', *Journal of Advanced Nursing*, 14, pp. 336–42.

Swansburg, R.C. 1990, *Management and Leadership for Nurse Managers*, Jones & Bartlett, Boston.

Swanson, K.M. 1991, 'Empirical development of a middle range theory of caring', *Nursing Research*, 40(3), pp. 161–66.

Tanner, C.A. 1986, 'Research on clinical judgement', in *Review of Research in Nursing Education*, vol. 1, ed. W.L. Holzemer, National League for Nursing, New York.

Tanner, C.A., Padrick, K.P., Westfall, U.E. & Putzier, D.J. 1987, 'Diagnostic reasoning strategies of nurses and nursing students', *Nursing Research*, 36 (6), pp. 358–63.

Tattersall, R.B. & Gale, A.M. (eds) 1990, *Diabetes Clinical Management*, Churchill Livingstone, Edinburgh.

Taylor, B. 1992, The phenomenon of ordinariness in nursing, unpublished PhD thesis, Faculty of Nursing, Deakin University, Geelong, Victoria.

Taylor, B.J. 1994, *Being Human: Ordinariness in Nursing*, Churchill-Livingstone, Melbourne.

The Australian Nurses Journal, Dec./Jan. 1993, 22(6).

The Australian Pocket Oxford Dictionary 1976, 1st Australian edn, OUP, Melbourne.

The Macquarie Dictionary 1981, The Macquarie Library, Macquarie University, NSW.

The Macquarie Dictionary 1987, The Macquarie Library, Macquarie University, NSW.

The Macquarie Dictionary, 1990, The Macquarie Library, Macquarie University, NSW.

The Macquarie Encyclopedic Dictionary 1990, The Macquarie Library, Macquarie University, NSW.

Thiele, J.E., Baldwin, J.H., Hyde, R.S., Sloan, B. & Strandquist, G.A. 1986, 'An investigation of decision theory: What are the effects of teaching cue recognition?', *Journal of Nursing Education*, 25(8), pp. 319–24.

Thomas, S. 1987, 'Nursing diagnosis: What is it?', *The Australian Journal of Advanced Nursing*, 4(3), pp. 41–48.

Thomas, S., Wearing, A. & Bennett, M. 1991, *Clinical Decision-making for Nurses and Health Professionals*, Harcourt Brace Jovanovich, Sydney.

Thompson, J.L. 1987, 'Critical scholarship: The critique of domination in nursing', *Advances in Nursing Science*, 10(1), pp. 27–38.

Tillich, P. 1952, *The Courage to Be*, Yale University Press, New Haven.

Toffler, A. 1970, *Future Shock*, Pan Books, London.

Toffler, A. 1981, *The Third Wave*, Pan Books, London.

Tomlinson, P. 1981, *Understanding Teaching: Interactive Educational Psychology*, McGraw-Hill, London.

Tomlinson, P. 1988, 'The teaching of skills: Modern cognitive perspectives', in *Cognitive Approaches in Special Education*, ed. D.A. Sugden, Falmer Press, London.

Tomlinson, P. 1995, *Understanding Mentoring: Reflective Strategies for School-based Teacher Preparation*, Open University Press, Buckingham, UK.

Torres, G. 1990, 'The place of concepts and theories within nursing', in *Nursing Theories: The Base for Professional Practice*, 3rd edn, ed. J. George, Appleton & Lange, Connecticut.

Turner, B.S. 1986, 'The vocabulary of complaints: Nursing, professionalism and job context', *Australian and New Zealand Journal of Sociology*, 22(3), pp. 368–86.

Urmson, J.O. & Ree, J. (eds) 1991, *The Concise Encyclopedia of Western Philosophy and Philosophers*, Unwin Hyman, London.

Vaughan, B. 1992, 'The nature of nursing knowledge', in *Knowledge for Nursing Practice*, eds K. Robinson & B. Vaughan, Butterworth-Heinemann, Sydney.

Wald, F.S. & Leonard, R.C. 1986, 'Towards development of nursing practice theory', in *Perspectives on Nursing Theory*, ed. L.H. Nicoll, Scott, Foresman & Co., London.

Walker, K. 1994, 'Research with/in nursing: "Troubling" the field', *Contemporary Nurse*, 3(4), pp. 162–68.

Walker, L.O. 1971, 'Toward a clearer understanding of the concept of nursing theory', *Nursing Research*, 29, pp. 428–35.

Walsh, M. & Ford, P. 1989, *Nursing Rituals, Research and Rational Actions,* Butterworth-Heinemann, Sydney.

Waters, K.R. 1994, 'Getting dressed in the early morning: Styles of staff/patient interaction on rehabilitation hospital wards for elderly people', *Journal of Advanced Nursing*, 19, pp. 239–48.

Watson, J. 1979, *The Philosophy and Science of Caring*, Little, Brown, Boston.

Watson, J. 1985, *Nursing: Human Science and Human Care: A Theory of Nursing*, Appelton Century Crofts, East Norwalk, Connecticut.

Weber, J. 1988, *Nurses' Handbook of Health Assessment*, J.B. Lippincott, Sydney.

Weiler, K. & Buckwater, K. 1990, 'Is nursing research used in practice?', in *Current Issues in Nursing*, eds J. McClosky & H. Grace, C.V. Mosby, St Louis.

Weiss, S.J. 1988, 'Touch', in *Annual Review of Nursing Research*, vol. 6, eds J.J. Fitzpatrick, R.L. Taunton & J.Q. Benoleil, Springer, New York, pp. 3–27.

Westfall, U., Tanner, C., Putzier, D. & Padrick, K. 1986, 'Activating clinical inferences:A component of diagnostic reasoning in nursing', *Research in Nursing and Health*, 9,pp. 269–77.

Whall, A.L. 1993, 'Let's get rid of all nursing theory', *Nursing Science Quarterly*, 6(4), pp. 164–65.

White, R. 1972, *The Role of the Nurse in Australia*, Report to accompany the Annotated Bibliography, prepared for the National Health and Medical Research Council (Nursing Subcommittee), Tertiary Education Research Centre, UNSW.

Wiedenbach, E. 1964, *Clinical Nursing: A Helping Art*, Springer-Verlag, New York.

Wiles, V.H. 1994, Making a difference: In celebration of nursing practice, Forty-second Annual Oration, New South Wales College of Nursing, Sydney.

Williams, A. 1994, Nurses' perceptions of high quality care, unpublished report, Department of Nursing Research, Sir Charles Gairdner Hospital, Perth, WA.

Wilson, H.S. 1989, *Research in Nursing*, 2nd edn, Addison-Wesley, Redwood City, California.

Wilson-Barnet, J. 1988, 'Nursing values: Exploring the clichés', *Journal of Advanced Nursing*, 13, pp. 790–96.

Winch, J. 1989, 'Why is health care for Aborigines so ineffective?', in *Issues in Australian Nursing 2*, eds G. Gray & R. Pratt, Churchill Livingstone, Melbourne.

Winkler, S.J. 1983, 'Parse's theory of nursing', in *Conceptual Models of Nursing: Analysis and Application*, eds J.J. Fitzpatrick & A. Whall, Brady Publications, Bowie.

Wolfer, J. 1993, 'Aspects of reality and ways of knowing in nursing: in search of an integrating paradigm', *Image*, 25(2), pp. 141–46.

Wood, P. 1990, *Nursing: Progress through Partnership 1921–1991*, AGPS, Canberra.

Woolley, N. 1990, 'Nursing diagnosis—Exploring the factors which may influence the reasoning process', *Journal of Advanced Nursing*, 15, pp. 110–17.

Wright, S. 1989, 'Defining the Nursing Development Unit', *Nursing Standard*, 4:7, 8 November, pp. 29–31.

Yeo, M. 1989, 'Integration of nursing theory and nursing ethics', *Advances in Nursing Science*, April, pp. 33–41.

Yuen, F.K.H. 1984, 'Integration of theory and practice–illusion or reality?', *Australian Journal of Advanced Nursing*, 1(3), pp. 11–15.

Yura, H. & Torres, G. 1975, *Today's Conceptual Framework within Baccalaureate Nursing Programs*, NLN, Pub. No. 15–1558, New York, pp. 17–25.

Yura, H., & Walsh, M. 1988, *The Nursing Process: Assessing, Planning, Implementing, Evaluating*, 5th edn, Appleton & Lange, Norwalk.

Ziegler, S.M. 1984, 'Nursing diagnosis—the state of the art as reflected in graduate students' work', in *Classification of Nursing Diagnoses: Proceedings of the Fifth Conference*, eds M.J. Kim, G.K. McFarlane & A.M. McLane, C.V. Mosby, St Louis.

Ziegler, S.M., Vaughan-Wrobel, B.C. & Erlen, J.A. 1986, *Nursing Process, Nursing Diagnosis, Nursing Knowledge: Avenues to Autonomy*, Prentice Hall, Sydney.

INDEX

O

P